Memories

Memories

My Life as an International Leader
in Health, Suffrage, and Peace

ALETTA
JACOBS

Edited by Harriet Feinberg
Translated by Annie Wright
Historical Afterword by Harriet Pass Freidenreich
Literary Afterword by Harriet Feinberg

THE FEMINIST PRESS
AT THE CITY UNIVERSITY OF NEW YORK

©1996 by The Feminist Press at The City University of New York

Editor's Foreword, Notes, "Patterns of Remembrance: A Literary Afterword," ©1996 by Harriet Feinberg

"Aletta Jacobs in Historical Perspective" ©1996 by Harriet Pass Freidenreich

Translation©1996 by Annie Wright

Published 1996 by The Feminist Press at The City University of New York, 311 East 94 Street, New York, NY 10128-5684

Originally published as *Herinneringen* (Amsterdam: Van Holkema and Warendorf, 1924)

00 99 98 97 96   1 2 3 4 5

Library of Congress Cataloging-in-Publication Data

Jacobs, Aletta H. (Aletta Henriette), 1854–1929.
    [Herinneringen. English]
  Memories: My Life as an International Leader in Women's Health, Suffrage, and Peace. / Aletta Jacobs: edited by Harriet Feinberg: translated by Annie Wright: afterword by Harriet Pass Freidenreich.
    p. cm.
  Includes bibliographical references and index.
  ISBN 1-55861-137-1.—ISBN 1-55861-138-X (alk. paper)
  1. Jacobs, Aletta H. (Aletta Henriette), 1854–1929. 2. Feminists—Netherlands—Biography.
3. Women physicians—Netherlands—Biography. 4. Women's rights—Netherlands—Biography.
I. Title.
HQ1657.J3A3313 1996
305.4′09492—dc20
[B]   95-35736
                                         CIP

This publication is made possible, in part, by public funds from the New York State Council on the Arts, and with the generous support of The Prins Bernhard Fonds and The Rosa Manus Fonds. The Feminist Press is also grateful for a grant from the John D. and Catherine T. MacArthur Foundation, and to Joanne Markell and Genevieve Vaughan.

Cover: Portrait of Aletta Jacobs by Isaac Israëls, 1919. Courtesy of the International Information Centre and Archives for the Women's Movement (IIAV), Amsterdam, the Netherlands; gift of Mathilde Cohen Tervaert-Israëls.

Cover and text design by Tina R. Malaney

Typeset by AeroType, Inc.

Printed in the United States of America with soy-based ink on acid-free paper by McNaughton & Gunn, Inc., Saline, Michigan.

CONTENTS

EDITOR'S FOREWORD

D utch physician, suffrage leader, and peace activist Aletta Jacobs was at work completing her life story in her home at 46 Van Aerssenstraat, The Hague, in the winter of 1923 to 1924. Approaching seventy, widowed, she sometimes felt herself a last leaf—the only one of her sibling group of eleven children still alive. Yet, having moved several years previously from Amsterdam to The Hague, she was now near many of the Broese van Groenous, her dear family-of-choice of these later years, and felt settled and welcome.[1] This large, multitalented family, in which, as in her own family, a progressive father had encouraged the development of his daughters along with his sons, had for years embraced her. They provided her with the friendship and energy of a younger generation and also sheltered her from the financial distress that had overtaken her in later life.

Feeling at home in The Hague, but barely recovered from a serious illness and hurrying to complete her life story in time for a full-blown seventieth birthday celebration, Aletta Jacobs could muse yet again over the piles of old clippings, letters, and scrapbooks she found herself so often mentioning, so often quoting. Here in her second-floor front room were the written evidences of a life of activism and caring. Here was the note giving Minister Thorbecke's permission for her to study medicine at Groningen University; here was a sheaf of obituaries for her beloved husband Carel Victor Gerritsen, felled by cancer at a triumphant moment in his political career; here was the scrapbook of press clippings young Hungarian feminists had put together as a gesture of thanks after she and Carrie Chapman Catt campaigned for woman suffrage in Budapest; here was Woodrow Wilson's note to Jane Addams about the 1915 encounter when she, Aletta Jacobs, had crossed the Atlantic in wartime to plead with him to mediate among the European belligerents.

This was just where she needed to be to complete the work. Her dear friend Miel Coops-Broese van Groenou had invited her to live with her, Richard, and the children, but she refused, writing, "To do the sort of work I am now doing, one has to create a sort of 'work sphere' around oneself, such as one can only do at home. If you could see me in my upstairs front room, sitting at my desk, which has in each little drawer a different sort of document that now and then I need, and two tablefuls of papers in back of me, with orders to Luise [apparently the maid] not to touch anything till I've put it away, then you'd know that only in one's own house can one do such a task."[2]

How was she to turn the heaps of papers and her memories into a written account of her life? How could she tell her story not only for her many Dutch friends and associates, and for the up-and-coming generation of Dutch women, but even for readers in the United States—for she had already engaged a translator? She so much hoped that, with the help of her friend Jane Addams, an American publisher could be found . . .

Not until I had submitted a proposal to The Feminist Press to edit an English translation of Aletta Jacobs's autobiography did I learn that I would be fulfilling a wish of hers. On October 29, 1923, Jacobs wrote to Jane Addams: "I shall now use the winter months to finish my memoirs so that they are ready before I die. There is here an English professor, who has lived in Holland for several years, he is translating it into English, so that the English copy will be ready at the same time as the Dutch" (15–1576).[3]

Jacobs was very ill during that winter before her seventieth birthday, but she did recover and complete the manuscript in time for the birthday celebration and the publication of *Herinneringen* (Memories). But she wrote to Addams on December 12, 1924, that the first translation had not come out well and that the manuscript was now in the hands of "a Dutchman living in London. He always answers my questions about it, 'that he is working on it and hopes to be ready in due time.' I am not sure it will ever be finished" (16–1547).

The Dutchman must eventually have finished, for in October 1925 Jacobs wrote to Addams (who apparently had expressed willingness to try her own publisher) that the manuscript had gone to two New York publishers, one of whom had returned it (17–0003). Adele Seltzer of Thomas Seltzer Publishers, who still had the manuscript, then wrote to Addams in January 1926 that "what we have to convince ourselves of first of all is whether there would be a large enough reading public for Dr. Jacob's [*sic*] memoirs here in America. . . . Do you think there would be as many as a thousand people? . . . Or has the book so much social value that an individual or group of people here would sponsor its publication?" (19–1383).

But despite reassurances by Addams and her suggestion that Jacobs's and Addams's good friend Cor Ramondt could edit the manuscript, Seltzer, sad to relate, not only never overcame her doubts that the book would sell, but kept it until 1928. Finally Addams asked Emily Balch to pick it up personally while she was in New York (19–1387).[4]

Jacobs died the following year. But plans to publish were not completely dead. On July 6, 1931, her long-time assistant and friend Rosa Manus wrote to Addams expressing pleasure at a new hope of publication by the University of

Chicago Press, and publication in the series Social Service Monographs was provisionally approved in August 1931. But alas, on July 31, 1933, Sophonisba Breckenridge wrote to Addams that she was returning the manuscript to Rosa Manus.[5] Then Manus passed the manuscript along to Carrie Chapman Catt, who surprisingly had up to that point never read it. Catt wrote down a number of comments and, in September 1933, sent it back to Addams and Breckenridge, expressing her hope for its publication: "It is very important that the lives and accomplishments of women who did as much as Dr. Jacobs did for several causes should be known to the world. . . . in order that our own women's history as told by ourselves may be passed on to other generations" (25–167). But at that point, after another flurry of notes back and forth, the momentum finally wound down (25–167, see also 25–228, 25–247, 25–311).

The publishers involved in this saga behaved in a manner not unknown to publishers past and present: they kept the manuscript a long time, expressed doubts as to whether it would sell, wanted an outside source to fund the printing, and finally said no. From a publisher's perspective, the life of a pacifist/suffragist associate of Addams and Catt—and a relatively unknown Dutch one at that—may not have been an entirely desirable venture. The early twenties were characterized by a witch-hunt atmosphere, an antipacifist, nationalistic, Red scare mentality. Jane Addams's reputation had gone into deep eclipse because of her pacifism and, moreover, Addams, Catt, and other reformers appeared in "spiderweb" charts of Bolsheviks.[6] The early thirties, with millions unemployed, was also not a fortuitous period to find funds for subsidizing book publication.

Then, too, there was simply the aging of Jacobs's U.S. friends, their health problems, and their many other preoccupations. By the time of the Chicago efforts, Jane Addams and Carrie Chapman Catt were in their mid-seventies. It is touching that they persisted as long as they did. Yet it is ironic that Jacobs, so quintessentially an internationalist, was unable in her last years to have her memoirs appear in a form that her English-speaking associates could read. Now, albeit in a different era, her words, in a new translation, can finally reach their intended readers.

HARRIET FEINBERG

ACKNOWLEDGMENTS

F irst I would like to thank and acknowledge two exceptional scholars of Dutch women's history without whom this volume would never have appeared. Mineke Bosch and Inge de Wilde have been unfailingly helpful and supportive, each drawing on her own extensive research on Aletta Jacobs to provide bibliography, materials otherwise hard to obtain, comments and suggestions, and drafts of her own work-in-progress.

I also particularly thank those who encouraged and advised me during the years when I was beginning research on Jacobs. These include Anne Wiltsher, whose moving book *Most Dangerous Women: Feminist Peace Campaigners of the Great War* first held up for me the broad canvas on which Jacobs acted, Margot Badran, Peter van den Dungen, Jacqueline van Voris, and E. M. Beekman, who provided advice on issues involved in planning a translation of Jacobs's autobiography. The members of my women's Arab-Jewish dialogue group have a special place, as our four-year conversation sparked and nurtured my backward look at women and peace in earlier times.

I am greatly indebted to Charlotte Loeb, who encouraged and advised me when I was learning Dutch in order to do research on Jacobs, carefully checked passages I translated for my article on Jacobs's time in the Middle East and for this volume, and helped me broaden my knowledge of Dutch culture.

With gratitude I acknowledge many others who provided answers to specific questions, read portions of this manuscript, helped resolve problematic passages, gave advice about funding, and aided my endeavors in other ways. They include Marian Aptroot, Andreas te Boekhorst, Mary Lynn McCree Bryan, Wendy Chmielewski of the Swarthmore College Peace Collection, Sandi Cooper, David Doughan of the Fawcett Library, Jacqueline Guéron, David Herlihy, Martina van Issertum, Ulla Jansz, Selma Leydesdorff, David Smith of the New York Public Library, J. Soetenhorst-de Savornin Lohman, Brita Stendahl, Richard J. Wolfe of the Countway Library of Medicine, Edith Wynner of the Schwimmer-Lloyd Papers at the New York Public Library, and Marius van der Veen. Lilian de Bruijn, Aniek de Poorter, and Heidi Hopper rendered conscientious and reliable research assistance.

At The Feminist Press, Florence Howe was enthusiastic about my proposal and turned it into a Press project; Susannah Driver provided insightful editing and important encouragement. Harriet Freidenreich contributed much more than her thoughtful essay; drawing on her broad background in European history and in geography, she carefully reviewed the entire manuscript. Publication would not have been possible without translation grants from the Prins Bernhard Foundation and the Rosa Manus Foundation and support from the Royal Netherlands Embassy.

The encouragement and support of dear friends and relatives was invaluable. My thanks to them is overflowing and ongoing.

TRANSLATOR'S NOTE

Translating *Memories* involved an intensely personal relationship with its author, Aletta Jacobs. For several months I worked each day on the initial draft, and frequently I felt as if Aletta were personally confiding her story to me. I began to recognize her "voice" every time I opened her book and switched on my word processor. In this I was lucky, because there is no automatic affinity between a translator and the person whose words must be seamlessly transformed from one language into another.

Memories was first published in 1924. Even then the language that Aletta Jacobs used was archaic, and reading the original text first involved learning a new vocabulary in which some of the commonest words were unfamiliar. Other words, although basically unchanged, looked unfamiliar because of their old-fashioned, quasi-Germanic spelling. As I struggled through the first pages, I almost expected Aletta to be as "fuddy-duddy" as her language. Yet I soon realized that she was as fiercely articulate as any modern woman and that many of the issues she was dealing with are still topical today. Here, I am particularly thinking of her adolescent breakdown when her parents tried to curb her adventurous instincts by coercing her into "suitable employment" as a seamstress. Of course, at that time no woman had ever entered a Dutch university, let alone qualified as a doctor of medicine. So it is to her father's eternal credit that he subsequently helped her to achieve these pioneering goals. Many women today are still struggling with precisely the same problems when they choose male-dominated careers in, for instance, science and technology, manual work, and religion.

There were countless moments when Aletta Jacobs astonished me with her incisive observations. But nothing moved me as much as her description in chapter 2 of the young prostitute dying of syphilis: "I . . . remember that no one ever visited that pale and beautiful girl, that in fact no one took any notice of her at all." Little has changed since these events took place. While translating *Memories*, I was also making daily hospital visits to a friend suffering from AIDS. The ward included a separate section for women who in Dutch are known as "heroin hookers." I could hear one of them groaning rhythmically in pain and terror while the other women yelled at her to "shut up!" After an hour of pretending that we were both deaf, my friend turned to me and said, "It's terrible, isn't it?"

The next day I returned to the hospital. But there was no more groaning. I asked what had happened and the nurse jerked her thumb toward an open door. A young woman was lying alone and comatose in a small room reserved to give some semblance of dignity to the final moments of life. A cloud of deep red hair framed her delicate face, which was as white as alabaster. The next day the room was empty. It is to her memory that I dedicate this translation.

ANNIE WRIGHT

NOTE

Jacobs used "the Netherlands" and "Holland" interchangeably, and "America" and "North America" to refer to the United States. Because this was common practice in her day, her terminology has been retained. She also alternated between "Carel" and "Gerritsen" in referring to Carel Gerritsen, her husband. As her personal preference, this has been retained. Except in full titles of specific events, "conference" or "meeting" is used rather than "congress," to conform with contemporary usage.—*Ed.*

CHRONOLOGY

1854, February 9	Born in Sappemeer
1871–1878	Studies medicine
1879, March 8	Receives medical doctorate
1879–1904	Practices medicine in Amsterdam
1880	Becomes acquainted with Carel Victor Gerritsen
1881	Father dies
1881	Founding member of Nieuw-Malthusiaansche Bond (NMB)
1882–1894	Holds free clinic for working women
1892, April 28	Marriage to Carel Victor Gerritsen
1893, September 9	Bears a child who lives only one day
1900	Translates *Women and Economics* by Charlotte Perkins Gilman into Dutch
1901	Founding member of Vrijzinnig Demo-cratische Bond (VDB)
1905, July 5	Gerritsen dies
1903–1919	Chairperson of the Vereeniging voor Vrouwenkiesrecht (VVVK)
1908	Organizes International Woman Suffrage Alliance conference in Amsterdam
1910	Translates *Women and Labor* by Olive Schreiner into Dutch

1911–1912	Travels with Carrie Chapman Catt through Africa and Asia
1915, April 28–May 1	International Congress of Women at The Hague
1918	Candidate for election to the Tweede Kamer (VDB slate)
1919	Suffrage is won for Dutch women
1924	*Herinneringen* (*Memories*) is published in the Netherlands
1929, August 10	Dies at Baarn, the Netherlands

FOREWORD (1924)

The author of these *Memories*, my distinguished cousin, has asked me to help launch her book with a word of introduction. I am delighted to be able to fulfill this request, because both individually and collectively these *Memories* reflect a woman whose whole life has been dedicated to a single cause: to serve the interests of women and to work for their political and social emancipation. The examples of her father and brother inspired her to study medicine, and, despite all the difficulties this entailed fifty years ago, she managed to gain admission to a university. She refused to be discouraged by obstacles or derision and pursued her studies calmly and diligently. Eventually she became a physician and then received her medical doctorate.[1] Thus prepared for professional life, she was determined to use her knowledge and gifts to help alleviate women's suffering and to liberate them from their inferior status. She focused her busy practice on limiting the burden of motherhood and she never allowed gossip or slander to intimidate or distract her from working to prevent unwanted pregnancies.

In fact, medicine was not the only way in which she served female interests; she advocated women's rights socially, politically, and in terms of government participation. The long and difficult struggle to attain female suffrage in this country owes much to Dr. Jacobs, and it is mainly due to her determination that women now have the right to vote. She has also championed peace, tirelessly working with prominent women abroad in the struggle against war. These *Memories* provide a simple but colorful outline of the rich and fruitful life of this courageous woman. They unpretentiously command respect and admiration for their strong and sympathetic author and constitute a shining example for today's youth of what knowledge, willpower, dedication, and endurance can achieve in the public interest.

J. OPPENHEIM[2]
The Hague, February 1924

PREFACE

D oes this book need an introduction? Not really, since it should speak for itself, but I would still like to take the opportunity to add a few general observations.

I can assure the reader that the mere idea of this book filled me with dread, that it took me ages to get down to work. There is a great difference between simply committing one's thoughts and memories to paper and having all that revealed to the public. But I finally gave in to the friendly encourage-ment I received both at home and abroad. However, there is one thing I must confess: when I first started to read through my old letters and papers and make notes so as to put everything into some kind of order, I became increasingly heartened by the idea that there was some real point in writing this book. Modern women and girls will be able to understand just how dull, how difficult and restricted life was for their grandmothers and mothers, and, particularly, for their maiden aunts. Hence, they will be more appreciative of the fact that they can enjoy the best of life now that women are able to lead a free and independent existence. In the following chapters, I don't harp on about how different life used to be, although the contrast between past and present does remain consistently important.

There is yet another reason why I decided to publish this book. Women's memoirs are comparatively rare in this country. Hence, future generations could easily conclude that during the great upheavals of the last fifty years women were never actively involved in the process of social reform.

I have decided not to attempt a complete account of everything I have experienced and encountered; otherwise this book would become far too bulky. Nonetheless, it does convey the level of disappointment, opposition, and innuendo I have had to endure, but also conveys how even in the most difficult of times I have enjoyed the support, friendship, and love of many principled men and women. Fortunately I am an exception to the well-known Dutch maxim that "pioneers come to nothing."

Now, in the evening of my life, I can look back with gratitude on an extraordinary career. I have encountered both sadness and joy. I have traveled throughout much of the world and, wherever I went, found kind and sincere friends, whom I remember with great fondness. Although I can no longer actively participate in the struggle for reform, I am both cheered and comforted by my extensive international correspondence, which keeps me abreast of developments in all corners of the world.

I am still more grateful that I have been able to witness the actualization of three factors vital to the improvement of women's lives and happiness. With my support, women's political and economic independence and planned parenthood have become a reality in the Netherlands. Hence, when my time comes, I will feel free to say that I have contributed to making the world I leave a better place for women than the world I entered.

ALETTA H. JACOBS

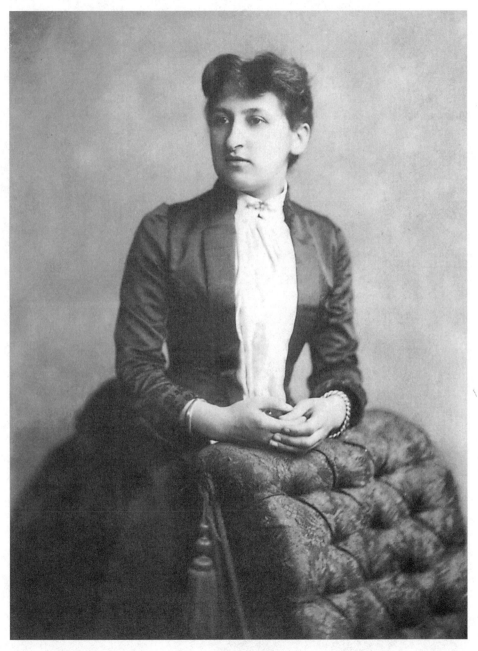

Aletta Jacobs, 1879.
University Museum, Groningen, the Netherlands

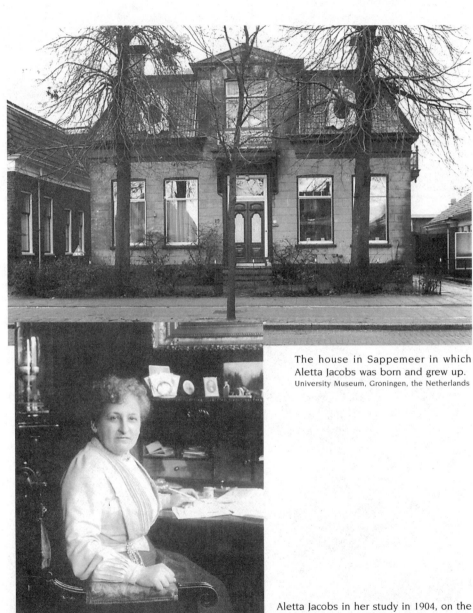

The house in Sappemeer in which
Aletta Jacobs was born and grew up.
University Museum, Groningen, the Netherlands

Aletta Jacobs in her study in 1904, on the
twenty-fifth anniversary of the conferment
of her medical doctorate.
University Museum, Groningen, the Netherlands

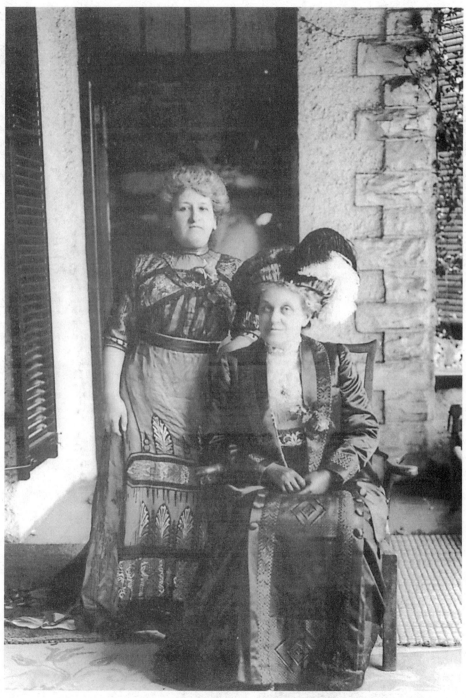

Aletta Jacobs and Carrie Chapman Catt in Capetown, South Africa, 1911.
University Museum, Groningen, the Netherlands

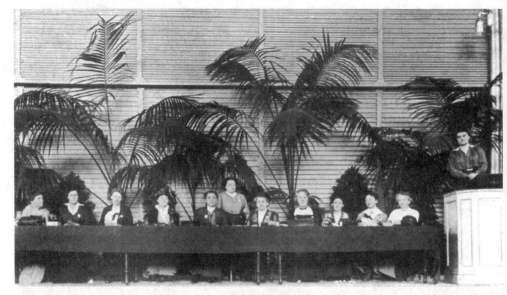

The International Congress of Women at The Hague, 1915. Left to right: Florence Holbrook (U.S.), Mia Boissevain (the Netherlands), Thova Daugaard (Denmark), Fannie Fern Andrews (U.S.), Jane Addams (U.S.), Rosa Manus (the Netherlands), Aletta Jacobs (the Netherlands), Chrystal Macmillan (Great Britain), Kathleen Courtney (Great Britain), Emma Hansson (Norway), Anna Kleman (Sweden), Rosika Schwimmer (Hungary).
International Information Centre and Archives for the Women's Movement (IIAV), Amsterdam, the Netherlands

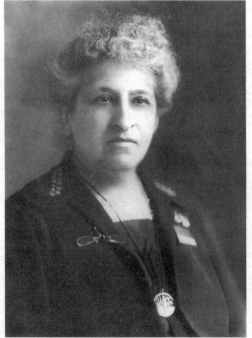

Aletta Jacobs wearing a brooch with a woman suffrage emblem (see page 170), Washington, D.C., 1925.
University Museum, Groningen, the Netherlands

ONE

CHILDHOOD YEARS

Parents and Children • My Early Childhood • How We Were Brought Up • School • Back Home with Mother • Wild Schemes • I Am Trained as a Seamstress • New Paths • My First Exam

A family with seven children rarely greets the advent of an eighth with great enthusiasm—still less so when the current youngest is already entering its fourth year and the parents confidently assume that their brood has reached its limit. It was indeed my doubtful privilege to enter the world on February 9, 1854, as the eighth child of the doctor's family in Sappemeer. Nonetheless my birth was the cause of sincere rejoicing.

My parents, Abraham Jacobs and Anna de Jongh, twenty-three-year-old newlyweds, had first set up house in 1840 in Kiel-Windeweer, a village in the province of Groningen where my father was starting work as the local doctor. His practice provided the only source of income for this otherwise penniless couple. This meant that, during the first years of her marriage, Mother had to manage all the household chores single-handedly—quite an undertaking at that time. She baked the bread, made the butter and cheese, did the washing, and cooked the sausages, preserves, and pickled meats; she also spun, sewed, and darned everything her young family wore. Often Father was away from home all day because most of his patients lived on remote farmsteads, which meant many long treks. When he returned at night, tired and footsore, Mother would help him prepare the medicines that, in those days, the country doctor was also expected to supply.

And each year saw a new addition to the Jacobs clan.

After their third child, Father and Mother realized that the village population would not increase at the same rate as their own burgeoning brood. Even in the long run, Father's limited practice could never support our ever growing number. So they decided to move to Sappemeer. Father was to serve as a physician to this large and prosperous community until 1878, when a heart disorder forced him to abandon his practice. The ledgers we later found among his possessions revealed that in Sappemeer we had to make ends meet on approximately two thousand guilders per year. One year, this amount was augmented by an extra thousand guilders, but there were also years when Father earned no more than fourteen hundred. Admittedly, money went further in the mid-nineteenth century, and life in a Groningen village was certainly cheaper than in a big city. Nevertheless, thrift was essential as the Jacobs family continued to expand.

Despite the fact that I ended up with a grand total of ten brothers and sisters, almost all of us received a thorough education, little of which was available locally. It therefore involved a substantial financial commitment, and Father and Mother were repeatedly advised to save for their old age rather than spend all they had on our schooling. But they simply replied that money invested in this way would yield the most interest. "The cultivation of knowledge for the sake of the common good is the highest of all pursuits" was a dictum that Father often gave us as a writing exercise.

The eldest of my six brothers followed in Father's footsteps, the second studied pharmacy, and the third, who died young, would have earned a doctorate in philosophy. The other three pursued military careers, much against my parents' wishes. One of them had even trained as an architect when he decided to become an officer. Of the five sisters, the eldest married a doctor at the age of nineteen, after briefly training to be a teacher. The second, Charlotte, was destined to become the first woman pharmacist in the Netherlands.[1] I studied medicine, and Frederika, my youngest sister, was the first woman to obtain her teaching certificate in mathematics and accounting. She was then immediately offered a position at the girls' college in The Hague. Just one of the eleven children—a girl—proved totally unsuited to any form of education. All attempts to prepare her for the outside world failed, more through her lack of ability than for want of our trying.

Beginning with the birth of their first child, my parents broke with the prevailing tradition that children should be named after members of the family. Mother felt that it was *her* right to choose the name. And because, like every mother, she was ambitious and had high expectations for her offspring, she felt that it was vital not to burden them with some ugly or discordant name. "After all, I could just as well call you something nice," she later used to say. And then she would tell us how she always wrote down the names she found in novels so that she had a selection ready for the next time a new Jacobs needed to be registered. There was just one exception to this rule, a son, born in 1850, whom Father called Johan Rudolf after Thorbecke, a statesman he greatly admired.[2]

There were various family stories about my birth. For instance, it was said that a few hours before the great event the five oldest children set off for a children's ball decked out in the dresses, trousers, and jackets Mother had washed and ironed that very day. She had carefully dressed the children herself, and when they returned bursting with excitement at about ten that evening they found a new baby sister lying in her crib, so tiny and delicate that at first the girls thought I was the doll Father had always promised them, a doll that could sleep and cry.

I heard this story so often that for years I thought I could actually remember it happening. And it hurt when my older brothers and sisters teased me about my overactive imagination. The stories about my birth always ended with the assurance that Father had greeted the advent of his eighth child with as much joy as he did the first.

That eighth child was to be his favorite. I could do no wrong in his eyes, and this was something my older brothers and sisters often turned to their advantage. If one of the children had some special request, I was usually the one to go and ask Father. I soon ceased being the youngest, as three new additions appeared at regular thirteen- to fourteen-month intervals. "The four little ones," as we were known in the family, formed what was virtually a separate club. I have no memory of dealing with any of the bigger children on equal terms, and I considered myself to be much more the sister of the little ones than of my older brothers and sisters.

Nonetheless, I always worshipped my oldest brother, Julius, who was thirteen years my senior. I have no memories of him before his student days in Groningen, when I knew him as a happy, fun-loving guest, who came to stay with us during his vacations and once turned up completely unannounced with a group of friends. As I have already explained, our financial circumstances could never provide Julius with an adequate student allowance, so he supplemented his income by teaching. He was popular among students and professors alike. And at home we would eagerly count down the days until his return. Sometimes he would regale us with an infinite repertoire of stories, tricks, and songs; sometimes he would chatter endlessly about his life in Groningen.

I worshipped my good, honest, and serious father and my happy-go-lucky brother with his constant high spirits. What's more, I wanted to be like them. I could listen to their conversations for hours on end. Mostly they talked about interesting cases at the Groningen hospital or about my father's practice. Of course I didn't understand half of what was being said, but I was so fascinated that I would instantly desert my friends and toys to listen to them talk.

At the age of six, I solemnly announced that I wanted to be a doctor, just like Dad and Julius. At that point I never imagined that this would be a particularly difficult choice for a girl. Why should it have been? At home the boys and the girls were treated the same: we went to the same school, attended the same classes, were given the same pocket money, and were assigned almost the same chores. Almost the same, because whereas the girls had to knit, sew, and darn, the boys' duties consisted of polishing the shoes and chopping the wood. There were no privileges and, just like the boys, the girls were expected to choose a profession. Of course my parents were greatly amused by my plans, but Father never tried to dissuade me and even actively encouraged me.

If, for whatever reason, I had the day off from school, I would accompany him on visits to patients on distant farmsteads. Later, there were countless occasions when I would reap the benefit of what Father had sown by conversing seriously with me as he made his rounds. In fact, my favorite memory of him combines the image of those country roads with the kindness of his gaze.

Although I loved being able to talk to Father about all sorts of things that were well beyond my experience, sometimes in the middle of a serious discussion I would suddenly find myself distracted by a flower, a field of turnips, or a brightly colored butterfly. Then, before Father knew it, I would vanish in a single leap across a ditch. Although I would later be thoroughly reprimanded, Father was always the first to burst out laughing at my heroic exploits once we reached the farm or returned home.

My repertoire consisted of more than just leaping over ditches. In climbing trees, swimming, rowing, or skating, I was a match for any boy. These activities are not at all uncommon nowadays, but in my time they were very unusual indeed. And when the villagers commented that I was "a real tomboy," it was not intended as a compliment. But although I certainly was a tomboy in some respects, in other ways I was very much a girl. I adored dolls. But I actually never played with them; rather, I spent hours and hours making their clothes. I not only sewed dresses and underwear, I also made hats and even tiny shoes. This is a hobby I still enjoy. After I completed my medical doctorate,[3] I spent some time in London, where I promptly bought myself a doll and some scraps of material. I spent my free time making clothes so that I could surprise my little nieces in Holland with a doll dressed just like the ladies Aunt Let had known in England. Later on when I had to convalesce after an illness and was forbidden to do anything strenuous, I found making dolls' clothes to be a most pleasant diversion. In fact, I was a real professional with handicrafts, and I usually made the lace cap of decorative tulle that our Sappemeer maid wore over her gleaming hair ornaments. I also enjoyed making strips of embroidery and tatting collars, which were all the rage then.

Home was dominated by an exemplary sense of order, and when I compare my parents' methods of bringing up children with those used today, I still feel that their beliefs were in many respects sound. No matter how demanding Father's practice was, he still found time for his children, carefully following both their physical development and their character formation. Each day, under his direction, we performed walking exercises in the long corridor at home: head up, elbows back, chest out. And, each day, we practiced on the gymnastic equipment in the playroom, which was the largest room in the house. Everything was childproof. The wooden chairs and the sturdy table were built to last, and we were allowed to romp to our hearts' content. We each had a cupboard for individual possessions that could be safely locked away. Once a week Mother would check that everything was kept tidy and there was no mess or dirt.

On winter evenings when dusk began to fall, Father would gather us little ones around the fire. With the youngest on his knee and the other three sitting at his feet, he would tell us about the lives of famous men and women or review a particular period of history. The following night we were each expected to describe in our own words what we had heard the day before. If Father was unable to be with us, Mother would take his place. She told us fairy tales or joined us in singing the songs we had learned at school. And with the little ones thus occupied, the older children could get on with their homework in a room that had been specially reserved for the purpose.

Although Father never joined a political party (neither the Social Democrats nor the Liberal Democrats were as yet organized nationally), he was nonetheless a true democrat.[4] I have already mentioned his admiration for Minister Thorbecke. But no matter how great his respect for this extraordinary statesman, he regretted that Thorbecke's brilliance and principles had never come to fruition because prevailing attitudes and the leading parties had always forced him to compromise.

My parents' progressive attitudes even extended to the system of punishments they devised for us. The rule was that the children were sent to bed two by two at half-hour intervals. Those being punished would be sent to bed thirty minutes earlier than their seniority demanded, with the comment, "You've acted like a child and now you're going to be treated like one." This form of punishment was strictly adhered to, and the worst of it was that the parental goodnight kiss was also withheld. That caused real grief. In my case, without my kiss I simply could not sleep. Fortunately Mother made the rounds at ten o'clock each evening, providing the perfect opportunity for the repentant sinner to make amends. Another example of my parents' system of punishment involved an elderberry tree in the back garden. We were forbidden to eat its fruit, and although Father had repeatedly told us the reason why, we were still unable to resist the temptation. One morning when the little ones thought that no one was looking, Father's orders were yet again ignored. When tea was served that afternoon, we were each presented with a covered plate. We were allowed to lift the lid only when everyone else had been served. It was then we discovered that our plates were filled to the brim with elderberries.

"Go on," said Father, "I want you finally to be able to enjoy yourselves to your hearts' content. Today you'll have nothing but elderberries."

Tears streamed from four pairs of eyes, and not one of us managed to gulp down a single berry. In the end, we were allowed to clear our plates for some real food, but from that day on the elderberry tree had completely lost its charm.

The rule was that Mother judged the minor misdemeanors. Father dealt with us only when we had been really wicked. Father never seemed to doubt our stories and as a result we could hide nothing from him. If one of us had been caught misbehaving, he would ask, "Well, what do you think: punishment or forgiveness?" and the perpetrator often meekly admitted that he or she did indeed deserve a small punishment.

The piggy bank played an important role in our upbringing. We were each given one on our fifth birthday. It contained a quarter, and it was our responsibility to ensure that the sum increased. Although we were in charge of our own capital, we also had to buy each other birthday presents and pay for any luxuries, such as silk sashes, bracelets, and necklaces with gold clasps for the girls and silk ties and silver watches for the boys. Every week, Mother gave two cents to each of the little ones and a bit more to the older children. We received a similar amount from Father. We had to keep this in our purses for a whole week, after which those who had succeeded in safeguarding all or part of their capital would have their pocket money replicated on the condition that the original three or four cents were transferred to the piggy bank. The test would then be repeated with the new sum. In addition, we could also earn money by doing jobs around the house. We were paid for everything we did for the family. Whoever knitted ten rows or hemmed a tea towel earned a cent. Darning socks brought in as much as one cent an hour. The boys received similar rewards for polishing shoes, chopping wood, or keeping the turf cellar in order.

Tending the garden was a major undertaking. It took up our free afternoons and many Sunday mornings as well. Weeding, raking, and tying the tall plants, we did everything for a reward of between five and twenty cents per crew, which consisted of all the children still living at home. One of the older brothers or sisters was voted responsible for providing a just division of both work and reward.

If we had heard of partial or general strikes, workers' demands, and the right to fair treatment, I suspect that the gardening would have led to a state of complete uproar. As it was, we were not always satisfied with our individual assignments and tried in vain to determine their price in advance. But the way things stood, the leader had absolute power, and we were to obey his or her commands without questioning.

However, the real problems started when we got paid. Sometimes, we simply refused to put up with the leaders' arbitrary division of the spoils, especially when it involved reserving an inordinate amount for him or herself or resulted in the little ones working for nothing. When this happened, we immediately approached the highest authority, and Father made sure that we didn't fall short, either by redistributing a part of the older children's wages or by giving us each an extra cent out of his own pocket.

One by one, we were sent to the village school, which was attended by boys and girls from all kinds of families, both rich and poor. I shared a desk with an orphan who lived at the workhouse among the sick, feebleminded, and senile. We two were always at the top of the class. In other circumstances, this intelligent child would probably have gone on to further education, but, as it was, she left school at twelve, became a maid, and later married a simple laborer.

The fact that I have always opposed the existence of private schools is based on my experience at the village school. I simply cannot understand the need to categorize small children. Mixed schools automatically confront the sons and daughters of the well-to-do with the hardships endured by working-class families. Conversely, if children from poorer backgrounds are left free to study alongside their wealthier friends, they learn much that will benefit them in later life. As an adult, in my own small way I have always actively supported the abolition of private schools.

I was thirteen when I left the village school, where I had generally been at the top of the class despite the attacks of malaria and the nosebleeds that had often forced me to stay home for anything from a few days to several weeks. During my last year at grade school, I also attended a crafts school where, every evening between five and seven, I learned knitting, crocheting, sewing, and other similar skills. Knitting was my favorite activity because I could read at the same time.

Once she left lower school, the only opportunity for a village girl to continue her education was at the local ladies' school. A high school had just recently opened but it was only for boys. The daughters of gentlemen farmers and prominent families inevitably attended the ladies' school, where they were taught handicrafts and a bit of French, but, above all, they learned "good manners."

I survived just two weeks of life at that fashionable school. They tried to teach me how to enter a room when visiting and I discovered that there was a difference between the way men shook hands with men and the way they shook hands with ladies. I had to learn how to curtsy properly, and, to my eternal discredit, I must admit that I was a less than able pupil. We learned to replace perfectly good Dutch words and expressions with their French equivalents, "because," as our teacher said, "it's more refined to use a little French now and then."

I found all this completely idiotic. "Isn't there something terribly wrong," I wondered, "with wasting your time on this kind of drivel?" I just couldn't see the point of all those classes. Equally I failed to understand why a young girl was supposed to lower her eyes if she passed a gentleman on the street and why in male company she was only to speak in response to questions. The ladies' school became a real nightmare. I felt I was getting dumber by the moment and after just two weeks I decided to call it quits. No matter what they said at home, no one could persuade me to return to school.

My parents were faced with a real dilemma. What were they to do with me? After lengthy deliberation, it was decided that during the day Mother would teach me housework and in the evenings I would learn French and German. I loved those evening lessons. My German progressed at such a rate that I was soon able to read it fluently. And, from that moment, I always had a German book with me, borrowed from Father's extensive collection, so that I could bury myself in some classic when nobody was looking. I tried reading and dusting at the same time, which resulted in many breakages and undusted corners. Mother was horrified and scolded me repeatedly. During that time, my respect for her diminished considerably. Mother simply did not understand me; she never understood the reason for my indifference, for my complete lack of ambition as a housekeeper. As for me, I felt bitterly unhappy at the prospect of living my life like all the other unmarried women in the village: housework in the mornings, knitting, sewing, and staring out the window in the afternoons, and taking a walk between 3 and 4 P.M. Only that, year in, year out. It was enough to drive one crazy, and I resolved to avoid this fate at all costs. But how? Sitting in a dark corner of the attic, I spent hours trying to think out how I could steer my life in a completely different direction. I began to think about the merchant marine captains who lived in the village and were some of my best friends.

If one of these master mariners were to smuggle me to America, I could dress as a boy and get myself a job as a coachman. I wasn't afraid of horses and I had driven a wagon for years. Once I had earned lots of money—and, of course, everyone earned lots of money in America—I could go to college. It seemed a simple enough plan. The one problem was that I was still so small, but, with childish optimism, I figured I would probably shoot up in the coming months.

I was increasingly fascinated by these plans. In fact, I was completely obsessed. I neglected my friends and preferred to be left to my own devices. Of course, my family soon noticed the change in me. The noisy, lively child had suddenly become silent and introverted. Father shook his head doubtfully and warned Mother not to be too strict with me.

"Perhaps we should let her study something outside of the home," Mother suggested in desperation. The idea was duly considered. Mother felt that I had some aptitude for dressmaking, a skill by which I could eventually earn my living. Father let himself be persuaded, and I was even in favor of the plan myself. Anything seemed better than this endless sweeping, dusting, and wash-ing of dishes. What's more, it was only a question of weeks. None of this would matter once I went to America.

So I was apprenticed to the village dressmaker. The fashions of 1868 decreed that skirts should be stitched from bottom to top with narrow strips of material cut on the bias. It was my job to hem these frills by hand. The sheer monotony of this mind-numbing work made me feel more depressed than ever. I slowly realized that the American plan was doomed to failure, yet I could see no other way out. I became more listless as each day passed; I was bored by everything. My malaria attacks returned, and I suffered terrible headaches, which I bore in silence. Illness, even death, seemed preferable to this misery.

Father was never out of touch with his children and he was probably more concerned with me and my future than I ever realized at the time. He suddenly summoned me one day during a visit of the Groningen medical inspector, Dr. L. Ali Cohen, who was a friend of the family.[5] "Show your written language work," said Father. I fetched my exercise books. The guest leafed through them and expressed his satisfaction. This unexpected praise was all too much for me. Beside myself with nervous rage, I grabbed the books, tore them into little pieces, and cried, "Who cares whether or not I do my best? I can never amount to anything because I'm a girl!"

Mother took my arm and as she led me from the room I heard her say to Father, "You have just witnessed one of her tantrums. The child's unmanageable."

A little later, Father summoned me once again. In a friendly tone, he calmly announced that I need never return to the sewing school. "We'll have you learn Greek and Latin," he said, "and then I'll discuss your future with Dr. Ali Cohen."

To calm me down Father took me out for a walk. On the way, I began to complain of a bad headache, and once we got back I felt so sick that I had to go to bed immediately. My nerves were in a terrible state and I was also suffering from anemia. Good food and a few months of rest were prescribed. During my illness, we were often visited by my eldest brother, who was by now a doctor in Groningen and working as Professor Rosenstein's clinical assistant as well.[6] He acted as if it were a foregone conclusion that I would study medicine. We spent many hours building castles in the air and dreaming of what it would be like if we had a joint practice in Groningen. Suddenly life seemed worth living again. I did my best to get fit and healthy, and after some months I was strong enough to begin Latin and Greek. Father was my teacher and Julius would come home now and then just to check my progress. I studied diligently and spent my free time outdoors. I walked on stilts, played with a hoop, did gymnastics, and rowed. I did everything I could to regain my health, "because," as Father kept saying, "you must remember that your future profession will take a great deal out of you physically."

In the autumn of 1869, Dr. Ali Cohen came to tell us that for the first time a girl had taken the admission examination to become a pharmacist's assistant.[7] He thought I should apply to take the same exam. If I passed, I would at least have proved that I was good at studying and I would also gain some useful knowledge for the future. Father and I agreed with him, and I decided to take the exam the very next year. My Latin was certainly good enough, but the curriculum included other subjects I was unable to study at home. Fortunately my second brother, Sam, had set up as a pharmacist in Arnhem just the year before. And Charlotte, who was later to become the first woman pharmacist in

Holland, was working as his housekeeper. The obvious solution was that I would join them and gain the experience necessary for the practical part of the exam. Brother Sam agreed that I should go and live with him, but on the condition that he was not to be dragged into helping out with my studies. Like most men of the day, he found it incomprehensible that I would rather become a pharmacist's assistant than a seamstress. However, these views were not shared by his assistant, who worked in the busy pharmacy morning, noon, and night. He helped me a great deal with my preparations for the exam.

My studies came to an abrupt end a few months later. My married sister's two children were suffering from measles and whooping cough. Their mother was expecting her third baby, and simply could not cope with both housework and nursing on her own. The sister who normally helped out at home was suddenly unavailable, and so, at the tender age of sixteen, I was dispatched to Drenthe to provide the necessary support. During those months I spent at my sister's, I found myself performing tasks that were simply beyond my physical capabilities. Yet I dismissed the suggestion that on that account I postpone taking the examination until the following year. I registered for the exam, along with a number of other women, as it later turned out, and was eventually told to be in Amsterdam on July 26, 1870.

In those days, the journey from Sappemeer to the capital was an event in itself for a young girl who was hardly more than a child. I was inundated with lurid stories about the dangers of the big city and the hazards of traveling, but I took no notice of them. Father reserved a room for me at a hotel on the Damrak that had been recommended by friends and I calmly embarked on the journey to the big and as yet unknown city.

Of the little group of female candidates, I turned out not only to be the youngest but also the smallest by far. In fact, I even had to stand on a footstool to prepare the prescriptions. The other entrants treated me with extreme disdain. A village girl in short skirts who turned up quite on her own, without even a father or brother to chaperone her, was evidently beyond the pale. Indeed, I found myself completely ignored during breaks, but fortunately the examiners turned out to be extremely friendly. Even now, after more than fifty years, I still remember their kindness with deep gratitude.

The exam was a great success. Not only did I pass—the examiners actively encouraged me to study to become a pharmacist, thereby implying that women would also be allowed to take the next round of examinations.

Armed with my diploma, I returned posthaste to Sappemeer, where my future plans were already under discussion. My supporters, including Dr. Ali Cohen and Professor Rosenstein, felt that I should follow the examiners' advice. I, of course, wanted to stick to my original plan. I thought to myself, "If a woman can become a pharmacist, then she's also capable of being a doctor." Nobody had ever tried it and, who knows, maybe it wasn't as impossible as everyone made out.

I finally won Julius over. The other men, including Father, feared that I was physically too frail for such arduous training. And it would take so many years to complete. My entire youth would be spent working and taking exams. I tried to counter these and many other objections, and finally I succeeded, so that the one remaining question was how to prepare me for the admissions exam. Two years of private tutoring in all the required subjects would be an expensive affair, and right up to the exam no one would be able to predict whether or not I would actually be accepted at the university. If I failed, I would have wasted a great deal of money, but, needless to say, all I wanted to do was get down to work immediately.

Many of the subjects were taught at the local high school, but that was only for boys. The headmaster, Mr. Renssen, however, had no objections to my attending. The school was allowed to admit only boy pupils, but there was no ban on girls sitting in on classes. With Thorbecke as minister, he decided it was worth taking the risk. And so it was that I became the first girl to attend a boys' high school. I had known most of the boys from grade school and I got on fine with the teachers as well.

While I was spending Christmas vacation in Groningen, Professor Rosenstein told me that the son of a fellow professor had also passed his student pharmacist's exam. He was using the diploma to try to gain exemption from the university admissions exam so that he could register to study math and physics. This was momentous news, since the sooner I could get started at university the happier I would be. And who better to ask permission from than that well-known liberal, Minister Thorbecke, who also happened to be in power at that time?

We carefully read through the Higher Education Act and concluded there was nothing that specifically forbade women from attending a university. This meant that granting my request would not involve having to change the law. But we decided to first wait and see how it worked out with the son of the Groningen professor.

Minister Thorbecke apparently attached little importance to the admissions exam, and when he granted the boy's request a few days later I immediately applied for exemption as well.[8] I returned to Sappemeer full of hope. But now that my dreams had almost come true, Father took to reiterating his previous objections with fresh conviction. He was worried that I was physically too weak, that even if I managed to finish my training I would be too frail for such a demanding career. Of course it would also involve a considerable financial commitment, and what would happen if, after a few years, I suddenly changed my mind and wanted to do something else? We argued for days on end, but meanwhile I waited, full of anticipation, for the minister's reply.

Finally, and much later than expected, I received a letter from The Hague. But there was no answer to my request, just a list of questions to which I had to respond. Minister Thorbecke wished to know how old I was, why I wanted to study, for what reason I had decided not to work toward the pharmacist's exam, and why I had requested exemption from the admissions examination.

I waited until February 9 to answer, because then I could say that I was seventeen. I answered the minister as honestly as possible but only after I had mailed my letter did I finally tell Father what had been going on. Although he scolded me for my high-handed action and was a little indignant about the fact that I had never mentioned the minister's letter, it was obvious that despite everything he greatly respected my self-reliance.

A few weeks later, the postman returned with a second letter from The Hague. This time it was addressed to Father. Minister Thorbecke informed him of our correspondence and expressed the opinion that I was too young to appreciate the consequences of my actions. Perhaps it would therefore be wiser to reject my request. I could go on studying for a few more years and still have time to change my mind.

Nonetheless, the letter stated that the minister would give his consent provided that Father also approved of my plans. Hence, the decision lay with the man who up until recently had always championed my choice of career. Father hesitated. He did not know what to do, so he asked Julius to come over from Groningen and suggested that I think things over once more.

"There's no point in thinking things over," I replied. "I know exactly what I want to do and I have known for ages."

Julius arrived and I was summoned to face the "triumvirate." First my father and brother described in lurid detail all the least appetizing aspects of a doctor's training, including anatomy lessons, vivisection, skin diseases, and the shameless conduct of some hospital patients. But that came as no great shock. Then Julius asked me whether I really believed that I was capable of taking the examinations. I reminded him of his endless complaining about the stupidity of many of the students he had prepared for these exams. If these young people still managed to get through, then why not me, especially as I was full of ambition and determined to study?

No sooner had Father, Julius, and I concluded our discussions, than Mother voiced her own objections, and these were harder to dismiss. She was convinced that the only reason I wanted to study was to get out of doing housework and felt it was essential for me to learn these domestic skills. She finally consented to my future career on the condition that I agreed to devote my holidays to household chores and that henceforth Father would treat me just like my sisters. If I needed a new dress, I would be given the money to buy the material, which I would then have to cut and sew myself. Of course, I was prepared to agree to anything and everything. What did I care about all those conditions now that I had practically achieved my goal? I promised Mother that during the holidays I would do whatever she wanted me to. I should perhaps add that what I eventually learned from her did indeed stand me in good stead in later life.

The outcome of our discussions was that Father wrote to Minister Thorbecke that he approved of my plans. At the beginning of April 1871, I received notice of my exemption from the admissions exam and that I was permitted to attend classes at the University of Groningen for the period of one year. The minister wrote that, after this probationary period, I was to request permanent permission to study. So, ultimately, the opening of the Dutch universities to women depended on my progress during this first year.

After talking with Professor Rosenstein, who was also rector that year, it was decided that I would begin to attend medical lectures right after the Easter holidays. I could thus use the short period preceding the summer vacation as a test period. Should reality fall short of my dreams, there was nothing lost, and, if it all worked out, the other students would already be used to my presence by the start of the new academic year. I had only two weeks to prepare, and that included making a new dress. There was no way I could attend lectures looking like a child. Out of the money that Father gave me, I bought a piece of black worsted and tailored a plain and unadorned dress, although the current fashion was for crinolines and frills. Also, my cupboard in the playroom was cleared out to make space for textbooks and my toys were handed over to the younger children. But I did keep one beautiful doll whose clothes I had made myself.

Since then I have been repeatedly asked whether at the time I was fully aware of what my entering a university was to symbolize to the women of Holland. Did I know that the issue of women's admission to higher education was also the subject of heated debate in a number of other countries?

Despite the fact that the opposite is suggested by various articles about me, I will now set the record straight by stating that when I went to Groningen I had virtually no idea of the consequences of what I was doing. How could I? I had been brought up in a village and knew little of the world at large. It is true that ours was a liberal household, but the newspaper was all that kept us in touch with outside events. I should also point out that one copy was shared with three other families and that the younger children never got a chance to read it at all. Combine that with the fact that the Dutch women's movement was still in its infancy and I think the reader will by now appreciate that this seventeen-year-old village girl was completely ignorant of the objectives later attributed to her.[9] My sole ambition was to complete my education and to go into practice with either Julius or my father.

When I first became a student I was little more than a child. I was frail and sexually undeveloped. The only difference between me and other children was a matter of willpower and the thirst for knowledge. It was only after graduation that I became involved in the struggle for female emancipation.

To conclude this first chapter, I would like to draw attention to one aspect of this story that was to have important consequences for Sappemeer. My youngest

sister, Frederika, was just fourteen when I left for Groningen. She had completed grade school and wanted to continue her education, although she had
yet to decide about a future career. Again we encountered the complete absence
of academic opportunity for the girls of our village. However, Frederika
followed my example and was allowed to sit in on classes at the high school for
boys, but this time at great expense. Both my youngest brothers were also sent
there because the fees were considerably lower for additional children from the
same family. Nonetheless, Father still resented having to pay out large sums of
money when the boys were accepted as regular pupils but Frederika was not.

Minister Thorbecke somehow discovered what was going on, with the result
that Father's request was granted and, in 1871, the high school opened its gates
to girl pupils under exactly the same conditions that applied to the boys. Things
remained this way until 1901, when this provision, which pertained only to the
village of Sappemeer, was withdrawn by Minister Abraham Kuyper. Girls
wanting to attend the local high school encountered the same restrictions that
applied to their counterparts elsewhere. But finally, in 1905, Minister Rink
reinstated the privileges that Thorbecke first bestowed on Sappemeer.

TWO

STUDENT YEARS

I Become a Student • My Experiences in and around the University • Provisional Permission Becomes Permanent Permission • A Candidate in Mathematics and Physical Sciences • I Pass My Second Exam with Honors • The Practice of Life • Disillusionment • Fresh Hope • I Begin Practicing • Amsterdam • I Achieve My Goal • My Country Practice • My Doctorate • London

April 20, 1871, was undoubtedly one of the most extraordinary days of my life. That was the day I left for the University of Groningen with my brother Julius, who was to introduce me to my future professors and fellow students. For the time being, I had only to attend math and physics lectures and classes in logic.

My first weeks at college have been described by Professor Salverda, who was then head of zoology and comparative anatomy at the University of Groningen.[1] Writing for the May 7, 1871, issue of *Ons Streven,* he comments, "Did Miss Jacobs encounter many difficulties? You should have asked me that *before* our new student was first introduced by her brother, Dr. Julius Jacobs, and then took her place alongside the rest of the class. I would have made no secret of the fact that I felt that initial step was going to need quite some courage, but she never hesitated for a second. And the way it worked out surpassed even my wildest dreams. I'm convinced that we'll soon get beyond any initial awkwardness. And I think it's important to add that Miss Jacobs's attitude has also been extremely helpful.

"It goes without saying that you need a certain delicacy in dealing with introductory subjects in an auditorium that includes the presence of a female student. And that's particularly true of zoology. But, apart from the fact that *'c'est le ton qui fait la musique,'* my comparative anatomy classes will also involve dealing with some aspects in a special way, meaning that on certain occasions Miss Jacobs will be advised not to attend those lectures, which will be taught to her on an individual basis.

"Of course, we will try to make Miss Jacobs's life as simple as possible. She spends the fifteen-minute interval between lectures in the empty hall or in an adjacent room and then proceeds to the next class where a place has been specially set aside for her.

"That's all I have to say for the time being. If everything continues as well as it has up till now, we can but hope and trust that Miss Jacobs's example will be followed both here and elsewhere."

I rarely exploited the privilege of separate classes. After my second individual lesson in comparative anatomy, I decided I had to speak to Professor Salverda, who was a most kindly and patient teacher. I had come to the conclusion that from the very start I should view myself as being the absolute equal of the young men whose student rights and duties I wished to share. It would be better all around if everyone immediately accepted my presence at lectures where, after all, scientific subjects were being dealt with in a scientific way. I had no desire for any preferential treatment whatsoever and that was why, rather than spend my free time in the empty lecture hall, I soon joined the other students to discuss the most interesting parts of our lectures.

In this respect, fortunately not only the professors but also the vast majority of students were both courteous and encouraging. This attitude is also demonstrated by an article that was published in the *Studenten Weekblad* of June 5, 1871. It was written by "O.," a Groningen student, in response to a piece penned by a certain "Theodoor" who was attending Leiden University. Theodoor had made certain insinuations about me and had advised the Groningen students to make my life so miserable that I would be forced to quit the university. My sudden departure would in turn discourage all the other women who were about to follow my example. Like a knight-errant, O. decided to champion my cause. He wrote,

"We are grateful for Miss Jacobs's confidence in us. She has made it clear that she knew there were no Theodoors at our university. The fact that we have not betrayed her trust is something we can be proud of at Groningen. That's why your words offend us and why I must take up the gauntlet on her behalf."

Kamerlingh Onnes later became a professor at Leiden University and his research in physics is of worldwide repute.[2] He apparently thought none the worse of me when years later I publicly thanked him for the way in which as a young student he had protected my interests and defended my rights.

Although I experienced no hostility from the people I was *directly* involved with, my attending the university caused considerable commotion in the country at large. Even the liberal newspapers repeatedly voiced their opposition. Ironically they were always the first to inform their readers when prevailing male opinion condemned or ridiculed female students abroad. Of course, it goes without saying that I would not be "spared" by the conservative and religious press. Those papers seemed convinced that Miss Jacobs had become a student just so she could meet members of the opposite sex! While it was impossible to suggest that I lavished excessive attention on my appearance, they even managed to spot some dangerous intent in my *simple* choice of clothing. The reason I dressed as I did was that I was determined to attract notice.

The worst of it was that the press even managed to influence the attitudes of my own family. Brother Sam, the pharmacist, had first dissociated himself from my academic aspirations when I stayed with him in Arnhem. He now accused Father of giving in to my every whim. As a result, the whole family felt dragged into the Aletta Jacobs affair. "There's something wrong," he argued, "with one child out of eleven being allowed to damage the prospects of all the others. You should have her doing the washing instead of packing her off to a university with a pile of books under her arm."

And my brother Johan, who had by then become a petty officer at the military school in Kampen, wrote that my ridiculous actions had made his life completely unbearable. His fellow soldiers had invented all kinds of insulting nicknames for me and, merely because I was his sister, everyone automatically assumed he shared my views. The situation got so bad that he finally announced to his class that he would have nothing more to do with me.

He kept this up for a year and a half. He never mentioned me in his letters, and when he was at home on leave he acted as if I simply did not exist. How often in those days I seemed to be surrounded by men saying, "Fortunately my daughters, or sisters, aren't like *that*."

Mine was no easy life. I got up at half-past five each morning because if I wanted to be on time for lectures I had to catch the six-thirty train from Sappemeer. The walk to the station was always windy and dusty, but it became virtually impassable when the weather was bad, particularly if it had snowed.

If I walked fast, it took only fifteen minutes to get to the station. Sometimes I saw the train approaching while I was still on my way, but the stationmaster always made sure that it didn't leave without me. And, thanks to the benevolence of the stationmaster and the ticket collectors, I was usually ushered into a first-class compartment although I had only a third-class season ticket. When I arrived in Groningen, it was still far too early for class. If the weather was bad, I would end up spending at least an hour in a drafty waiting room. But if it was dry I could go to the local botanical gardens where I learned much from the old gardener who worked there.

Our lectures were usually over by 4 P.M. I would return to Sappemeer as quickly as possible, gulp down a meal, which had been kept warm for me, and proceed to one of the private lessons I was taking in math, physics, and a number of other subjects. Then, after tidying up my lecture notes, I was finally able to relax.

Sometimes severe headaches forced me to let up for a few days. With infinite compassion, Mother would spend the whole day applying cold compresses to my burning forehead. Even at night she never left my bedside. She was more convinced than ever that I was suffering because of a dreadful error in judgment for which my father and I were jointly responsible. And whenever I had almost recovered, she would again try to persuade me to abandon my studies.

Rumors began circulating in the spring of 1872 that Thorbecke was suffering from a serious illness and that his life was in danger. The minister's death could have had disastrous consequences for me as I had not yet been granted permanent permission to complete my education. What would happen if Thorbecke's successor opposed my cause? After consulting my professors, I quickly took exams in those subjects where my knowledge was already sufficient. I immediately sent the written proof of my successful results to the minister with the request that he should no longer withhold my permanent permission for further education.

Two days after Thorbecke's death, on June 5, 1872, I received the permission, complete with a funereal black border. It was dated May 30, 1872, and an accompanying letter informed me that the granting of this request had been one of the minister's last official acts.

This valuable document filled me with an enormous sense of relief. I could now calmly prepare for my first academic examination, which I passed *non sine laude* (with honors) on October 17, 1872. It also meant that from that point on I would be officially regarded as being a "candidate in mathematics and physical sciences."

Miss H. J. Schaap, who was the sister-in-law of the painter Jozef Israëls, wrote in *Ons Streven* of October 10, 1872,[3]

"This afternoon at two o'clock, the small auditorium of the Academy Building was the scene of a unique event for these simple surroundings. For it was in this hall that an exam was taken by a young lady whose name was the subject of much debate just some eighteen months ago. I am, of course, referring to Miss Aletta Jacobs of Sappemeer.

"She entered our university as a medical student in 1871 and followed the lectures with great enthusiasm. Gifted with a fine intellect and plenty of willpower, she has managed with relative ease to overcome the obstacles encountered in her struggle to become a pioneer, an undertaking which is still unusual for a woman in this country. Today she has been able to reap the benefit of her labors, having gained honors in her philosophy exam, which precedes the study of medicine.

"It is no wonder that this exam attracted a horde of curious students, yet there were just two women present, one being the author of this piece.

"Leaving the spacious entrance hall, which was filled with students, we entered a small room where the candidate waited with her father for the moment when the bell would signal the examination's commencement. She was completely calm, talking and laughing as usual. The bell went off, and Miss Jacobs and her father entered the auditorium where the exam was to take place, the rest of us trailing in after her. With complete composure, she sat down at the green table facing the professors of the philosophy faculty. The public settled down and the exam was soon underway.

"To make a long story short, there were four examiners specializing in botany, advanced mathematics, physics, and chemistry. Not once did Miss Jacobs lose her customary directness, and she responded to her examiners' questions with brief but well-thought-out answers.

"After an examination lasting about an hour and a quarter, Miss Jacobs was asked to leave the auditorium for a moment, during which the faculty decided to award her the degree she so obviously deserved. And, a little later, this future doctor discovered to her absolute delight that she was now officially a 'Candidate in Mathematics and Physics,' which is preparatory to the study of medicine. Her efforts also received the additional accolade of *non sine laude*.

"The building resounded with students' cheers that reflected the way in which they too have participated in the success of their female classmate.

"Let's hope that others follow her example and that she is not simply one of a kind."

After the success of my first examination, I was inundated with letters of congratulation from all over the country. People I had never heard of, and would never hear of again, invited me into their homes or to their country estates where I could relax after all my hard work. I replied thanking them politely but wrote that I was not planning to take a holiday at this point in time. My next goal was to take my medical degree. And it was a matter of "the sooner the better."

Out of all the messages, there was one letter that particularly attracted the attention of both Father and myself. It was postmarked Amersfoort and signed by a C. V. Gerritsen. Neither the handwriting nor the contents gave any clue as to whether this letter had been written by a man or a woman. But it conveyed a real sense of joy that a Dutch girl had proved that she too could succeed at a university and wished me luck in my future studies both personally and for the sake of the women of Holland.

An Amersfoort family now living in Groningen was finally able to unravel this mystery. The letter had been written by a man. My informants told me that he was about twenty-three and had caused his parents great distress. When I asked what exactly he had done, they told me that he came from a religious family but refused to go to church, that the controversial writer Multatuli had been his guest, and that they had even been seen together in public![4] C. V. Gerritsen was also rumored to have written a pamphlet inciting working-class discontent, which he had distributed to all interested parties entirely free of charge.

Although Father could hardly *object* to all this, for reasons of prudence he nonetheless advised me not to answer this letter. I completely disagreed with him. What was wrong with a young man expressing his beliefs? Why should he attend church if he was not religious? Certainly it would be hypocritical to go just for the sake of his parents. Many of the most important people in Holland admired Multatuli, and, although I had not read his books myself, I knew many sensible young men who positively worshipped him. As far as the workers were concerned, Father himself always said, "Their lot will never improve until they can bear it no longer."

After some consideration and despite Father's advice, I finally decided to answer the letter. I never suspected for one moment that it would lead to a deep and loving friendship.

When I think back over the years, the period spent preparing for my medical exams now strikes me as being the most difficult of my entire life. I often felt dissatisfied with myself and wondered if it would not have been wiser to have followed Mother's advice and stick to housekeeping like other girls. Yet I did not find studying difficult, and housework hardly seemed an attractive alternative. There were other, deeper reasons for this mood. Opposite my parents' house, and on the other side of the waters of the Winschoterdiep, was a shipyard with a couple of modest dwellings. A young couple with a year-old baby lived in one of these houses. I could watch them from the study. Sometimes, in the afternoons when my attention wandered from digesting my boring anatomy notes, I would look up to see the young woman holding the child in her arms, waiting for her husband's return. As he approached, she would place the child on the ground so that he could toddle toward his father. The man would put the delighted baby on his shoulders, and the happy parents would head back home together. To have a child like that, to bring it up far from the rest of the world, seemed to me to be the greatest of all joys. But, since I had become a student, I was always hearing and reading about what an example I was to other women, and I realized that I had no alternative but to follow my chosen path.

Only much later did I realize that then I had been in the process of changing from a child to a woman and feeling the first stirrings of sexuality. These feelings included a strong desire for motherhood, although I never thought in terms of a man, the child's father. I later discovered that these experiences cause many young girls to abandon their education. They do not realize that this sense of dissatisfaction is in no way connected with their studies. Even girls who do not choose to study find themselves with exactly the same longings because almost every normal woman wants to have a baby at some point in her life. The fact that this urge cannot be fulfilled causes actual suffering, which would not occur in a *well*-ordered society. Our immoral conception of sexuality means that *respectable* motherhood must be confined exclusively to the sanctity of marriage.

I found anatomy unbelievably dull, especially the first part, which deals with bones and muscles. But I realized that I was just going to have to struggle through it, preferably as quickly as possible. The circulatory organs were marginally more interesting, and I was completely fascinated by the brain. I wanted to learn far more than was actually required for my medical degree. However, at that time little was known about the finer details of cerebral anatomy so many of my questions simply went unanswered.

The horrors of my first dissecting room class will stay with me forever. In my mind's eye, the unknown corpse was still a living person. Cutting into it was like committing a murder. And when I was given one of its arms to prepare, I had to summon up all my willpower to get on with the job and not show how I felt about it. The dead body and the bloody arm haunted for me ages, both night and day. I was unable to eat meat and wherever I went I seemed to be pursued by the stench of cadavers. My sole comfort was that none of my fellow-students realized what I was going through. They had expected at least a fainting fit and were forced to admit that I had braved the secrets of the dissecting room with manly determination.

Anatomy was never to be one of my favorite subjects; however, I was completely fascinated by my physiology lectures. I would have loved to continue studying this science even after I had taken my degree, but it proved difficult to combine with my plans for the future. Moreover, I found it hard to come to terms with experimenting on living animals, and was totally incapable, for instance, of cutting the head off a frog. Fortunately Mr. Plugge, our kindly assistant, would surreptitiously perform that part of the exercise for me whenever the need arose.

On April 23, 1874 (and hence within the statutory two years), I took the first of my qualifying exams and once again I passed non sine laude.

By now it was high time that I took a rest. My temperature would shoot up once every three days, thoroughly undermining my whole system. I was ordered to take a "complete break and a change of air." After dutifully promising not to do anything until September, I left for Lochem where my brother Julius had set up his practice some years previously (in late 1871). Nonetheless, I brought my new textbooks in case I recovered sooner than expected.

Everything worked out as I had hoped it would. My fever attacks slowly subsided, and after three months they had disappeared altogether. And, thanks to the Gelderland air, I felt much stronger and healthier than when I had first arrived in Lochem. Sometimes I took out my books. Julius helped me with my work, and by the time lectures resumed in September I already had some idea of what lay ahead.

I moved to Groningen at the beginning of the term. My new home was a small back room above a carpenter's yard on the Turftorenstraat. Now I could finally get down to the part of my training that attracted me most: the practical lessons with real patients. To be honest, I was generally as interested in the patients themselves as I was in their illnesses. And I was particularly fascinated by the lives of the women I treated.

It is possible that this was the point at which my feminist and democratic beliefs first began to take root. I certainly had plenty of opportunities to witness the hardships endured by working-class women and to see how little government and philanthropic support was available for families when the wife and mother was absent because of illness. For my part, I tried to alleviate the suffering of hospital patients by contacting their families and, if necessary, providing active support. In this way, working with patients not only taught me about disease but also much about society itself. I learned how our absurd marriage laws caused blatant inequality between husbands and wives. I discovered social injustice: despite the general increase in prosperity, many families could never rise beyond a certain level. I encountered the consequences of child neglect and began to realize why, despite the ability to achieve, many boys and girls are doomed to a life of poverty. And, I gradually became aware of abuses in society, which, although I did not as yet understand them fully, were to obsess me until I later decided to find out everything I could about them.

I also began to realize what it was like to be a prostitute in our society by treating a twenty-eight-year-old woman who was admitted to the hospital in the final stages of syphilis. Above her bed hung the standard sheet of paper used to record patients' particulars. It stated that she was a "meretrix," a word I had never heard before. I was made none the wiser by its dictionary definition, "a woman of the streets." So I asked my old friend Dr. Ali Cohen to enlighten me on this subject. Previously he had always done his utmost to satisfy my curiosity, but this time his answer was evasive, and he suggested that I should have nothing to do with this woman. I cannot recall whether or not I obeyed his advice at first, but I do remember that no one ever visited that pale and beautiful girl, that no one actually took any notice of her at all. Finally a sense of empathy drove me to bring her some flowers. The more I saw of her, the more she felt she could trust me. And when she realized that I really was interested in her, she began to tell me the story of her life, which I later discovered was typical of so many other prostitutes. She was an orphan from Amsterdam who had been seduced at the age of nineteen by a gentleman of means. Knowing no way out, she went from bad to worse and from brothel to brothel until she finally ended up in the hospital, a safe and peaceful haven that she would never leave alive.

My bedside visits did not pass unnoticed, and one day the assistant physician discreetly advised me to terminate all contact because otherwise I would be the target of malicious gossip and ill feeling. I responded by telling him a little about this woman's life and I assured him that nothing would keep me from helping her through the last days of her life. My words obviously impressed him. He promised not only to assist me but also to inform the other students of my views.

And soon afterward my unfortunate patient was released from her mortal suffering.

Another current form of abuse was brought to my attention in a somewhat cruder fashion. One day, one of the professors asked me to accompany him and his assistant to a back room of the hospital where nine poorly dressed women were awaiting our arrival. One by one, they were curtly ordered to strip and to lie down on a wooden table. Both men treated these women like objects and inspected them without actually bothering to touch them. There followed a brief discussion, after which seven of the women were told to leave and the other two were instructed to have themselves admitted to the hospital. The seven women left in the company of an insolent-looking fellow who had been waiting for them. I felt furious at the cynicism with which these women had been treated—altogether their examination had lasted less than twenty minutes—and by the peculiar manner in which seven of them had been dismissed. I wanted to know exactly what was going on, why these women were being treated in this way, why two of them were detained, and what was going to happen to the others. Sensing my consternation, the professor apologized for having asked me to attend this examination. Because I had talked so much with the prostitute on the ward, he assumed that I would automatically understand what was happening. He felt that it might help me in my future career to know something about the regulation of prostitution.

He was quite right, for I was later to become deeply involved in the battle against brothels and against the regulation of prostitution in the Netherlands.[5] That afternoon in Groningen proved to me that regulation provides absolutely no guarantee against infection, that the process humiliates both patient and doctor, and that a civilized land should tolerate brothels no more than it would permit slave markets.

Armed with an increasing understanding of both medicine and society, my plan was to begin working for my clinical finals. Unfortunately I suffered a recurrence of malaria—complete with secondary symptoms—in the early spring of 1876. I felt dull and listless and was plagued by a constant dry cough. Concerned about my symptoms, one of my professors decided to give me a thorough examination. I was slowly, painstakingly percussed and auscultated. He then tried to persuade me to give up my studies for, even if I passed my examinations, I would never be strong enough to maintain an active medical practice. Would it not be wiser, given the state of my health, to concentrate on the enjoyment of life?

It was obvious that the professor had diagnosed pulmonary tuberculosis, as he was later to inform my father in writing. At the time no one believed that it was possible to cure this disease, not even when discovered in its earliest stages. With the professor's words still ringing in my ears, I returned to my room, packed my bags, and left for Sappemeer to inform my parents about my condition.

I arrived home in a state of complete despondency. I had overestimated my strength and had tried to do far more than I was capable of. Lying in bed that night, I finally reached my decision: what point was there in prolonging an empty and meaningless life?

In the dead of night, at about two o'clock, I crept into Father's pharmacy looking for the key to the poisons cabinet. No sooner did I lay my hand on it than the door swung open and Father was standing in front of me still fully dressed. He said in a calm voice, "That's just what I thought you would do, but we should talk about it first." He then told me how, even in his own practice, some cases simply defy diagnosis. He mentioned the current difficulty in determining the early stages of tuberculosis and suggested that I go to Professor Rosenstein in Leiden for a second opinion. If his diagnosis concurred with the Groningen professor's, then I still had time to decide what I wanted to do about my future.

It took Father two days to make arrangements regarding his work, and then we left for Leiden. Later I found out that those two days were also necessary for Professor Rosenstein to receive a detailed letter from Father describing my symptoms. Rosenstein also examined me with painstaking care, and then announced that he had found nothing seriously wrong with me. My cough was simply a nervous cough. I should return to work so that I could take the next round of exams as soon as possible. After that, he advised an immediate change of air to give me the best possible chance to recover from the malaria and regain my health and strength.

This advice cheered me up no end. I tackled my studies with renewed vigor and passed my exams just before the beginning of the summer holidays. Two days later, I left for Lochem, and this time my books stayed safely at home. I wanted to make sure that I returned 100 percent healthy.

Even in those days I soon realized how quickly people would adjust to the idea of being treated by a woman doctor. I often replaced my brother in an emergency and there was never any problem, regardless of whether the patient was a woman in childbirth, a young boy, or an elderly person. I was accepted with complete confidence and was sometimes even asked to continue treating the patient. Once, many years later, when I lectured on woman suffrage in Lochem, a young man gave me a bunch of flowers on behalf of his parents to thank me for treating them in the summer of 1876.

Because my brother Julius, who was by that time married, left shortly after my visit for the Dutch East Indies, I was never again to have the opportunity of practicing in Lochem.

Now that my health had greatly improved with the change of air, it was decided that I should take my clinical finals at a different university. We first thought of Leiden because of Professor Rosenstein. But no sooner had news of our plans leaked out than two of the local professors bluntly informed me that they could survive quite well without my presence. I did not let this announce-ment influence my decision, but I nonetheless felt far more attracted by the prospect of Amsterdam, where the hospital was bigger and the social life brighter. However, I was warned that my classes would also be attended by military students training to become medical corps officers, who had a reputation for being extremely crude. This objection failed to make much of an impression on me, and I should also add that it was never a problem in practice. Once I had received assurances that the Amsterdam City Council would in no way object to my attending the university, I rented a small room from a widow who lived near the hospital.

On October 2, 1876, the dean of Amsterdam University, Professor Jorissen, registered me as a medical student at the Athenaeum Illustre. The same day I went to meet the medical professors whose lectures I was to attend.

I first went to see Professor Stokvis, and it soon became apparent that my visit was more than simply a matter of courtesy.[6] The professor greeted me with an air of surprise, and one of his first questions concerned my youth. He found it hard to believe that at the age of twenty-three a woman's experiences could drive her to seek solace in such a demanding subject as medicine. Now it was my turn to feel astonished, and my astonishment grew by the moment as I heard the stories that had been circulating in Amsterdam about the unhappy love affair for which I had substituted my medical training. The other professors also expressed amazement at my appearance. One of them asked me sympathetically if it was possible to be so young and already a widow. I assured the professors that not only was I not a widow but that I had yet to fall in love.

The next morning, I was met by a throng of students at the hospital entrance. These young men formed two parallel lines through which I was forced to pass. Maybe they thought that this would intimidate me. I acted as if I did not understand what was going on. I greeted the students and calmly walked between the two rows toward the lecture hall. The ice was finally broken. A student then introduced himself and offered to help me. Others followed suit, and soon both professors and students were completely accustomed to my presence. To the very end of my student years, I encountered nothing but politeness and helpfulness from everyone, whether it was in the dissecting room or on the maternity ward at night.

Amsterdam taught me how to stand on my own two feet. In Groningen it was as if I were still tied to Mother's apron strings. Moreover there were always friends and acquaintances whom I could consult whenever I needed advice. But when I first lived in Amsterdam I was completely on my own; I knew no one. And life in the hospital was even more rudimentary than in Groningen. There was no such thing as a well-trained nurse in those days. After the doctors had made their rounds, the female patients were left to the tender mercies of the "hospital maids," and the male patients to the "hospital servants." These "maids" were women whose backgrounds prevented them from entering normal domestic service. They were rude, uncouth, and often dissolute creatures, and yet were considered good enough to work in a hospital. It goes without saying that these circumstances gave Amsterdam's poorer inhabitants little reason to choose to learn the skills of hospital nursing. Sometimes I would take personal responsibility for the care of a seriously ill patient, and I spent many nights in the hospital with my textbooks. I soon learned by experience that it was a good idea to stay inside the wards at night. The scenes that took place in the corridors between the maids and the servants defied description. In short, they were disgusting.[7]

It was a harsh winter that year (1876/1877). The ponds in the Vondelpark were covered with thick ice for days on end. Because I had learned to skate when I was very young (like most children in Groningen and Friesland), I was able to enjoy this healthy winter sport to my heart's content.

I caused quite a sensation because at that time women did not skate in Amsterdam. There was always a band of curious onlookers every afternoon I went skating in the Vondelpark with a group of students or with the sisters of colleagues who also happened to come from the north. It even got into the papers, with the result that Amsterdam women also took to skates.

I slowly got to know a few families who would invite me into their homes on Sunday afternoons so that, after much studying, I could relax in a pleasant environment like any other young woman my age. My Amsterdam acquaintances treated me warmly, and I still remember the many happy hours I spent enjoying their hospitality.

One of the reasons I had chosen to complete my training in Amsterdam concerned the state examining board for clinical finals. Each year it entirely reconstituted itself and met in a different university town. In 1877, the board was to move to Amsterdam and would mainly consist of local professors. Groups of students would begin taking the first part of their finals in the spring of that year. I had registered with one of the first of these groups so that in the autumn I could take the second part of my finals, which would, of course, be adjudicated by the same board. I looked forward eagerly to April 12, when I was to take the written part of the examination. At that time, I was never afraid of failing, yet in the days preceding the exam I began to feel a sense of unease. I began to dread whatever lay in store for me. There was a gap of a few days between the written and oral parts of the examination during which I felt increasingly miserable despite reassurances that I had done well so far. I knew that fear was not the cause of my problems. The day before my oral exam, I felt so wretched that I asked one of the examiners if I could postpone the date.

The good man was highly amused and quickly diagnosed a bad case of exam nerves. "I wouldn't back out if I were you," he said. "Get a grip on yourself and turn up tomorrow as agreed." And I dutifully did what he said, although I felt extremely unwell.

By this stage, my results hardly seemed to matter anymore. I collected my diploma and accepted the congratulations of both professors and students with a feeling of complete indifference. Without thinking, I set off for the house of Mrs. Godefroy, a close friend who was holding a dinner in my honor. But, by the time I arrived, I felt so ill that I had to go to bed immediately. The doctor was sent for, and he was so concerned about my condition that he decided to consult Professor Stokvis. Stokvis also seemed alarmed. He insisted that I needed round-the-clock care and managed to find a nurse for me from one of the private hospitals. The next day, they diagnosed that I was probably suffering from typhus. Father was sent a telegram asking him to come at once. There was no question of my being transferred to a hospital. I simply had to stay with Mrs. Godefroy. Father came as soon as he could. He also brought my sister Charlotte, who, after my brother Sam had married, had returned home to train as a pharmacist and had already taken her first exam.

I was to stay with my friend Mrs. Godefroy for a full four months. Nothing was too much trouble for her, and she made sure that I got plenty of peace and quiet. Charlotte nursed me devotedly, and my doctor was none other than Professor Stokvis himself.

I suffered several intestinal hemorrhages and other serious relapses. Telegrams were immediately dispatched to Sappemeer that made one fear the worst. Father would once again make an anguished journey to the distant capital while Mother stayed at home in a state of complete despair. Friends and acquaintances remained in touch throughout my illness, with one young man even making inquiries several times a week, although he refused to leave his name. "She doesn't know me yet," was his excuse. It was only much later that I discovered that my loyal well-wisher was none other than C. V. Gerritsen from Amersfoort.

I had become ill in mid-April, and it was not until August that Professor Stokvis finally allowed me to travel to Sappemeer. Weak, and completely bald, I arrived to be greeted by the entire village. Everyone had been deeply concerned for my parents and was overjoyed at the news of my recovery.

Although my hair grew back and I gradually regained my strength, for the time being there was no question of resuming my studies. It was only after the winter holidays that I was allowed to return to Amsterdam to prepare for the second part of my finals, which would be held in Utrecht. Secretly I had hoped that I would be included in one of the later groups, but that was not to be. On March 15, 1878, I was informed I had an appointment five days later with the medical examining board in Utrecht.

It was during this exam that I first encountered professors who openly opposed the idea of women doctors. Two gentlemen treated me in a way that was simply unfair. Fortunately, several other Utrecht professors as well as my teachers from Amsterdam actively protected me from these two examiners' remarks and behavior. Indeed, it was only because of this protection that I was able to complete the exam at all.

I felt a profound sense of happiness when I finally received my medical degree on April 2, 1878. Now there would be no more examinations. Although I still had to write my thesis, at that stage there was no real risk of failure. Of course, there was much celebrating at home. Father was so happy that, for the first time in his life, he committed pen to paper and wrote a poem in my honor. He presented it to me when I arrived home, and I have guarded it all these years like a sacred text.

FOR MY DAUGHTER ALETTA HENRIETTE JACOBS
On Passing Her Clinical Finals
April 3, 1878

Not for you the housewife's role,
Her duties, her aspirations.
Your soul has sought a higher goal,
Its meaning and destinations.

Yet still it was within your might
To choose a fate and find it worth
Your yearning to work and fight,
Your life's one aim upon this earth.

And I it was who heard your plea,
Who took your side and gave you heed.
I it was who helped you study
and gave you courage to succeed.

Now you've done with education
and gained a doctor's degree.
Through strength and dedication,
You've reached a female apogee.

Saving woman and tiny mite
From illness's crushing load
is now your job, your sacred fight,
your deepest urge and chosen road.[8]

When I returned home, I had originally planned to prepare for my medical doctorate in Groningen. This involved writing a thesis. Much to my disappointment, lack of materials and of the necessary guidance meant that I was unable to cover any subject relevant to my subsequent field of activity. Partly because Professor Kooyker had specifically asked to be my supervisor, I finally decided to write "On the Localization of Physiological and Pathological Symptoms in the Cerebrum."[9]

I slogged through the available literature on this subject at home, where I also did much of my written work. Everything went well until one sunny August afternoon in 1878, when Father suddenly suffered an apoplectic stroke that left him temporarily paralyzed on one side of his body and blind in one eye.

This misfortune caused great consternation in the Jacobs household. Father was vital to all our lives: he still supported a large family and was doctor to a great many patients. I felt I should assume responsibility for his practice as long as necessary, and this was a view that was apparently shared by the farmers of Sappemeer. I was received with respect wherever I went. My authority over my patients and their environment was such that I could take immediate and decisive action whenever needed. I remember early one Sunday morning being called out to attend a woman who was expecting her first child. The farmstead where she lived was several hours away, and the farmer came to fetch me in an open cart. As we lurched along the country lanes, he told me that his wife had been in labor for the last two days. The woman next door had tried to help, but since the previous day something had been hanging out of his wife's body and the neighbor had no idea what to do about it. She had pulled and pulled but it refused to budge. I realized that this was to be an extremely complicated birth and was grateful that Father had advised me to take his instruments.

We talked until we reached our destination and then went straight to the room where the pregnant woman was lying in an old-fashioned box bed. The atmosphere was suffocating. And no wonder: men were smoking and women were drinking brandy. They had been sitting there for the last two days without ever thinking of letting in a little fresh air. I had to act immediately and with a complete sense of authority. Both concerned family members and curious friends and neighbors were ordered to leave at once, the brandy bottle was sent to the cellar, and, much to the horror of those who had stayed to help, I threw all the windows wide open. The table was cleared, and I had a bed made up on it for the exhausted woman because the box bed was simply too high for me to help her. Once I began to examine her, I discovered to my dismay that an extremely swollen arm was hanging out of her body. The neighbor-*cum*-midwife was incensed when she saw my attempts to reinsert that weak little arm. As a woman with years of experience, she felt it her duty to prevent this mere beginner from making such a dreadful blunder. I had to ask the farmer to have her removed. She eventually slunk off full of indignation and after warning me repeatedly that it would not be her fault if the whole thing went wrong. The woman finally gave birth early that evening. The child was dead, but I at least had the satisfaction of having saved its mother's life.

The following example is also typical of the medical practice I had so unexpectedly taken over.

One evening I was called to an inn just outside the village because a man had had an accident. I rushed over immediately and found the bar so filled with smoke that it was impossible to make out its customers. Once again, my first task was to open the windows and ask all those who were not directly involved to vacate the premises. There was an unconscious man lying on the ground, covered with blood. Apparently he had been driving an empty cart to the village in an extremely inebriated condition. He had fallen somewhere near the inn and had been dragged for some distance by his cart. I examined him and found that nothing had been broken. I stitched him up and cleaned and dressed his wounds, after which some farmers put him, still unconscious, into his cart and drove him home.

In medical terms there was nothing particularly remarkable about this case. But the whole experience did wonders for my self-confidence when I saw how both tipsy customers and curious onlookers had obeyed my orders without a moment's hesitation.

Obviously I had had no time to work on my thesis while Father was ill. And, I wondered, what was the point of completing it? After all, just being an ordinary doctor was good enough for the village practice. I wrote explaining these views to Professor Stokvis and other friends in Amsterdam. I added that, now that the typhus had run its course, I was sure that I was physically strong enough to practice in the country. My friends were horrified to think that all my training would end up invested in a simple country practice! They insisted I get my medical doctorate and set myself up in Amsterdam. Professor Stokvis had an additional suggestion, "First the doctorate and then some time abroad so you can also learn a little about the world at large." I thought these were wonderful ideas. I knew that my friends meant well, but I also realized that I simply did not have the financial resources to follow their suggestions.

However, I was soon to have an unexpected windfall. One of Professor Stokvis's patients who was suffering from terminal tuberculosis had asked me to visit him. When I stopped by, he suddenly handed me a thousand guilders, which I was to use for a trip abroad after I had completed my doctorate.

Meanwhile Father had also been consulted, with the result that I was to give up the practice in Sappemeer and get back to my thesis. I was awarded my doctorate on March 8, 1879, in front of a large crowd of spectators. The *Groningen Courant* of March 10, 1879, reported that "last Saturday, our university was the scene of a doctoral ceremony that will surely go down in its annals as an extraordinary and as yet unique event. For it was on this day that Miss *Aletta Henriëtte Jacobs* of Sappemeer (who passed her finals just a year ago) was promoted to *medicinae doctor* after defending her thesis *On the Localization of Physiological and Pathological Symptoms in the Cerebrum*. This thesis, complete with two illustrations, has been dedicated to H. R. H. the Dowager Princess Hendrik of the Netherlands. Before Miss Jacobs's supervisor, Professor Kooyker, conferred the degree, Assistant Dean Professor van Bell, who stood in for the absent dean, Professor van der Wijk, gave a speech in which he underlined the fact that the first Dutch woman to gain her medical doctorate had been able to do so at the University of Groningen. He also stated that the strength of mind demonstrated by this first doctor *feminini generis* should provide plenty of incentive for future doctors *masculini generis*! Needless to say the ceremony attracted so many members of the public (of both sexes) that not all of them could fit into the auditorium."

Among those who later came up to shake my hand was the governor of the province of Groningen, Mr. L. Graaf van Heiden Reinestein. He told me that when I had started my medical training, Minister Thorbecke had specifically asked him to keep an eye on me and report back on my progress both in my chosen subject and in my private life. The governor had continued to fulfill this request even after Thorbecke's death. "I have always kept track of you," he said, "and I'm delighted to be able to compliment you on the way in which you have fulfilled what must have often been a difficult task."

The liberal newspapers of the day also reported and commented upon the events surrounding my doctorate in great detail.

I had decided to go to London even before I completed my doctorate. I chose the English capital rather than Vienna or Paris because I had read in British women's magazines about how professors, doctors, and students were actively sabotaging women's attempts to study medicine in England. I already knew from reading the newspapers that it was mainly Russian and American women who studied medicine in Vienna and Paris.[10]

My parents were not at all pleased about my plans to visit London. They had never seen the sea, anticipated the journey with a sense of impending doom, and were horrified to think of their daughter living in a great metropolis about which they knew nothing. They did their utmost to make me change my mind, but I stood my ground and refused to be talked out of my original plans.

Professor Stokvis kindly contacted Mrs. Rennefeld, the widow of the principal of the Amsterdam Drama School, and asked her to find me a room. He also gave me letters of introduction to a number of London professors. Meanwhile, C. V. Gerritsen had found out from the newspapers that I was to leave for England. He wrote me immediately and offered to introduce me to some of his English friends. I received the letter the day before I was due to leave. Mrs. Rennefeld had already rented a room for me from a widow who lived in her neighborhood. I immediately sent my London address to my unknown friend, asking him to mail me his letters of introduction.

Before embarking on the sea voyage, I spent several days in Amsterdam visiting friends and looking for a house for my parents. Father had decided to sell our home, and the practice in Sappemeer, and move to the capital in the spring. For several reasons, we all felt that this was a wise decision. He had suffered a number of subsequent strokes, which, although much less severe than the first one, still ruled out any possibility of his resuming his practice. Charlotte was in the process of preparing for the last of her pharmacy exams, and Amsterdam would be the ideal place for her to study. My younger brother, Eduard, who was later to become mayor of Lonneker and of Almelo, was at that time an infantry officer in Amsterdam. I was also planning to settle there once I returned from London. My youngest sister, Frederika, had passed her teaching certificate in mathematics and accounting and was teaching at the girls' college in The Hague. Once my parents had moved to Amsterdam, she would be able to visit them for several days each week. Apart from Emma, who always lived at home, the other children had all gone their own ways and most of them were married. In those days it was easy to find suitable accommodation, so I was able to leave for London on March 14, 1880, with an easy mind.

Friends waved me off from Rotterdam, and I embarked on my travels in the best of spirits. Everything went smoothly. In Vlissingen I was given a splendid cabin all to myself. Despite being at sea, I slept soundly that night, and the next morning, for the first time in my life, I set foot on foreign soil.

THREE

MY STAY IN LONDON

My Arrival • New Friends • Study and Relaxation • I Return to the Netherlands •
The Medical Conference in Amsterdam • A Practice in the Capital

I n Sappemeer, I had been bombarded with dreadful stories about London coachmen dumping young girls onto deserted streets at the wrong address. Although these tall tales made little impression on me, I nonetheless made a point of carefully studying a map of the British capital before I left so that when I arrived in London, I already had some idea of how to get to the lodgings that Mrs. Rennefeld had found for me. And, in any case, the coachman, whom I had chosen at random, seemed to harbor no evil intentions. He took me by the shortest route to the address I had given him, and I scarcely had arrived before Mrs. Rennefeld rushed out to welcome me. She helped me to unpack and to arrange my belongings into some semblance of coziness. Then we went to meet her family, with whom she lived. I was received with great warmth and spent the rest of the day with them. I even got to meet the world famous painter Alma-Tadema![1] I fit in with remarkable ease, and when I returned to my lodgings that evening I felt as if I had been living there for ages.

The next morning I was again greeted by a pleasant surprise. I was eating breakfast when two young ladies came to pay their respects. They told me that they were medical students and friends of C. V. Gerritsen, from Amersfoort, who had sent them an elaborate telegram asking them to look after me. And so they had come to offer their help. We soon became firm friends and left a few hours later for the women's medical school on Henrietta Street where they introduced me to the male professors and more of the female students.[2] During that first visit, I was repeatedly invited to attend classes at the school. After Henrietta Street, we went to visit Dr. Drysdale, who, although I saw relatively little of him in London, was to be a great influence on my later life. It was through him that I first met Annie Besant, who was at that time collaborating with Charles Bradlaugh on speeches and articles promoting freethinking. I was also to meet Bradlaugh and his daughters.

For those unfamiliar with the prominent personalities of the day, Charles Bradlaugh (1833–1891) had embarked on his crusade against Christianity when he was just seventeen, with a pamphlet called "A Few Words on the Christian Creed" (1850). While I was in London, he, like Dr. Drysdale, was an active supporter of Malthusian theory. And it was through these individuals that I came to meet other men and women whose campaign for "motherhood by choice" and whose theories concerning the "voluntary limiting of families" had caused an uproar in the sanctimonious England of the day.

So, before I had a chance to explain myself or decide what I actually thought, I found myself surrounded by radicals of the scientific, political, and ethical worlds whose sole aim was to counter conservatism and hypocrisy. I attended meetings where Bradlaugh and his small group of followers discussed contemporary politics. On Sundays I went to the Fabian Society, which was still in its infancy, and I also followed the meetings of various working-class groups.

I should perhaps point out here that although the Fabian Society was completely socialist in outlook, it never sought to incite working-class unrest. Its members mainly came, and continue to come, from the intellectual middle classes. They believe in promoting greater social awareness among the ruling classes. The society's name is derived from Fabius Cunctator, a Roman consul famed for his wise tactics during the war against Hannibal.[3]

My evenings were thus filled with different meetings, which I attended after many long hours of intensive work. I spent my mornings at the large children's hospital on Great Ormond Street where I first worked in the busy outpatient clinic and then accompanied the doctors on their rounds of the wards. In the afternoons, I went to one of the women's hospitals where I both attended the theoretical lessons of a well-known professor and also applied that theory in practice. Remarkably, although English women students had to overcome countless obstacles to be admitted into these hospitals, for me all the doors seemed to swing open of their own accord.

At that time, there was a real sense of tension between the very few English women doctors and their male counterparts. The professional organization had refused to admit women as members and women were barred from medical meetings. By contrast, I encountered nothing but affability wherever I went. Married doctors invited me to visit their families and, whenever I

met them, unmarried doctors were courtesy itself. I have never fully understood the reason for this disparity. Of course, everyone knew that I would
eventually return to Holland and therefore could not be viewed as a potential
competitor. But neither were the American women students who came to
complete their training in London. Yet they were treated in a way that
was anything but friendly. Perhaps my favorable treatment was due to my youth
and to the fact that, although I was so young, I was quite obviously dedicated to
my work.

Of all the hospitals I visited in London, my favorite was the women's
hospital that had just been established on Marylebone Road.[4] It was run by Mrs.
Garrett Anderson, who also happened to be the first woman doctor in England.
The few female doctors who worked with her had, without exception, studied
abroad (and mostly in Paris). As the youngest of them was on the wrong side of
forty, I was considered a mere baby at the age of twenty-five. Nonetheless, I was
greeted with great warmth and felt completely at home among these women. I
particularly liked Mrs. Garrett Anderson, who was not only interested in
medicine but also maintained an open-minded attitude toward society in
general. I was also greatly impressed with her sister, Mrs. Millicent Fawcett, who
at that time was president of the English woman suffrage organization. Thanks
to my friendship with these women, I was frequently invited to "drawing room
meetings" where lectures on woman suffrage would be held before an audience
of forty or fifty well-to-do women.[5]

Of course, I hardly needed any convincing. To me it was obvious, and had
been for years, that women were entitled to the same political rights as men. Yet
I enjoyed attending these meetings because it gave me the opportunity of
familiarizing myself with the arguments used to propagate this aim. My first
contact with the early supporters of woman suffrage in England dates from this
period and subsequently led to many close friendships.

I later wrote an article about this part of my life for *Gedenkboek 1894–
1919* (Commemorations 1894–1919), published by the Dutch woman suffrage
organization.[6]

I returned to Holland earlier than I had originally intended. From September 8 to 15, 1879, there was to be a conference in Amsterdam on the advancement of medical science, attended by many of the English professors and
doctors I knew.[7] At their recommendation, I decided first to go to Amsterdam
and then to resume my studies in London after the conference had ended.
However, this was not to be. During the conference, I received so many requests
from Amsterdam families asking me to replace their regular doctor and I was
approached by so many mothers wanting me to supervise the health of their
children that it seemed to me wiser not to return abroad.

Thanks to the conference, my name was on everyone's lips. It occurred to me that I should take advantage of this unexpected and unsolicited publicity and so I immediately decided to set up practice in Amsterdam.

I was constantly in the papers during the conference. Numerous articles pointed out that the conference board of management, which was headed by Professor Donders, actively appreciated my presence at every event of any significance. For instance, the *Algemeen Handelsblad* of September 9, 1879, ran an article under the headline "Doctors at the City Hall" about a reception at the Prinsenhof given by the City Council for conference participants on the first evening:

"The chamberlain announced the guests in a commanding voice and the gentlemen visitors went through the usual formalities with the mayor and City Council. The hall was packed by 9 P.M. but new guests continued to arrive.

"Then a name was announced that attracted everyone's attention, 'Dr Aletta Jacobs!' and the first Dutch woman doctor made the most unassuming entrance imaginable. But the mayor received her like no other guest. He not only bowed, but as head of the city he welcomed Miss Jacobs to Amsterdam's council chambers with great warmth and sympathy."

Even forty years later, there is one other evening I remember with particular vividness that had been organized in honor of the foreign guests. The program included two tableaux vivants. The first tableau, representing the present and the past, showed Lister doing battle with Ambroise Paré. The hall erupted with instant applause, which turned into a standing ovation for the English innovator, who also happened to be present in the audience. People shouted and cheered until finally Lister appeared on stage to acknowledge this tribute.[8]

The second tableau, "Future," was a representation of Rembrandt's *Anatomy Class* with one major difference: all the male figures had been replaced by women. The *Algemeen Handelsblad* of September 16, 1879, described it thus:

"The woman teaching, Professor Tulp, was a well-known woman doctor. Of course, it was not really her, but the clothes, figure, and face were sufficiently convincing that everyone guessed her name and it was the turn of Dr. Aletta Jacobs to receive a round of sympathetic applause."

I even got into the foreign papers. Dr. Petithan, who published a report about the conference in the French medical journal *Le Scalpel*, described me as follows:[9]

"At the fourth conclusion, I seized the opportunity to pay tribute to those women who have chosen to train as doctors, and who have been so impressively represented at the conference by Aletta Jacobs. I said that it is the duty of women doctors to educate their sisters about the laws of hygiene, which are far too frequently ignored.

"It would be hard to imagine a more charming practitioner than this attractive, twenty-five-year-old Jewish girl who followed the discussion of even the most delicate of subjects with the utmost tact and seriousness. Yet she always remained gracious, as was the case when, as a mark of respect, she presented me with a copy of her erudite thesis."

I am now old and gray, but I would like to conclude this chapter by confiding to my female readers that during the conference, and afterward, doctors from every corner of Europe made proposals of marriage to me. And I must admit that these offers certainly boosted my ego. But my heart remained unmoved.

FOUR

THE EARLY YEARS OF MY PRACTICE

A Pioneer in All Respects • What Amsterdam Was Like Forty Years Ago • I Meet Carel Victor Gerritsen • New Friendships • Doctor to the Working Classes • A Heavy Blow

I began to practice as a doctor immediately after the conference ended. I set up my office on the Herengracht, near the Koningsplein, in the house of a widow from whom I had rented a few rooms. Each evening, at around six o'clock, I would walk to my parents' house on the Ferdinand Bolstraat where we would eat supper together.

From the very first day, I was seeing so many patients that I could feel completely confident about the future. Office hours were between 1 P.M. and 3 P.M., and I also made house calls each morning and afternoon.

To keep track of the foreign medical journals, I decided to become a member of the Leesmuseum on the Rokin.[1] I had regularly visited the Groningen Leesmuseum, and in London I had spent much of my free time in the British Museum. So, time permitting, why should I deny myself in Amsterdam the same pleasure of browsing through those books and magazines I did not personally own? Hence, one fine day I set off for the Leesmuseum to inquire about the rules and regulations of applying for membership. How could such a simple question cause such consternation! I was informed that I had come to a *gentlemen's* Leesmuseum. I was also told that I was the first woman ever to attempt to become a member. They tried to persuade me to abandon my plans by suggesting that, as a woman, I ran the risk of being blackballed. If, against all odds, this did not happen, then many of the men would resign rather than risk a great deal of unpleasantness at home. I had to admit that I simply did not understand the connection between the two facts. They then explained to me that members' wives would view the Leesmuseum in a very different light were they to know that their husbands would be likely to meet women there. Despite all these objections, I decided that nothing was going to stop me. I immediately approached a few of the members, explained that the museum's collection of books and magazines was vital for my future development, and asked them whether they would be willing to propose me for membership. Fortunately, they agreed, with the result that my candidacy was put to the vote.

Nowadays, the women and young girls who visit the Leesmuseum without the slightest problem will probably find it hard to believe that a number of Amsterdam ladies felt compelled to write letters, mostly unsigned, informing me that I had had the impudence to apply for membership in an establishment that had been set up by men and for men. Two of these ladies even went so far as to confront me in my own home. I calmly ignored all this fuss and was not particularly surprised to discover that my membership application had been accepted. I should immediately add that no one ever bothered me at the Leesmuseum, where I was to spend many happy hours.

Once I had set up practice, I began to receive many visits from my fellow doctors. They declared that they wanted to help me in whatever way they could, and I do believe that they were quite sincere in their intentions. But unfortunately their views and mine were diametrically opposed and inevitably my colleagues' interest waned once it became clear that I did not appreciate their suggestions. Certainly it would have been far more sensible of me not to spoil the illusion that I would follow their good advice, but dissembling is something that I am innately incapable of. Both then and later I would have spared myself a great deal of unpleasantness had I learned to keep my thoughts to myself.

Looking back, I can vividly remember how these visitors made my blood boil. They would say things like "You should stick to gynecology," despite the fact that none of them was an obstetrician. And they would calmly assure me that I could then count on the complete cooperation of every doctor in Amsterdam. Others advised, "Make sure that you charge a lot less than the usual rates to show that you're not pretending to be the equal of your male counterparts." They would stare at me with astonishment when I told them that I did indeed intend to present myself as the absolute equal of every other doctor in Amsterdam. And their astonishment changed to exasperation when I indignantly declared that, despite growing up with brothers and attending both school and college with boys, I had never detected even the slightest sign of male intellectual superiority.

In this context, I would like to describe an amusing experience concerning payment that happened during the first years of my practice. After a lengthy treatment, I was able to reassure the wife of an Amsterdam city notable that she was now cured of a serious gynecological complaint from which she had suffered for years. I mailed my bill at the beginning of the year, as was the custom of the time. A few days later, I was unexpectedly visited by my ex-patient's husband. I can still see him marching into my consulting room with my bill clutched between the thumb and forefinger of his left hand. I can still hear the irritated tone with which he reproached me for sending a bill as high as any male doctor's.

"Whatever possessed you to do such a thing!" he shouted indignantly. "I can quite assure you that no one would ever dream of paying women the same as men."

To me, the fact that an important member of the Amsterdam business world should object to my asking the standard rate seemed so silly that even his tone of voice failed to annoy me.

"And," I calmly replied, "did you ever dream of asking a cheaper but less reputable doctor to treat your wife? I suspect that at that point in time your sole concern was with *effective* treatment. I thought this was the reason you decided to consult the only woman doctor in Holland."

"So have you come here," I continued, "to complain in all seriousness about a bill based on rates that have been established by my male counterparts? You should count yourself lucky that I stick to the rules instead of exploiting my exalted position as the first Dutch woman doctor to charge more than other practitioners."

I have completely forgotten my visitor's immediate reaction to this philippic, but what I do remember is that his wife came to pay the bill a few days later and that she apologized profusely for her husband's behavior.

I cannot begin to count the obstacles that had to be overcome during the early years of my practice as an independent woman doctor. Yet how times have changed! If I compare contemporary society with life forty years ago, I can well imagine that these stories must seem unbelievable to young people today. I am thinking of incidents that in themselves were no more than minor details but provided an intense satisfaction at triumphing against all odds.

For instance, I wonder if the hundreds of women who stroll along the Kalverstraat each day ever stop to think that forty years ago this busy shopping street was strictly off limits for "ladies" between the hours of noon and 4 p.m. It was at these times that the gentlemen brokers would enter and leave the Stock Exchange and any woman seen frequenting the Dam Square or sauntering along the Kalverstraat was invariably a prostitute. No woman of untarnished reputation would be foolhardy enough to visit the Kalverstraat in the afternoon. She knew that she risked all manner of unpleasantness, that her conduct would be severely criticized over the gentlemen's cocktails and at the ladies' sewing circles. Needless to say I rebelled against this convention from the very start. I demanded the right to use the Kalverstraat as I needed it and when I needed it, day or night. Anyone who has followed the story of my life so far will take this as a matter of course. However, I decided to go one step further. Whenever I had the opportunity, I called on other women to follow my example. In this way we would put a stop to a disgraceful situation where, to put it bluntly, women were being bought and sold in broad daylight and in the center of the nation's capital. It brought dishonor to the woman and entailed obvious dangers for the man. So, at least for the sake of public decency, I felt that it was vital that those women who had always avoided the Kalverstraat in the afternoon should now make a point of going there during Stock Exchange business hours.

Today, working women and young female students simply take it for granted that they are free to wander through the streets at any hour, day or night. They will find it difficult to understand exactly what was implied forty years ago by a woman simply walking down a public street during the afternoon or evening. Neither the public nor the police was used to such an occurrence; in fact even the men who had been appointed by the government to ensure the safety of the streets were known to neglect their duty in this respect.

Every evening after supper, I would leave my parents' house between seven and eight to return to my lodgings. I had been repeatedly followed by a particular gentleman, and one night he even went so far as to grab me in a most improper way. All this took place right in front of a policeman to whom, of course, I immediately complained. Instead of protecting me against my assailant, this maintainer of public law and order simply looked at me and snarled, "If you stayed at home at night, you wouldn't get pestered like that." Although I was utterly incensed, I decided to let the matter rest for the time being. But soon afterward I was provided with an ideal opportunity to air this and other grievances.

One evening, I was returning just after midnight from visiting a patient. The carriage that brought me back to my lodgings had already left when I discovered a letter upstairs urgently requesting me to visit a scarlet fever patient who lived on the Herengracht, near the Thorbeckeplein.

The telephone was yet to be invented, so there was no question of ordering a coach. In any case, it would take only five minutes to walk to where the child lived. So I set out on foot. The street was completely silent and deserted. The only person I met was a policeman, who was obviously looking me over. I saw him again as I was returning home from my house call. The man had the impertinence to grab me, and I actually had to defend myself, say who I was, and inform him that I intended to report his conduct. The next morning I asked to speak with the chief superintendent and told him of my unfortunate experiences with his subordinates. He was most grateful for the information and correctly maintained that the primary task of the police was to maintain public safety on the streets—and that meant for women too. I left his office with the assurance that I would have no further reason for complaint about the Amsterdam police force, a prophecy that remains true to this very day.

Remembering those ridiculous conventions of an era that must now seem positively antediluvian reminds me of one particular custom: that only men sat in the stalls of the City Theater while all women were confined to the boxes or balconies above. As far as I was able to ascertain, there were no printed or written rules on this subject; it was simply a matter of custom, and one to which theatergoers always adhered.

Between acts and during the intermission, those in the stalls would openly train their opera glasses on the occupants of the boxes and the balconies to make sure they got the best view possible. I have no idea whether the objects of their exertions ever complained, but I certainly do remember that one fine day the theater management decreed, "Unescorted women will no longer be admitted to this theater." Those "ladies" lacking the convenient chaperonage of a husband or brother would actually employ the services of an Amsterdam "porter." His company was paid for by the hour, the price also being determined by whether he wore a cap or a top hat. It was as a woman and not as a doctor that I felt myself compelled to protest against this decision. Although I went to the theater relatively rarely, I did not want my few visits to involve the additional company of a "porter," especially since I felt perfectly capable of looking after myself.

I immediately wrote a strongly worded protest against the management's decision and also took the opportunity to point out how silly it was to segregate the sexes so strictly in the City Theater. The answer I received from the management board informed me that the decision was not intended to apply to ladies such as myself but to those women whose clothes or conduct were liable to give offense.

The sheer stupidity of this stance was eventually demonstrated one evening when the wife of a prominent local figure was nearly ejected from the theater because some of the attendants considered her clothes to be simply too outrageous. This blunder was averted just in the nick of time. Since then, as far as I know, women have been able to visit the City Theater without further ado.

Shortly after I set up practice, Father received a visit from the young man who, despite the fact that we had never met, had proved his friendship at every turn. Carel Victor Gerritsen came to ask if there would be any objection to his making my acquaintance. Our visitor made such a good impression on Father that he invited him to call whenever he wished and he correctly surmised that I would appreciate the opportunity of thanking Mr. Gerritsen in person for his kindness throughout the years. Because I was at my parents' home only during mealtimes, Father suggested that Gerritsen make an appointment to visit me during an afternoon or evening at the Herengracht.

To be quite honest, I had never given this friendly stranger a second thought, despite writing to thank him for the congratulations he always sent after my exams, and even though I actively appreciated Mr. Gerritsen's introductions, which were so helpful during my stay in London.

By contrast, I had always been part of Gerritsen's life. He had followed all the various stages of my training and he was present during the oral part of my doctorate. His diffidence was the reason why, unlike so many others, he felt unable to congratulate me in person. Still, I was pleased finally to be able to meet this young man who had shown so much interest in me. But it was to take quite some time before our newfound friendship would blossom into love.

Obviously, my circle of friends and acquaintances expanded as I became more involved with public life. Women such as Hélène Mercier, Catharina Alberdingk Thym, Cornélie Huygens, and Elise Haighton all expressed a wish to meet me.[2] I had previously known of them only through their writing, but the friendships we forged were to last a lifetime.

In fact, I not only attracted the attention of the prominent women of the day; I was also warmly received by men such as B. H. Heldt, who was leader of the Dutch General Trade Union, Dr. W. Doorenbos, the spiritual father of the 1880s literary movement, and others whose names are too many to mention.[3] My development, both political and social, owes much to my contact with these eminent men and women.

Through Heldt, I was introduced to other members of the trade union's board of management, whose wives I also met in time. In talking to them, I began to realize that the working classes urgently needed to be educated about matters of hygiene, particularly with regard to child care. Heldt helped me greatly. In the winter of 1880, he made available several rooms in the union's building (which was above a bar on the corner of the Spuistraat and the Kattegat) so that I could offer a course for women. My students came twice a week to learn the rudiments of hygiene and how babies should be cared for. One result of these classes was that I decided to hold a free clinic two mornings a week, in the same room, for penniless women and children, a practice I was to continue for fourteen years. The management board repeatedly showed their appreciation of my efforts, and when the union moved to a larger building, called d'Geelvinck, located on the Singel, I was immediately provided with two spacious and well-lighted rooms. However, the fact that these rooms were located on an upper floor proved to be an insurmountable problem for many of the sick women and children. Hence, when a widow in the Tichelstraat offered me two rooms for a very cheap rent, I decided to seize the opportunity and move. But from the moment I went to the Jordaan, I began to gradually lose contact with the Dutch General Trade Union.

Twice a week for fourteen long years I treated needy women from all walks of life. And there was never a shortage of patients. I eventually terminated the clinic after a protracted illness that prevented me from working for many weeks. During this period, the widow decided to live with one of her daughters, and thus that space was no longer available for my clinic.

Shortly after I had established my practice in Amsterdam, a number of people began to set up an association "to stimulate political life and promote social interests," which was to be called the Union. Once again I was the first woman to apply for membership, and it even took some time before my example was followed by others. This new association's meetings enabled me to acquaint myself with the important social issues of the day. It was so unusual for women to attend public meetings that the newspapers made a point of mentioning my presence, a practice that continued until I specifically asked the journalists in question not to include my name as I found it a hindrance.

My free clinics in the Jordaan brought me into contact with the poorer sections of Amsterdam society. If women or children were too sick to come during office hours, I would often visit them at home. And what misery I encountered there! But more than by the desperate poverty of so many families, the scandalous living conditions in the city's poorest districts shocked me. How did people survive in these slums? How could the government let them exist?

Finally, a mixture of compassion and sheer indignation forced me to confide in Hélène Mercier, who I knew was deeply concerned with the distress of the poor. During her years of protracted illness, this woman of immense social awareness had read much about the lives and labor conditions of the working classes abroad but had seen next to nothing of the shocking conditions in her own backyard. After listening to my stories, she asked if she could sometimes accompany me on my rounds of poor districts, a request I willingly granted, although I took care to shield my physically weak and highly strung friend from the worst of the squalor. Our slum visits were to inspire her to write a widely influential article in the *Sociaal Weekblad*. The fact that living conditions have slowly improved in Amsterdam is in part due to the publicity created by Hélène Mercier.

In May 1881, I was dealt a heavy blow that robbed me of the will to work for months on end and blunted my desire to continue developing.

My dear father died suddenly and completely unexpectedly. A stroke killed him in a matter of seconds. I will never forget how I felt standing by his deathbed. How bitterly aware I was of my loss. Each afternoon, I had always discussed my patients with Father, and we would also debate every conceivable social issue. I often disagreed with him but, even when his opinion was diametrically opposed to my own, I still enjoyed listening to him argue. And, of course, I knew he sometimes deliberately took the opposite position, since his awareness of the difficulties I was likely to face prevented him from encouraging my beliefs. Love and concern for his child, which was how he always saw me, forced him to confront me with a different point of view.

I often ignored Father's suggestions. But the very thought that he was always there to be consulted as a source of sensible and selfless advice when I was in doubt gave me a great inner strength.

It was a long time before I could adjust to the fact of this irreparable loss.

FIVE

PLANNED MOTHERHOOD

Women's Suffering • A Remedy Is Found • Rowing Against the Tide • Hours of Doubt and Days of Struggle • My Efforts Are Rewarded

W hen I was a student, and particularly when I worked at Amsterdam Hospital, I was haunted by the suffering caused by frequent pregnancies, which, for various reasons, can have a disastrous effect on a woman's life.

In my long conversations with a variety of women in the delivery room, they explained to me that they found it impossible to prevent pregnancy when sexual abstinence was the only method available. Women who produced sickly babies or stillbirths, for whom birth meant yet another brush with death, kept on returning to the delivery room. Families that were already large enough, considering the mother's physical condition and the parents' circumstances, simply continued to expand. I spent hours wrestling with this problem without any solution in sight. Sometimes I discussed the issue with my fellow students. "Yes," they would coolly reply, "that's what's called a woman's destiny" or "Thank God, there's no way of preventing pregnancy. If there were, then the whole world would soon collapse through underpopulation."

Chance, which always plays an important role in our lives, had brought me into contact with a group of individuals in London who were involved with exactly the same issue that I had so often thought about on my own. While I was England, people such as Annie Besant, Dr. Drysdale, and the publisher Truelove had repeatedly risked prosecution for discussing the issue of family planning in public and allowing these views to be published. Some years previously, a book *by a doctor of medicine* called *Elements of Social Science*, with the subheading *Physical, Sexual, and Natural Religion*, had been published.[1] It was later translated into German, French, Dutch, Italian, and Portuguese. The author, who had been a student of both Malthus and John Stuart Mill, attempted to prove that the world's population naturally multiplies at a geometric rate of 1, 2, 4, 8, 16, 32, et cetera, whereas during the same period of time essential resources increase in only an arithmetic progression of 1, 2, 3, 4, 5, 6, et cetera. The sequel to this scientific work made it quite clear that the author sympathized with Malthus in terms of what these predictions implied both for families and for society in general, yet he took an opposing viewpoint so far as preventing overpopulation was concerned. For social and medical reasons, this "doctor of medicine" rejected Malthus's belief in "late marriage and sexual abstinence before marriage." And he argued for the introduction of contraception.

When I first read this book, I already knew both its author and the publisher and was also acquainted with many of the people who promoted, wrote, and spoke on behalf of this doctrine. I had great respect for these men and women whose sole aim in life was to make the world a better place, even at the cost of their own happiness. I admired their ideals, which included a strong sense of social justice.

Despite the fact that I disagreed with the economic theory on which their principles were based, which may simply have been because I knew too little about the subject, I nonetheless understood from a medical and sociomedical point of view the immense importance to humanity of the means they believed in to achieve their goal. The availability of contraception would prevent immeasurable suffering. I had learned that much from the pregnant women I had met in Amsterdam Hospital and from all the newborn babies whose births were greeted by anything but joy and whose very existence was a burden both to their families and to society in general. There remained only the question of which contraceptives were effective in preventing unwanted pregnancy. I felt unable to come up with any definitive answer. Doubting that the existing means were reliable or even suitable for use, I was uncertain as to whether they could damage users' health. In the end, I was forced to admit that I had reached an impasse. My contact was with groups that included the book's author and with others who described themselves as Neo-Malthusians because they followed Malthus's ideas yet chose to employ their own means to combat this social ill. Although they had provided me with much theoretical knowledge, I had no way of transforming theory into practice.

When I first returned to the Netherlands, the pressure of other matters had forced me to set this concern, which had so obsessed me in London, aside. But my free clinics for poor and destitute women brought me into close contact with this issue. My renewed concern was simply a consequence of treating daily the direct results of unwanted pregnancies that ultimately produced children who were a material and ethical burden not only to their parents but also to society in general.

During my search for a remedy for this state of affairs, I chanced upon an article in early 1882 in a German medical journal that had been written by Dr. Mensinga from Flensburg.[2] He recommended the use of a pessary for the kinds of cases I was dealing with. This purely scientific article made such an impression on me that I immediately wrote to its author. A lengthy exchange of letters followed, in which Dr. Mensinga informed me fully about the way in which pessaries should be used. He also sent me a number of specimens. Although Dr. Mensinga had assured me that they were effective and in no way jeopardized users' health, I decided that I had to have them tested before I could provide any personal recommendation.

For social, moral, and medical reasons, women from different social classes had often asked me for some form of contraception. I had always had to fend off these requests without providing adequate explanation or advice. Eventually I sent letters to a number of women whose need was greatest. I told them that I believed I had found a means to help them, but before I could fully recommend it, they would have to agree to regular examinations during the first months of its use. Some of these women eventually agreed to the experiment, and the results were such that, some months later, I was able to announce that I could provide a safe and effective contraceptive.

Although I deemed it unnecessary to advertise my wares, I felt duty-bound to announce that I was now able to prescribe contraception for those women wishing to avoid pregnancy on social, moral, or medical grounds.

Not for one moment did I delude myself that I would be supported by many of my fellow doctors. I knew that they were deeply conventional and also that they were ignorant of society and social issues. Hence, I expected very little cooperation. On the other hand, I had never imagined that I would create such a furor. But in fact I incurred the wrath of the entire medical establishment. Even those who privately agreed with me carefully kept it to themselves for fear that they would receive the same treatment. These were difficult times for me, and I sorely missed the one man in whom I had always been able to confide. Sadly, my father was gone, and the few friends I trusted simply lacked the medical and sociological knowledge to be able to understand the importance of my work for humanity. I discussed this issue so often with them that they finally suggested, with the best of intentions, that I should publicly admit I had made a mistake and state that I would no longer provide this treatment. Fortunately I had never doubted my actions; otherwise I might indeed have followed their advice. But I was too deeply influenced by what I had seen and by my belief that this work would benefit humanity.

As the only woman doctor in Holland, I often found it difficult and painful to row against the tide of lies and slander spread by my male counterparts.

However, the absolute conviction that I was doing the right thing, and the awareness that this whole situation concerned not only individual suffering but also the interests of society at large, gave me the strength to stand by my point of view. But, even so, I was sometimes assailed by doubts. I would wander aimlessly around the Vondelpark, oblivious to my surroundings and wrestling with the dreadful thought that maybe, despite everything, I had made a mistake. Could the availability of contraception ultimately lead to a world without children? Would it cause adultery? And, if the birth rate fell, would the country's economic position be threatened? I was obsessed by these questions and wanted to find answers, though I was a layman as far as economics was concerned. But I kept thinking that the longing to have a child is so strong in most normal women that only for the most serious reasons would they choose to avoid motherhood. Of course, I thought, contraception would certainly lower the number of unwanted pregnancies and hence should be welcomed for many social, sociological, and individual reasons. If there were fewer unwanted babies, the race would advance, which in turn would lead to greater social well-being and human happiness. Studying this subject in great depth finally convinced me that I had taken the right course of action. I already felt what Nietzsche later so eloquently wrote: not propagating the race, but raising the level of humanity, must be the aim of existence.[3]

These experiences thoroughly undermined my trust in other people. Of course, I knew in advance that those narrow minded in outlook and suspicious of all innovation were bound to disagree with my way of thinking. I also reasoned that my opponents would include both those whose religious beliefs were directly contradicted by my opinions and those who were quite simply ignorant of social problems. But this did not bother me. In fact, through what I said and wrote, I even hoped to convert a few of them. But not for a single moment did I expect the level of hostility and obstructiveness I encountered from my fellow doctors (and particularly from the obstetricians and gynecologists whose livelihood I apparently threatened). Had they cast doubt on the contraceptive's reliability, they would have at least been forced to confront its social implications. I, in turn, could have defended my views, and an honest discussion would have ensued based on differences of opinion and experience. The issue of contraception was also later occasionally broached by the *Geneeskundig Tijdschrift* (Medical Journal). And whenever this happened I joined in the debate, with the result that I eventually emerged victorious. However at first my opponents were quite willing to resort to spreading stories that were entirely untrue. They accused me of promoting abortion and of leading an immoral life. How I wished I could refute these lies in public! But I never got the chance. These tales were never related to me directly. On the very few occasions that I managed to unearth the original source, the culprit was invariably either an obstetrician or a gynecologist. I would always confront him and demand an explanation for his behavior, but usually he would shrug it all off with some remark about contraception being the same as abortion. Of course, such reasoning was totally illogical because, as everyone knows, while the former is legal, the latter is a criminal act. For the rest, the people who opposed me in this manner were generally careful not to air their questionable opinions in public.

The more my practice expanded, the more I was viewed as a formidable competitor, which meant that ever-increasing numbers of colleagues were siding with my opponents. Unable to defend myself, I simply continued to live my life and tried to perform my work openly and as honestly as possible.

It was an age steeped in hypocrisy! I am particularly thinking of those clergymen who would denounce contraception from the pulpit and then pack their wives off to my office. I also remember women who were only too pleased to use the means I prescribed for them yet never lost a chance to condemn me at every tea party and sewing circle. And, while publicly denouncing my work, some doctors would still expect me to instruct them in the practical application of birth control! Fortunately these irritating experiences were more than made up for by the gratitude of a great many women and the warmth and friendship of a number of people in high places.

This was also the time when my friendship with Carel Victor Gerritsen was really starting to blossom. Previously, I had seen relatively little of him. When he returned from visits to London, he would convey the greetings of mutual friends, but our paths seldom crossed apart from that. He sided with me unequivocally in the fight for contraception. He also made clear his admiration for the courage I had had to muster in my lone struggle against prejudice, insinuations, and vilification. Carel Victor Gerritsen was the first and for a long time the only Dutchman with whom I could discuss this issue in the knowledge that my words and opinions would meet with a clear and honest response.

It was at about this time that a Neo-Malthusian union was first set up in Holland. Like its English equivalent, it was based on economic principles. In my opinion, this made the group far too secretive, and I was unable to offer it my full support. I have no real sympathy for the work of the Dutch Neo-Malthusian Union. Although I did join at first, I soon canceled my membership and I have never since felt the slightest inclination to help boost its numbers.[4] Of course, no one was under the illusion that this implied I had changed my mind about the benefits of contraception. On the contrary, the events of my later life were still further proof that my views were valid, that these means, just like any expedient against physical or social ills, must be openly prescribed by licensed practitioners, in this case by doctors who should support their use. Unfortunately, these days the reverse is true, with birth control often supplied secretly by people who are unqualified.

Now that I have reached the end of my life, I at least have the satisfaction of seeing that prominent men and women, the stars of the scientific world, have finally recognized the need to control overpopulation, and not simply from an economic viewpoint but also for sociomedical and eugenic reasons. In the years since I retired from active practice, I have received frequent visits from foreign professors and doctors inquiring about my experiences in this field. The 1920 Christmas issue of the *Pictorial Review* published an article by an American journalist about this part of my life's work.[5] As a result, I was inundated by mail from North and South America, Canada and Australia. There were so many letters that I was simply unable to answer each one personally and had to enlist the help of the magazine's editorial staff.

Sickness prevented me from attending the Congress for Birth Control held in London from July 11 to 15, 1922.[6] However, once it had ended a number of foreigners visited me in The Hague to learn more about my deep commitment to the cause all those years ago. Such eminent men as John Maynard Keynes, Havelock Ellis, Edward Carpenter, Harold Cox, Knut Wicksell, Edward Wester-marck, and H. G. Wells attended the conference and openly recognized the value of planned motherhood. The medical section of this conference was attended by 164 doctors from various countries, including Lord Dawson, per-sonal physician to the King of England, and Sir Arbuthnot Lane, one of the first surgeons in London. They clearly recommended the use of contraception wherever family planning is necessary. Hence, this issue has been brought to the attention of those people able to ensure its full realization.

Let me conclude this chapter by pointing out that after all these years there is still no better form of contraception than the Mensinga pessary I always prescribed.

SIX

THE CAMPAIGN FOR WOMAN SUFFRAGE

How It Began • My Public Activities • Why My Request Was Turned Down • Contact with Foreign Sisters • The Founding of the Dutch Association for Woman Suffrage • My First Speaking Engagement • The Founding of the International Woman Suffrage Alliance • My First Foreign Tour

I n the previous chapter, I described my often bitter campaign to highlight certain medical issues. I intend to devote this chapter to my involvement in the movement for woman suffrage. I have already mentioned that I wrote an article for *Gedenkboek 1894–1919* (Commemorations 1894–1919) published by the Dutch Association for Woman Suffrage. I would now like to illustrate how this fight for political enfranchisement was to occupy both my time and my energy for a great many years and to leave an indelible mark on my entire life.

Although some readers may find it hard to believe, I was already a committed supporter of woman suffrage at fourteen. There was a reason for this. Whenever he had the time, Father would read aloud to Mother and my older sisters during afternoon tea in Sappemeer. The women would sew and listen to an interesting newspaper article or to a book that had just been published. One day in 1868, Father was reading the Dutch translation of John Stuart Mill's *The Subjection of Women*.[1] Although this was not particularly intended for my consumption, I followed at least a part of his argument. In fact, I was so fascinated by what I heard that I later took the pamphlet from the bookshelf up to the corner of the attic where I retreated whenever I needed to think or read in private. I have no idea how much of John Stuart Mill's principles I actually understood, but I do remember that I was impressed by their basic message:

woman is the slave of man; he makes the laws, she obeys them. As a child I was obsessed with freedom and independence, and so it was no wonder that I was alternately inspired, depressed, and terrified by the title of the Dutch version: *The Slavery of Woman*. It became my personal touchstone, intensifying everything I saw, heard, or discovered. Girls did not become doctors. I was told that universities were only for boys. When I thought about all this, I realized that men not only made laws; they also had the power to reserve every privilege for themselves and to perpetuate women's subordinate role. I knew that this had to change, but as yet I had no idea how.

Even in those days, I copied down or kept a scrapbook of everything I read about electoral suffrage and laws that concerned women. When that political visionary, Minister Thorbecke, first granted me permission to study at Groningen University, I was struck by the fact that I still had to survive a trial period of a year before I finally could apply for permanent permission. "Why," I asked myself, "do I have to prove myself worthy of being registered as a medical student when even the dumbest and most loutish of boys is automatically granted it just for the asking?"[2]

Shortly after I gained admittance to the University of Groningen, one of the faculty, Professor B. D. H. Tellegen, published a pamphlet called *Woman's Future*.[3] The author succinctly described the legal subordination of women in general, and of married women in particular, and argued for a fairer form of legislation. It affected me deeply. I still have my copy, which I always quote whenever I am called on to defend our right to vote.

Although during my training I had little opportunity to involve myself with social issues other than those that directly affected me, I faithfully collected every newspaper article I could find on woman suffrage. Just before I took my doctoral exam, I discovered an article dated April 22, 1877, maintaining that the section of the constitution concerning enfranchisement needed to be revised. The idea put forth was that male suffrage should be greatly extended, but the revision should stipulate that all voters had to be of the male gender. Although I was supposed to be working flat out for my exam, somehow I could not get this article out of my head. What was the point of deliberately excluding women from enfranchisement in a country where they could not vote anyway? After finishing my training, I left for London where I first met English suffrage workers, who were to be a great inspiration to me.

Returning to Holland in late 1879, I noticed that virtually every day newspaper articles argued for constitutional reform and a broader franchise. Even at that time, an increasing number of voices were being heard in support of universal suffrage. But there was little general interest in political or social issues; although such matters were now and then discussed publicly, as yet there was no question of holding regular gatherings. Whenever the opportunity presented itself, I attended meetings where political and economic issues were discussed, and for a long time I was the only female member of the audience. During the discussion, I would often ask if universal suffrage would also mean votes for women. No one bothered to take my idea seriously, and my question was greeted by general ridicule. In fact, when the speaker answered each of the debaters in turn, my question would be summarily dismissed with a joke.

In 1882, I happened upon a pamphlet written by the premier of Holland, J. Heemskerk, father of the present (1923) minister of justice. His Excellency argued that, as it stood, the constitution did not specifically deny women the right to vote. This information gave me an entirely new perspective. "If the law does not actively prevent us from voting," I reasoned, "then why can't we exercise that right?" Why, if I fulfilled all the necessary conditions for enfranchisement, was I not sent a ballot like everyone else? But whenever I sought an answer to these questions, I received only contradictory responses. Feeling distinctly frustrated, I knew there was no point in this approach. Finally, on November 30, 1882, I consulted Mr. S. van Houten, a member of the Dutch parliament known for his feminist views.[4]

He advised me, "Take this case to the highest authorities. This is a vital issue for the Supreme Court, which has yet to render a decision." The idea appealed to me, and when Mr. van Houten explained the procedure, I decided to go ahead. When the new voter registration list was published in 1883, I checked to see whether my name had been included. Of course, I knew in advance that this would be a complete waste of time. However, I wanted to comply with all the formalities. Once I knew for certain that my name had indeed been omitted, I sent a letter, dated March 22, 1883, to the mayor and councilmen of Amsterdam. It requested my inclusion on the registration list, since I had fulfilled the legally stipulated conditions for enfranchisement, as proof of which I enclosed all the necessary evidence.

There was to be a council meeting that very day. Both mayor and councilmen seemed to find my letter extraordinarily amusing. It was read aloud to the general mirth of all. Neither the council nor its individual members seemed to appreciate its gravity and importance. They found my actions so ridiculous they did not bother to follow the usual legal formality under which answers to such requests must bear an official signature.

More than a week after I had submitted my petition, I was informed by letter that *"[my] request had been refused because the petitioner has appealed to the letter of the law, which, according to the spirit of our Constitution, does not extend suffrage to women. If one wishes to challenge the spirit of the law, then the question is whether women are considered to enjoy full citizenship and civil rights. And as far as these rights are concerned, women are excluded from guardianship except in terms of their own children."*

Not a single council lawyer opposed this reply, which lacked any legal basis. My action was attacked in all the daily newspapers, both large and small. "She challenged the council just so that she could get her name in the papers," was how one journalist put it. Other newspapers proclaimed that I "completely misunderstood the women of Holland." These gentlemen wrote that "the Dutch woman is quite happy with her appointed task. She has no desire to meddle with politics." The *Algemeen Handelsblad* even felt compelled to inform me that "a woman who claims the right to vote must first learn to respect the law."

I was deeply shocked that none of the women's magazines of the day seemed to understand the importance of woman suffrage. Without exception, they sided with those who denounced my efforts. They even went so far as to declare that I was doing women a real disservice. "Dr. Jacobs should stick to being a doctor" was one of their comments, supplemented by the inevitable jibe, "As if she hasn't already done enough with that."

I received my rejection from the city's mayor and councilmen so late that I scarcely had time to enter an appeal at the Amsterdam District Court before the legally stipulated period had expired. The court announced its verdict on April 13, 1883. It stated that *"it could never have been the intention of the Dutch legislature to allow woman suffrage."* This was followed by the announcement that I would be expected to pay the full costs of the case.

Not only was I now being attacked in the press but many private individuals, both men and women, also felt compelled to send letters and cards bearing the grossest insults and insinuations. I received only one note of sympathy. Three men wrote to say how much they admired my courage and tenacity. They encouraged me to continue my fight and subtly suggested that they would be prepared to shoulder all my legal expenses. I was touched by their kindness, but told them that the costs involved were extremely modest and that fortunately I could easily cover them myself. For the rest, I was upset by the general resentment caused by what seemed to me such a simple and obvious request. At times I felt deeply unhappy. Nonetheless, I was aware that I had to see this issue, now awaiting the Supreme Court's decision, through to its conclusion.

On May 18, 1883, the Supreme Court quashed my appeal against the district court's decision for the ludicrous reason that each of these impartial gentlemen had come to the inescapable conclusion that there was simply no other way out. The first reason offered to explain why women were denied the right to vote was that *"they do not have full citizenship or civil rights,"* because *"they lack the right to vote."* Further, "Dutch citizens and residents should be understood as referring exclusively to men because any other interpretation would have automatically been mentioned as such." And finally, *"Husbands and fathers pay taxes for their wives and underage children, a fact that unequivocally proves married women are excluded from enfranchisement."* These legal eminences had omitted the fact that widows and unmarried women most certainly did pay taxes both for themselves and for their underage children. It was for these and similar reasons that my appeal was rejected by the Supreme Court.

Shortly after this verdict, a member of the Supreme Court whom I knew personally wrote me to say that I should not view this judgment as being final. He advised me to go through the same legal process the following year, but this time in collaboration with other taxpaying women, preferably residing in different cities. He felt that I had a chance of succeeding this time. His idea appealed to me, but I immediately encountered great difficulty in finding women willing to fight the proposed constitutional reform that would add the adjective "male" before "Dutch citizen" whenever enfranchisement was mentioned. Were that to pass as law, there would be no question of woman suffrage in the foreseeable future.

To be able to vote at that time, one had to pay fairly high taxes. Since married women were not seen as contributing to the national economy, it proved extremely difficult to find women able to participate in the plan mentioned above. I wrote to all the likely candidates to invite them to collaborate with me during the following year. But the answers I received were so discouraging that I soon abandoned this strategy, convinced that my female compatriots did not understand the importance of suffrage.

In March 1885, Minister Heemskerk announced his planned constitutional reforms, and his proposed revisions concerning enfranchisement were immediately endorsed. The new constitution was introduced two years later, in 1887. This meant that from that point onward women's exclusion from suffrage had become a fait accompli. The constitution explicitly stated that only *male* Dutch citizens and *male* residents were granted active and passive suffrage.[5] The newspapers had made such a fuss about my attempts to achieve woman suffrage under the old constitution that my efforts were mentioned even in the foreign press. This publicity brought me into contact with kindred spirits in both the New World and the Old, with women who, like me, were fighting for their rights and who wrote me to convey their support and sympathy. The first of these women were Baroness Alexandra van Gripenberg from Helsinki in Finland and Gina Krog from Oslo in Norway.[6] They asked me for information about the Dutch women's movement and about my future plans concerning woman suffrage.

The English campaigners, most of whom I had met during my stay in London, urged me not to neglect or abandon the fight until I had achieved my goal. What they did not know was that, with the introduction of the new law, there was not the slightest chance of reform in the near future, especially since mine was a one-woman campaign. The North American suffrage workers soon contacted me as well, and from that time on I have corresponded regularly with leaders of women's movements in many different countries. I met most of them in person when my husband and I took part in the first international women's conference [of the ICW], which was held in London in 1899. During our two weeks in the British capital, we stayed with the young Herbert Samuel and his wife.[7] Little did we suspect that our host was later to become Sir Herbert and the first high commissioner of Palestine.

At the 1899 conference, I was warmly greeted by all those who knew me by name. But most of the women were amazed to see me in person because I was so much younger than they had expected. Susan B. Anthony, who was by then almost eighty, was the first to ask whether I really was the same Aletta Jacobs whose medical training she had followed in the newspapers of twenty years ago. And when I answered that question affirmatively, she wanted to know everything about my training, my practice, and my campaign for woman suffrage. I will describe this conference in a later chapter. But for now, I will limit myself to my enfranchisement work.

In 1893, seven women from the board of the Free Women's Movement made it known that they intended to set up an association whose aim would be the promotion of woman suffrage.[8] I had just been through a difficult birth and the child that I had brought into the world had survived for only one day. As a result of the birth, I needed an operation in the near future. Yet, despite feeling weak and depressed, I immediately sent a message of support, and when I was invited to join the committee to formulate the association's rules and statutes, I realized that this was one obligation I simply could not shirk. At first, I refused to assume any leadership role. Only in 1895 did I become head of the Amsterdam section and later, in 1903, decide to accept the association's leadership. For me, both running a section and being president of the Association for Woman Suffrage were easy tasks. I did not find it difficult to write articles about women's enfranchisement for newspapers and magazines and I never had any qualms about petitioning the government or approaching influential people. But whenever I had to speak in public, I needed to muster all my willpower to overcome my natural diffidence. I gave my first speech about woman suffrage shortly after the association was set up, in the winter of 1894–95. The Rotterdam section had asked my husband to give a lecture and he had agreed. But, the day before, he discovered that he urgently needed to attend to business in the north. "I'm afraid that I'm not going to be able to manage Rotterdam tomorrow," he said as he left. "Shall I send them a telegram to cancel the meeting?" I asked. "Cancel? Of course not. You're going to go in my place!"

I was less than enthusiastic about this idea, but, on the other hand, I realized that I had to overcome my shyness at some point. Maybe it was a question of simply jumping in feet first. After some consideration, I contacted the Rotterdam board to inform them that Mr. C. V. Gerritsen was unable to fulfill his speaking engagement but that I would attend in his place. Despite my nervousness, the evening was a great success, so great that after the meeting I was approached by a member of parliament who said, "Dr. Jacobs, you convinced me tonight. From now on, you can count on me as a supporter of woman suffrage."

My later speeches were also successful, yet I have always regarded speaking engagements as being the most difficult and unpleasant aspect of my career as a feminist. With lectures, I have often made the mistake of overestimating my audience. Here I am particularly thinking of the lectures held in 1900 in connection with my Dutch translation of Charlotte Perkins Gilman's *Women and Economics*.[9] In this book, the writer attempts to prove that many social problems are to a large extent due to married women's economic dependence. I encountered so much resistance and sheer incomprehension, in discussing her ideas, that I eventually had to drop the whole subject. I am also thinking of a lecture in which I tried to demonstrate the way that militarism has perpetuated woman's subordinate role. My words provoked a storm of protest that included a barrage of hate mail.

As I mentioned earlier, I took over the leadership of the Association for Woman Suffrage in 1903 and remained its president until votes for women became a legal reality.

The struggle for women's enfranchisement was just as difficult in Holland as it was in any other country. At first we were treated with mockery and derision. The press and public opinion twisted our words and obscured the facts. Then came a period of gossip and insinuation. And when we continued our campaign, despite all these obstacles, we found ourselves surrounded by a conspiracy of silence. However, the press eventually had to resign itself to the way things were going and, once we finally achieved our goal, newspapers of every persuasion blithely declared that they had of course supported woman suffrage from the very beginning.

The Association for Woman Suffrage campaigned for twenty-five years before Dutch women were finally granted the right to vote. And, during that quarter of a century, we traveled around the entire country, from north to south and from east to west. We visited even the most remote areas to argue our cause.

I quickly decided that a younger association member should accompany me on my travels. At first I let her speak for just a few minutes so that she could work gradually up to longer periods of time. And while I initially took charge of the discussion, I would come to entrust her with this part of the speaking engage-ment as well. This was how I trained our speakers, many of whom were to achieve a far greater eloquence than their teacher. Often it was simply a matter of helping them overcome their initial shyness and of arming them with all the necessary arguments. Then we could let them stand on their own two feet. And of course we were always delighted to add a new campaigner to our number. It gave us the satisfaction of knowing that younger members were out there spreading the same message that had originally drawn us into the fray. Readers who are particularly interested in this aspect of our work and who would like to know more about its success should consult *Gedenkboek 1894–1919* (Commemo-rations 1894–1919), which contains a wealth of detail.

Apart from campaigning in Holland, I also worked for the International Woman Suffrage Alliance, although I never held office in it. During the 1899 conference of the International Council of Women in London, the German delegates, Dr. Anita Augspurg and Lida Gustava Heymann, inspired a number of progressive women of various nationalities to consider the possibility of founding a second organization. Its main aim would be the introduction of woman suffrage in every country with a constitutional government. I was invited to attend the discussions as the Dutch representative. This initial meeting confirmed that this organization was definitely needed, and those present agreed to keep in contact with each other.

Three years later, the need for this organization was confirmed at a meeting in Washington. In a resolution, representatives of various countries again declared their solidarity and their intention to work toward the organization's realization. Mrs. Carrie Chapman Catt was to convey information to all the countries involved. It was her job to provide information and to receive reports about the current state of affairs in each individual nation. From then on, once every three months, I sent a brief report to America about the recent achievements of the Dutch Association for Woman Suffrage and about the progress of the enfranchisement movement in Holland. I was also responsible for publishing all the news I received from abroad in the association's monthly magazine. The International Woman Suffrage Alliance was formally established in Berlin in 1904. The Netherlands was one of the six founding members.[10]

A year previously, in 1903, I had accompanied my husband to Vienna where he was attending the meeting of the Interparliamentary Union.[11] I had devoted a part of my stay in the Austrian capital to contacting local suffrage workers. In terms of my interests, the situation in Austria was extremely depressing. Not only were women forbidden by law to join political organizations; they were also forbidden to attend political gatherings, or meetings where political issues would be discussed. Yet this whole situation had developed into a simple case of "where there's a will there's a way." My Viennese contacts decided to take advantage of my presence and asked me to address a private group of invited guests where I was to describe the work of the Women's Council in Holland and to emphasize the need for woman suffrage. During my lecture, I mentioned the influence of the Association for Moral Advancement on the Women's Council and especially its work to combat prostitution.[12] Scarcely had I uttered the word "prostitute" than one particular lady made a great show of taking her two daughters by the arm and marching out of the hall in a state of high fury! And yet this was a woman who was apparently progressive enough to be sent an invitation to the meeting. As a result of my lecture, a number of Viennese women asked me to help them set up a committee for woman suffrage. This was to serve instead of an association, which would at that time have been illegal.[13]

We left Vienna for Budapest where I was to meet Rosika Schwimmer, whom I knew of through her journalism.[14] Still young, she was already the leader of an association for working women. Most of its members were teachers, clerks, and salesgirls. The organization's aim was to create a network of women to serve their mutual material and intellectual interests.

The president asked me to address her members on the subject of working women in the Netherlands. This I did, but in addition I tried to convince my audience that their organization would make real headway only when women had achieved their civil rights and thus could ensure the passage of legislation to safeguard their interests as well as those of their male counterparts. My attempt to jolt the awareness of these Hungarian women was not without its consequences. Austrian and Hungarian women were to attend the 1904 meeting in Berlin that I mentioned earlier. And when the International Woman Suffrage Alliance was set up, both the Austrian Committee for Woman Suffrage and the Hungarian Feminist Association soon became affiliated organizations.

The first international conference of the newly formed alliance was held in Denmark in 1906. It was decided that two representatives would be sent to Austria-Hungary to help the local women in their fight for woman suffrage. This task was eventually assigned to Mrs. Chapman Catt, the president of the International Alliance for Woman Suffrage, and myself. And so we left in September of that year for Austria-Hungary.

Prague was our first port of call. I knew the city and was friendly with a number of prominent women there. Bearing this in mind, I was sure that my traveling companion and I would soon feel at home. But not for one moment did I suspect that we would be inundated with visitors, both male and female. We were never once alone during the three days in Prague; quite honestly, we never had a moment to catch our breath.

Of course we had expected to be met at the station and escorted to our hotel. But what followed caught us off-guard. Our welcoming committee of Austro-Germans immediately launched into unflattering descriptions of their Czech counterparts and urged us to speak only German. No sooner had they left than a group of Czech women arrived to pay their respects with the ulterior motive of suggesting that we should take absolutely no notice of the opposing camp.[15]

It was no easy task to get across the message that we intended to remain completely neutral, that we refused to take sides. Exhausted from all this negotiating, we attended a busy meeting the following evening where we stressed the need for woman suffrage and for women to organize themselves in order to achieve that goal.

It turned out to be an extremely topical subject because universal male enfranchisement was currently under debate in the Austrian parliament. We took our seats on the platform alongside two men and a woman. The hall was almost completely packed, and we could not understand why the chairman, a university professor, kept delaying his introductory speech. Then a high-ranking police official entered wearing his full regalia. He marched right up to us and, after being formally introduced, he sat down next to me. The chairman immediately brought the meeting to order, briefly introduced the evening's speakers, and called on Mrs. Chapman Catt to deliver her lecture.

"What on earth is that policeman doing here," I wondered. He obviously did not speak much English because despite the wit of my companion's speech, his face remained deadpan throughout. He sat motionless on his chair and stared straight ahead into the audience. After I mounted the podium and began my lecture in German, I suddenly realized the reason for his presence. Whatever I said, whether it was perfectly innocuous or somewhat risky (in terms of the Austrian public), he copied down with such gusto that I could hardly keep a straight face and I was constantly reminded of Beckmesser in *Die Meistersinger*.[16]

During our Prague sojourn, we were also able to confer with the Czech women in private so that in the end we could leave the city with the knowledge that neither side had been antagonized. We were due to leave for Brünn [Brno, Moravia] at about one in the afternoon, where we had a speaking engagement the following day. Because we wanted a couple of hours to ourselves, we had taken leave of our friends and acquaintances the previous evening and urged them not to go to any further trouble on our behalf. In the morning, we visited the city, which was full of interesting sights. Then we left by coach for the station as our time of departure drew near. We were never to discover whether our coachman had played a trick on us and had misdirected the porter, who had taken our bags, or whether the porter had simply misunderstood us. One thing was certain: we were put onto the wrong train, which left the moment we took our seats. So it was already too late when the ticket collector informed us of our mistake. We had to wait until we reached the next station, more than an hour away on this express train. After several tedious hours in a small station where literally nothing could be purchased, we were reduced to quelling our hunger with the chocolates we had tucked away in our bags. A train finally arrived at six, and we were back in Prague by eight. Since we had no desire to spend another night there, we asked whether it was possible to continue to Brünn. The night train did not go as far as Brünn, but it would at least take us out of Prague. And, stupidly, we decided to go as far as we could. Once we had left Prague, we settled down in our compartment and were soon sound asleep. At about one in the morning, the train braked abruptly several times, decelerated, and finally stopped altogether. We waited five minutes, ten minutes, and then decided to see what was happening. The train seemed completely deserted. It was pitch-black outside, with no station in sight. We finally spotted a man with a lantern walking alongside the tracks. We called to him and after a while he headed toward us and told us that the train had gone into a siding.

"Can we spend the night in the carriage?" we asked anxiously.

"Impossible," he replied. The carriages were to be cleared out, and he did not know what was to happen with the train the next day. The man was civil enough to take our two heaviest bags, and we carried the rest ourselves as we followed him and his lantern, trudging across the tracks and toward the station way off in the distance. All the doors were shut, and there was no one on the platform or in the building. Fortunately our guide knew of a safe place to store our largest suitcases, and we left for the nearest town once they were carefully stowed away. Soon we had reached an inn. The railroad worker opened the door and we found ourselves in a large barroom thick with black smoke and men with beer mugs. The whole scene was extraordinarily grim. Our guide approached the two women behind the bar, and even they looked less than agreeable. But when he asked if we could stay, their answer was affirmative. And as we were wondering whether this was such a good idea after all, one of the women told us to follow her. She took us through a back door to a shed and pointed to a ladder up which we clambered to find an attic with six bedsteads. There were also a couple of bowls of water on a wooden table and a large but rather grubby towel. In short, this was the most rudimentary guestroom either of us had ever seen! And of course there was no question of locking your door at night. The bedding looked as if it had been in use for weeks, even months. At this point, we were uncertain whether we should be thankful for small mercies or wondering what would happen next!

I immediately decided to sit up all night but Mrs. Chapman Catt was so exhausted that she lay down on one of the bedsteads and wrapped herself from head to toe in a cloak. By dawn, she was well rested, so we washed ourselves as best we could and clambered back down the ladder. It was so early that the barroom was completely deserted. We rattled around until one of the women finally appeared in a state of complete disarray. When we told her that we wanted to leave, she said that there was no point because it was too early. Even the station was closed. She suggested that we sit there and offered to bring us coffee and fresh bread as soon as the baker had opened. And this she did. Once we had opened the door and let in a little fresh air, the barroom no longer seemed so disagreeable.

The day was well underway by the time we had consumed the coffee and fresh bread and left for the station in time for the first train to Brünn at nine. Since we would reach our destination by midday, we immediately sent a telegram to the group that had organized the meeting. We knew that our appointment was at six, which would give us plenty of time to relax and rest. We faithfully promised each other that we would see no one before the meeting. Easier said than done! We arrived to a welcome from an entire ladies' committee. A number of open carriages in front of the station took us through the city as a sort of mobile advertisement for the evening's events. Apart from the women, we also met a man of Austro-German origin who was now acting as the Dutch consul. He had decided to take us under his wing, which, we were told, was a good idea. It turned out that the papers had published detailed reports of my speech in Prague, which apparently contained passages that approached the limits of what was then legally acceptable in Austria. There was barely any mention of Mrs. Catt's speech; presumably because English was not the forte of most Prague reporters, they did not venture beyond generalities. Our friendly consul advised me to be more careful that evening, because, as he said, "You've already said some pretty strong stuff."

"Like what?" I asked, more than a little curious.

And then I was told that I had insulted the Austrian premier. I had quoted a newspaper report that when woman suffrage was brought up in the Austrian parliament the president stated that it was simply a novelty that had never caught on.

At the meeting I had commented, "You'd expect a president to know what he's talking about. But the Austrian premier seems to be an exception to the rule because it has apparently escaped his notice that Australia and some North American states have already introduced woman suffrage."

With the best will in the world, I failed to understand why this remark constituted a threat to the Austrian state. The consul thought differently and beseeched me not to repeat this statement.

Fresh ordeals awaited us after the carriage tour of Brünn. The consul and his family especially wanted us to lunch with them that very afternoon. No matter how hospitable his intentions, Mrs. Catt and I were determined to avoid these duties because we yearned for a hot bath and a bed or sofa on which to rest our aching limbs. Our protests were fruitless. We were obliged to follow the preordained itinerary, the only concession a stop at the hotel to freshen up. The consul arrived half an hour later and drove us by car to his house. And there we had lunch. Every member of his family seemed positively charming, and I am convinced that they must have found us poor company. We were so exhausted that we could hardly eat, and neither of us felt like talking.

As I now sit writing, I can still envisage the whole scene. One of the daughters was herself the mother of several children. She had read *The Century of the Child* by Ellen Key, which was extremely popular at that time, and asked our opinion of every chapter.[17] The rest of the family, also well acquainted with the author's ideas, wanted to know what we thought of the book. Hardly in the mood for a debate, I simply concurred with their views. Years later, I still felt immediate irritation at the mere mention of Ellen Key and *The Century of the Child*. Instantly, it brought back memories of that disastrous afternoon in Brünn.

The meeting started at six and finished at approximately nine o'clock. However, even at that hour our hope of finally being left alone to relax was not to be fulfilled. Delighted with their organizational skills, the committee members proudly informed us that a simple supper would be served in an adjacent hall. There we found ourselves surrounded by a group of Czech men and women whose sole aim was to enlighten us about the unjust way in which they were treated by the Austrians. Once we reached our hotel, we decided to take the first train to Vienna the next morning, and to deliberately remain incognito. That was clearly the only way we would get some well-earned breathing space.

Fortunately, the Viennese women had organized a program that was not taxing and allowed us to see the city's sights. At that time, the Austrian parliament was debating the issue of broader enfranchisement. But even the most progressive of parliamentarians had abandoned the demand for woman suffrage and campaigned exclusively for male enfranchisement. I brought this up at a meeting attended by several members of parliament and advised all the women present to refuse to help in achieving this goal. I tried to explain that it would do nothing to further their cause should these plans become law. In fact, universal male suffrage would make their struggle even harder to sustain because at present they could at least count on the support of those men who, like themselves, were denied their civil rights. In the future, they would find themselves isolated and battling to convince even more men than ever of the justice of their cause. Although the Austrian men had sworn to campaign on behalf of woman suffrage, once universal male suffrage became law, I knew from the experience of women in other countries not to attach the slightest significance to these promises.

My words provoked a storm of protest. Everyone wanted to join in the discussion. Although I no longer remember how many people were involved, I do recall that Victor Adler, an extremely progressive member of parliament and a friend to women, put in a few strong words on my behalf.[18] He came and sat next to me at the supper that concluded the meeting so that he could continue the discussion with me. Not only the men but also many of the Austrian women seemed to disagree with me. They repeatedly assured me that the men in this country would be an exception to the rule and would keep their promises.

In the end history proved me right. After many invitations from the Austrian Committee for Woman Suffrage, I eventually returned to Vienna in 1913 for a speaking engagement where I made a point of mentioning my prediction of 1906. Universal male enfranchisement had been introduced some seven years earlier, while women were still forbidden to organize themselves politically and were banned from attending political meetings.[19] Some of the audience responded to my words with thunderous applause while others, including most of the men present, reacted with indignation. Both sides were heard in the morning papers: some who supported my views strongly criticized the men for their disloyalty, while others described me as a foreigner making a seditious speech.

I now return to our campaign tour of 1906. After Vienna, we visited Budapest, where we had a whole series of speaking engagements. Initially this seemed a daunting task, but thanks to the support of the local suffrage workers and their excellent organization, it was possible to move through our program at a steady and sensible pace. Our duties included a Sunday afternoon spent addressing an audience of working-class men and women in the main room of the town hall. We spoke at meetings with reduced admission fees and also at those where six crowns were charged, which was a lot of money in those days. We responded to an invitation from the Freemasons to explain our views concerning woman suffrage to their members. In addition, we also argued our cause at afternoon tea parties where we met those women who preferred not to attend meetings. Moreover, we gave press interviews virtually every day, not only about votes for women but also on a number of other topical issues. Needless to say, these opportunities were used mainly to draw attention to our own cause. Budapest newspapers and magazines ran a great many articles about Mrs. Catt and me, illustrated with portraits and caricatures, some of which were more successful than others. The young women who had invited us and supported the campaign for woman suffrage thoughtfully collected all our press clippings and bound them in fine leather as a souvenir of our time in their city.

Returning from my first foreign campaign, I immediately threw myself into preparations for the first international women's conference ever held in the Netherlands, which took place in June 1908.[20]

SEVEN

MY WORK ON BEHALF OF SALESGIRLS

The Effects of Standing for a Long Time • My Attempts to Introduce Improvements • My Meeting with the State Commission • My Colleagues Refuse to Cooperate • An Appeal to the Women of Holland • Public Opinion • My Hopes Are Fulfilled

I moved to Amsterdam to begin practicing as the first woman doctor in the country and fortunately I soon found myself with a flourishing practice. Many women came during my office hours, including a large number of salesgirls who often reported similar symptoms. I almost always found that they were suffering from gynecological problems that I could only ascribe to the effects of being forced to stand each day for hours on end. At that time, shops in the major cities stayed open until eleven at night. With the working day starting at 8 A.M., salesgirls had no alternative but to stand behind their counters for exceptionally long periods of time with only the briefest of rests for meals.

Each time I encountered these cases, which could so easily have been prevented but would now entail a lifetime of suffering, I resolved to do whatever I could to improve the girls' working conditions. I was naive enough to believe that shopkeepers and department store owners prevented their staff from sitting simply because they were ignorant of the risks involved in standing for a protracted period of time. I felt that it was up to me to enlighten these employers and I never for one moment doubted that I would succeed. How wrong I was!

I spent several consecutive afternoons visiting these men and informing them of the fact that the human body was simply not designed to spend long periods standing in one spot. My message fell almost exclusively on deaf ears. The vast majority of these businessmen raised all kinds of objections against the ways in which I wanted to combat this evil. I was bombarded with so much blind prejudice and so many arguments based on self-interest that I eventually realized there was no point in going on in this manner. Hence, I decided to adopt a new strategy that would involve the government.

First I wrote an article for the *Sociaal Weekblad* that included detailed descriptions of some of my patients. Of course, I carefully omitted both the girls' names and those of the shops where they worked. But I did explain clearly and carefully the cause of these women's condition and how it could easily be prevented.

Much to my disappointment, the article was returned a few days later. The editor wrote to say that he had shown it to two other doctors who agreed that the medical condition described in these cases could in no way be ascribed to protracted standing, and that he was not prepared to publish my article unless I revealed the names and addresses of both the shop girls and their employers. If I complied, the matter could be further investigated. If I did not, then my article simply could not be published.

Needless to say, I had no intention of fulfilling these demands. I could under no circumstances reveal the girls' names or those of the shops where they worked.

There was no alternative but to allow the situation to continue and wait patiently for an opportunity for change. I could expect nothing of the girls themselves. For what could they do, powerless as they were? As yet there were no trade unions representing the interests of working women and, in any case, how could these girls attend meetings when they were forced to work until eleven at night?

My chance came in 1886, by which time "social justice" had become a fashionable phrase. I cannot say with any certainty whether this term created or reflected a new way of thinking. But one way or another, the terminology existed, and when the government set up a commission under the leadership of Mr. Verniers van der Loeff and Mr. Goeman Borgesius to investigate working conditions in factories and other locations, I felt that it should also examine the salesgirls' plight. So I approached the commission to report on the problems experienced by many women as a result of working in shops and department stores.

Initially its members did not seem to appreciate my concern. "Shops and department stores," read the response to my request, did not qualify as a "place of work," at least according to their interpretation. However, some time later I received a letter informing me that the commission was nonetheless prepared to hear me out. And of course I responded immediately.

During my talks with the commission on January 7, 1887, it soon became apparent that its members had no interest in the working conditions found in shops and stores. Rather they were hoping I could provide them with additional information to support the exclusion of women from factories and other locations, a campaign that was gaining momentum at the time. Needless to say, I refused to cooperate. The commission's chairman asked me whether I had already contacted the health inspector to discuss the possibility of introducing some form of seating for salesgirls. To be honest, I had not, but his question certainly provided me with a good idea. But before I pursued this course of action, I decided to wait for the commission's verdict, although I never for one moment supposed that its contents would result in legal reform along the lines I had suggested.

Meanwhile, I encountered a series of new cases that were similar to those I had already diagnosed. I also received a constant stream of letters from the parents of salesgirls who begged me not to abandon their cause because their daughters were working in conditions that had to be improved. A group of these young women even wrote to tell me that their situation was virtually unbearable.

I decided to contact the Amsterdam health inspector at once. In reply to my letter, he informed me that "shopkeepers cannot be forced to introduce seating arrangements for their employees; and only a reduction of working hours would provide these girls with more opportunity to rest."

This letter also referred me to the inspector of labor. I wrote immediately and to my great satisfaction he not only understood the issue's importance but was also prepared to cooperate fully. Because he felt that the shopkeepers would be unwilling to break with tradition, the inspector argued that all my efforts would be in vain unless they acquired the appropriate legal backing. To achieve this, he suggested that the parties involved should launch a campaign that would include the active support of myself and my colleagues. At once I made a number of copies of the letter the salesgirls had sent to me. I mailed them to those doctors who seemed most likely to respond, together with a request from me to join me in taking action. I quoted the inspector of labor at great length, pointing out that this kind of campaign would probably be the most effective in a number of different ways.

Once again the results of trying to involve my colleagues in a social issue were disappointing, to say the least. Two doctors wrote that they were not prepared to respond to my request; the others did not reply at all.

In January 1894, I published an appeal to the women of Holland in all the newspapers and sent additional copies to every women's association in the country:

> Shopkeepers claim that the health of many young girls is being sacrificed to unreasonable demands by you, the customer.

They maintain that on entering a shop you expect assistants to be standing ready to serve you.

To avoid offense or disappointment, shopkeepers are careful to make sure that there are no chairs or benches behind their counters. Hence, employees are obliged "to be on their toes" at all times during business hours. This means that a large number of salesgirls must stay on their feet for between twelve and fourteen hours a day, with only the shortest of breaks for meals.

The detrimental effects this can have on the female body are also demonstrated by the fact that a number of health inspectors have urged the minister to allow schoolmistresses to conduct their lessons seated, although, in their case, they are only required to teach five hours a day with a two-hour break for lunch.

You should consult your doctor if you wish to know what happens to women who spend most of their life on their feet. Since I set up my practice in Amsterdam, I have had a constant stream of patients suffering from conditions in which protracted standing has destroyed both their health and their zest for living.

The way in which salesgirls themselves experience these risks is amply expressed by a letter I recently received. It reads,

Dear Madam,

This letter is an appeal to you from the women and girls whose job it is to serve customers in shops from eight in the morning until between nine and eleven at night. We must stand at all times except for the occasional half-hour spent taking refreshment. For other people, it is one of Life's pleasures to be able to move around after being seated for a long time and for us too, no matter how tired and exhausted we are, it is a relief to be able to walk up and down after standing for hours on end. But it is particularly during that period which requires no further explanation that most of us are in a state of constant pain; there are few of us that do not suffer from those complaints so familiar to you in the course of your work. Naturally, a great many salesgirls do not even respond honestly to your inquiries because their livelihood is at stake.

In their ignorance of female physiology, our employers make no distinction between male and female employees. They forbid us to sit and enforce their ban by not providing chairs. Of course, we realize that we must stand when there are people in the shop, even when we see them approaching the door. Our employer's business is the main thing; but we are not allowed to sit at all, even when there is nothing to do. This rule is not simply tyrannical, it is literally killing us. The conditions we now suffer from make us fear for the future, yet our employers insist on this regime. This is simply a terrible state of affairs. We believe that you can help us both as a doctor and, more important, as a woman. You can assist us to maintain our health and you can restore it. We know that you can help us and, please, we beg you to listen to our plea. With your involvement, the employers could finally be convinced to allow us to sit and to provide us with chairs. They have always been immune to persuasion, but now they can be confronted with the fact that their interests are causing actual physical suffering. Please believe us, Madam, all that is needed is an advertisement to unite women in a boycott of those shops that do not provide chairs for their female staff and our grievances would be solved immediately. There is little point in conducting a survey of salesgirls because they can be laid off without warning, and many, especially the less educated, would prefer to work themselves to death than lose their livelihoods and face privation. Madam, you can help us; you can convince the ladies who patronize our employers that action must be taken. It is not that we are lazy or yearn for a life of leisure, we are simply aware that as each day passes we are becoming increasingly exhausted from ailments invisible to the layman and about which we dare not inform our employers. Sitting is allowed in shops run and owned by women. They, at least, are in a position to judge. Madam, once again we beg you to help us! Yours, et cetera.

Women of Holland! Repeated attempts have failed to eliminate the just grievances of these economically disadvantaged women. So I ask for your intervention. Let us make it absolutely clear that we in no way support this barbarous custom, as is claimed by shopkeepers themselves.

Hence, whenever you enter a shop where there is no form of seating behind the counter, you should inform the shopkeeper that your future patronage depends on his installing the necessary facilities.

In this way, you will soon enjoy the satisfaction of knowing that you have helped eradicate injustice and have eased the burden of countless women.

DR. ALETTA H. JACOBS

Amsterdam, January 18, 1894

This appeal did indeed succeed in arousing public interest. In a number of towns, women's committees were set up to inform the local shopkeepers that they supported my crusade to provide shop staff with seating facilities.

In Rotterdam, two hundred women signed the following letter, which was sent to the city's shopkeepers,

Doubtless you have already seen Dr. A. Jacobs's appeal, which was recently published in a number of daily newspapers. It again drew our attention to a much discussed issue: the dangers incurred by women and girls from standing for long periods of time.

Some of our number argued that we should follow Dr. Jacobs's advice and make it known that, from now on, we would only frequent those shops where female staff were permitted to sit—but, after further consideration, we decided that such measures were neither necessary nor desirable.

They are unnecessary because many shopkeepers already provide their staff with chairs. They are undesirable because we prefer that the freedom we demand for ourselves should also be extended to others.

Moreover, we flatter ourselves that employers will permit their salesgirls to sit quite simply because they know that it pleases their clientele.

The aim of this letter is to express openly and emphatically that the undersigned desire the salesgirls of Rotterdam to be provided with adequate seating arrangements. We further consider that the necessity of this measure has been amply elucidated by Dr. Jacobs and other experts and have therefore included no further explanation for its desirability, trusting instead in your benevolent cooperation.

The trade magazine *De Manufacturier* discussed my manifesto, which was viewed in a positive light in several successive issues. Without either denying the facts or overlooking my good intentions, the editor felt that the whole issue had to be considered from both sides, with the shopkeepers' objections also taken into account. The magazine argued that the public at large simply demands too much. Customers expect salesgirls to be standing ready to serve them. What is more, there is not enough space behind a counter to allow for any form of seating arrangement.

My appeal was included in its entirety in the January 25, 1894, issue of the police magazine *Het geïllustreerd Politienieuws*. In a detailed footnote, the editor expressed his support but felt that since few other women would risk involvement, the only hope was that the government would take up this issue and change labor laws to protect the salesgirls of Holland. To demonstrate the magazine's sympathy for my campaign on behalf of thousands of young women, a photograph was included in the same issue that showed a number of salesgirls delivering a petition to the Queen Regent to request the government's support for the movement so honorably begun by Dr. Aletta Jacobs.

Once again the national newspapers completely failed to appreciate the importance of this issue. The *Amsterdamse Courant* of January 29, 1894, declared that, because of my appeal, it had carried out its own investigation as to whether and to what extent it was possible to implement my suggestions. In fact, the paper had approached the owners of large department stores and not the salesgirls themselves. I have the results in front of me right now. Rereading these reports so many years later, I find these men describing our movement as "a grossly exaggerated and morbid affair, something no sensible person would waste his time on." One boss proudly declared that "in my shop, the girls work from 9 to 12 A.M., then they take a half-hour break; they work from 12:30 to 4:30 P.M., then they take another half-hour break; after that, they work from 5 to 6 P.M., with yet another half-hour break; and then straight through to 9 P.M., when the shop closes. That's hardly what you could call arduous."

Another businessman wrote, "I simply do not believe all those ridiculous old wives' tales about salesgirls standing around and getting all kinds of ailments. My girls are healthy and they look it. If some lady decides to tell us she no longer intends to patronize our shop, then our reaction will quite simply be, 'Go somewhere else; no one is going to tell us how to run our business. We do the best we can for our customers, for our staff, and for ourselves.' "

Yet another shopkeeper tried to suggest that the letter I quoted had not actually been written by the salesgirls themselves. "It's just some kind of advertisement for this cause."

After everything I had heard from them, and from nonpatients, I was not at all surprised that employers reacted in this way. But I was both astonished and irritated by the statements of two anonymous doctors who were brought in by a newspaper as specialists in gynecology. One boldly stated, "The patients that Miss Jacobs is referring to are all married women who have had two or three children." However, he did declare that these women—and everyone else for that matter—should be allowed to sit down at work. "But the fact that they have to stand is not the disaster Dr. Jacobs makes it out to be. Otherwise we'll have to do without nurses, since they spend much more time on their feet and their work is more exhausting." The other doctor wrote, "To come to any sound conclusion, one would first have to study the symptoms of girls whose work includes protracted standing and then consider to what extent these same symptoms are also prevalent among other groups of girls."

No matter how stupid these and similar statements seemed, I decided to return to this issue once more to make it quite clear that salesgirls must be given ample periods of rest.

Meanwhile, increasing numbers of shopkeepers were responding to my demands and various groups were campaigning for the legal stipulation of an earlier closing time and the provision of seating arrangements for shop staff. This continued until 1902 when the minister for internal affairs announced that plans were being made for the introduction of a law to enforce the provision of seating arrangements for salesgirls.

In Amsterdam, a committee had been lobbying for some time for a law concerning the closing times of shops and department stores. On December 20, 1902, it published an announcement in *de Telegraaf*, from which I quote the following:

Our committee has approached the doctors of Amsterdam to acquire expert evidence to prove our point that standing for long periods of time adversely affects the health of female employees. However, we have to report the following about a questionnaire that was circulated for this purpose,

"Despite repeated attempts, we have failed to receive an adequate number of replies. The attitude of Amsterdam doctors is (to put it mildly) incomprehensible. When a similar survey was carried out in Berlin, local doctors made a point of replying. The results were subsequently published in the *Handlungs-Gehilfenblatt* of the *Centralverband der Handlungs-Gehilfinnen Deutschlands*.

For the time being, the committee has had to make do with a report about health insurance for Berlin salesclerks, which clearly shows that the vast majority of doctors are well aware of the damage caused by prolonged periods of standing. They consequently recognized the importance, in terms of national standards of health, of salesclerks being provided with seating to be used during those periods when they are not involved with serving customers."

Does the above not make it all too clear how little Amsterdam doctors cared about social issues and how little awareness they had of their obligation to prevent illness whenever possible? I had worked a great many years for this cause when finally, in 1902, the government began to express interest and I was asked to address members of parliament about the importance for thousands of young girls of the introduction of a law to enforce my demands. I had then completed my task and enjoyed the satisfaction of knowing that, twenty years after I had first drawn attention to the importance of allowing salesgirls to sit behind their counters, a law had finally been passed to require the provision of seating arrangements.

EIGHT

MY INVOLVEMENT WITH PACIFISM AND ANTIMILITARISM

My Pacifist Sympathies • Contact with Bertha Von Suttner • My Meetings with William Stead and Bjørnstjerne Bjørnson • The Boer War • Disillusionment • The 1915 International Congress of Women in The Hague • Contact with the Governments of Various Countries • Travel in Times of War • I Visit America • The Congress in Zurich (May 1919) • A Revealing Trip to Germany • Work on Behalf of the Prisoners of War in Siberia • Impressions of Germany in 1920 • The Proposed Reform of the Peace Treaty • The 1922 International Women's Congress in The Hague

Although I can hardly claim to have done pioneering work for either pacifism or antimilitarism, I can honestly say that I detest war and view the armed forces as being an unmitigated evil. I probably absorbed these opinions from my father. Even as a child, I knew that, after completing his training, Father had terminated his government contract to serve as a military doctor as soon as he possibly could. The only reason he had signed up in the first place was in the hope of being able to speed up his wedding plans. But since his views and those of the military authorities were diametrically opposed, he decided to leave at the first opportunity.

Strangely enough, despite the antimilitary ideals he tried to instill in his children, three of his six sons chose army careers, although he had created ample opportunity for all six to continue their education elsewhere. It started with Johan, who was a natural soldier and gave up philosophy in favor of the army. He also tried to convince his younger brothers and sisters that the well-being of the nation depended to a great extent on its military might. His words certainly impressed my two youngest brothers. A combination of Johan's influence and their school books, which portrayed soldiers as being the only worthwhile heroes, led them to believe that there was no better or more honorable career than a soldier's.

As I mentioned at the beginning of this book, one of my brothers began training as an architect before switching to the military academy in Kampen, where he was later joined by my youngest brother. I often talked with these two and actively challenged their opinions. I frequently felt compelled to express my indignation at the degrading military discipline that required unconditional obedience to commanding officers even when those in the lower ranks were clearly their moral superiors.

This blind obedience, this impersonal devotion, completely contradicted my own sense of self-respect. It provoked feelings that were basically pro-democratic, although I was not yet able to describe them as such, and also offended my dearly held belief in freedom. It made my blood boil to see the sergeant testing the corporal's obedience, which was something that happened even at home.

I gradually became aware of the link between militarism and war during the Franco-Prussian War (1870–1871) when, like so many other children, I spent endless evenings unraveling old linen so that the lint could be sent to the military hospitals of both countries to be used for bandaging wounded soldiers. At that time, medicine was extremely primitive in comparison to what was available during the Great War. Yet men of science still can do little to ease the impact of brute force.

Even then, I had a strong sense that war was fundamentally inhuman. When the Netherlands shelled Atjeh, I openly expressed my sympathy for the local people and refused to view that war as being in any way justifiable.[1] Here I would like to pay homage to my late brother Dr. Julius Jacobs, who died in 1895 in Makasser [Ujung Pandang]. As a medical officer, he was involved in the Atjeh war, but despite that experience, or more likely because of it, he was essentially a pacifist. At a time when the Atjeh people were constantly referred to as "filthy pigs," he viewed them as being a heroic enemy force. His respect was evident in books he wrote such as *Eenigen tijd onder Baliërs* (Among the Balinese, 1883), but even more so in a major ethnological-medical work published by the Royal Dutch Geographical Society, called *Het Familie- en Kampongleven in Groot-Atjeh* (Family and Kampong Life in Great Atjeh, Leiden: E. J. Brill, 1894).[2] I never saw him again after he moved abroad, but, since we corresponded regularly, I was well aware of his thinking. He was convinced that the needless war with Atjeh was a disgrace to our country and that it had been launched purely as means of defending Dutch interests.

As I said before, I cannot claim to be a pioneering pacifist. The Dutch peace associations required no more of their members than a small annual contribution, and there was little active campaigning.

In 1898, Holland hosted its first international peace conference, in which I chose to participate.[3] It was here I met the Austrian peace apostle, Bertha von Suttner, with whom I had been corresponding for some time.[4] During this meeting, von Suttner, who wrote the bestselling *Die Waffen Nieder* (*Lay Down Your Arms*), bluntly informed me that I had made the wrong choice in life. She suggested that I should dedicate myself 100 percent to peace work and should delegate my suffrage campaigning to someone else, as she considered this work to be unworthy of me.

In turn, I pointed out that Bertha von Suttner's ideals could be realized only when women had achieved full civil rights. The philosophy of peace would gain government recognition when women's opinions were also being expressed in parliaments everywhere. In my view, women had to achieve full emancipation before they could make any meaningful contribution to the peace campaign.

Anyone familiar with the work of both Bertha von Suttner and myself will realize that we failed to convince each other. *She* continued to regard the preaching of world peace as her chosen task and *I* just kept on working for woman suffrage.

In the summer of 1899, I accompanied my husband to Christiania [Oslo] where he was attending the meeting of the Interparliamentary Union. We ended up staying in the same hotel as the von Suttners, and it was over the breakfast table that Frau von Suttner and I continued the discussion we had begun in The Hague about which was more urgent: woman suffrage or peace? Finally I suggested a compromise, "When you're campaigning for peace you could also make a point of supporting woman suffrage, and while I'm defending our right to political equality I will in turn emphasize the close links between this issue and that of world peace."

But my eminent opponent found it impossible to accept my suggestion. In her opinion, it was a case of confusing two entirely separate ideals, "You can work either for women's emancipation or for world peace, but not for both at the same time. Each issue demands total commitment and is just too important to be dealt with in passing."

It proved impossible to bridge the gap that separated us. And when, during the meeting, I addressed a group of peace apostles and influential statesman on the subject of woman suffrage, I was soon to find myself confronted with an angry Frau von Suttner.

At the farewell dinner held for the foreign guests by the Norwegian board of the Interparliamentary Union, it was my honor to be accompanied by the minister of the interior, Mr. Quam, a privilege that was doubtless due to my acquaintance with Mrs. Quam, the leader of the Norwegian suffrage movement.[5] Probably this was also the reason I had been asked to respond to a toast given by the president of the Odelsting [Parliament], Mr. Horst. He toasted the women, whose presence, he said, had not simply endorsed the meeting's aims but had imbued its festivities with an additional luster. I had already tried in vain to persuade Bertha von Suttner to take over my task, but my letter asking her to express thanks on behalf of all the women present had been answered with a flat refusal. So there was no alternative but to perform this duty myself. I began by thanking Mr. Horst for his courteous words. I also thanked the Norwegian commission on behalf of those women who had listened to the conference from the balconies and had found their seats supplied with boxes of the most delicious candy. I then pointed out that in planning for the realization of world peace, none of the conference participants had stopped to consider the outstanding contribution that would be made as a result of women's emancipation. I continued, "We women would have gladly foregone our complimentary candies if only we had been permitted to participate in your discussions as your political equals." And I ended by expressing the hope that Norway would set an example for the rest of Europe by granting woman suffrage. This act would introduce an element into political life that would lead to international disputes being settled through arbitration rather than the use of force.

My speech was greeted with thunderous applause. However, Bertha von Suttner made clear her displeasure at my using a peace conference dinner as a platform for woman suffrage. She felt I had definitely gone too far. But I should point out to those who knew Bertha von Suttner personally that her resentment was short-lived. In fact, after experiencing the events of the next few years, she even admitted to me that wars will be prevented only when women have a direct influence on the world's governments.

She later attended a peace conference in the Netherlands in 1913.[6] This was a year before her death, and she was already in obvious decline. Nonetheless, she was quite prepared to address a public meeting of the Dutch Association for Woman Suffrage and delivered a dazzling speech on women's political emancipation that is doubtless still remembered by all those present. That audience will also recall her absolute belief in the power to combat war that would be unleashed once women gained their civil rights.

One of the people who complimented me on my speech in Christiania was the already world-famous journalist William Stead.[7] Over the years, a great many readers both at home and abroad have followed his vehement and articulate crusade for lasting peace, his articles on improving the penal code, and his essays on feminism.

Stead was to become a good friend of mine; we started corresponding from the first time we met. Many of my readers will recall that this formidable apostle of peace was one of the many passengers who sailed for the New World in 1912 on the brand-new ocean liner *Titanic* and who, as a result of its collision with an iceberg, found their final resting place at the bottom of the sea.

Writing about the men and women who attended the farewell dinner in Christiania inevitably reminds me of Bjørnstjerne Bjørnson, the great Norwegian who at the same farewell dinner delivered a speech that was based on the saying "Those who wish to combat war should begin by fighting the continuing lies of politics and diplomacy."[8]

My husband and I had the privilege that evening of meeting Mr. and Mrs. Bjørnson in person. We mentioned in passing that we intended to stay on for some time in Norway once the conference had ended. We wanted to travel in this spectacular country, already known to us from a previous visit. No sooner had they heard that than the Bjørnsons invited us to stay at their country residence, which was in fact a farmstead, in Olestad. So when we decided to visit Gausdal, where Olestad was located, we wrote to Mr. and Mrs. Bjørnson to say that we would like to stay with them.

You can imagine our amazement at being welcomed not only with the Netherlands' flag flying high above the house but also by two of our hosts' grandchildren standing at the entrance to greet us in Dutch.

I thoroughly enjoyed both this reception and my stay with the Bjørnson family. This visit gave us the chance to get to know and admire this man, who was at the center of Christiania life. We talked for hours about the subjects we cared most about. So much was happening at that time that deeply affected this man, who valued truth above all. England's actions in the Transvaal had outraged everyone who worked for truth and peace.[9] In Rennes, Émile Zola was arguing his case concerning Dreyfus, the Jewish officer who had been wrongly accused of treason.[10] Several phone calls a day brought Bjørnson the latest developments from Reuters in Christiania.

"What's happening in Rennes?" I asked once, when he had just hung up after one of these calls. He exploded with indignation. "Not one of the generals or ex-ministers has the moral courage to admit he has been misled or has made a mistake. They're just trying to save their own skins by perpetuating all those lies." Bjørnson felt that the Dreyfus affair was based on a lie, as was the unequal struggle between the mighty British nation and the tiny Boer state.

I still fondly remember my stay with Mr. and Mrs. Bjørnson and I often look through the books he inscribed and gave to me when I left.

The war between England and South Africa broke out soon after we returned to Holland. I had already publicly declared my support for that handful of brave Boers, and whenever possible I spoke or wrote on their behalf.[11] When the Peace Through Justice Association organized public meetings in every major Dutch city to mark the Russian tsar's message of peace, I was asked to prepare and lead one such gathering in Amsterdam, an opportunity I seized to denounce England's current actions.[12] One tangible result of this was that the English government refused me entry to South Africa, where I had intended to provide medical aid for women and children in the internment camps. I planned to pay for this out of my own pocket and expected no assurances of my safety. I later wondered if it would have been more sensible to express my opinions a little less forcibly. Then perhaps I would have been able to help the women and children of the Transvaal—but most probably they would have refused me entry anyway. England had every reason to wish to exclude outsiders from the internment camps, where conditions prevailed that were to the eternal disgrace of the British nation.

I did little work for pacifism in the years following the war although I always accompanied my husband whenever he attended the meetings of the Inter-parliamentary Union. But my main aim was to make contact with various governments' members of parliament in order to further the cause of woman suffrage. The excursions and parties that were extensions of these meetings provided me with ideal opportunities.

But there was another reason why I was not directly involved in the pacifist crusade. I simply felt that there was more important and urgent work to be done elsewhere. In my view, the major powers would not dare to declare war if they felt that they could not rely on their people's support. At that time, I was so idealistic I even believed that in Germany, a military state par excellence, the people were simply too highly developed to allow its participation in a European war. That war broke out now and then in the Balkans or in the Far East was, in my opinion, because of the fact that these regions were still at an early stage of development. Pacifism was not likely to have much influence before the local population achieved a higher level of civilization.

Sadly, history proved me wrong. Not for a moment had I imagined that we might be on the brink of a world war until a friend wrote in April 1914 from Russia to tell me that her country was in the process of mobilization and that there was an atmosphere of fear and tension in the political circles in which she moved. My reaction to her somber predictions was so casual that I wrote back to invite her to visit Scheveningen with me. "A sea breeze will soon blow away all those cobwebs!" I wrote. Similarly, when, at about the same time, I received advice from Vienna to dispose of any Austrian documents I might possess because of the imminent threat of war, I assumed that this was a standard announcement rather than a serious warning.

I first felt a sense of dread after attending the conference of the International Council of Women in Rome. Along with other delegates, I was warned not to speak German or any similar-sounding language in public, for I was liable to attract all manner of unpleasantness.

Following the conference, I spent several weeks on Capri and Anacapri with the eminent American preacher Miss Anna Howard Shaw, who has addressed the women of Holland on several memorable occasions, and her companion, Miss Lucy E. Anthony.[13] The last thing I thought about was war.

Refreshed by my Italian holiday, I returned home briefly before leaving for London where the international board of the International Woman Suffrage Alliance was to meet with the presidents of the affiliated national associations at the beginning of July. No one mentioned the possibility of war, not even when we were invited by British MPs for tea on the terrace of the houses of Parliament.

I returned from London to find a telegram from Olive Schreiner, the South African author of world-famous books such as *The Story of an African Farm* and *Dreams*.[14] She had written to say that she was returning from Germany and would like to stay with me for a few days. My older readers will doubtless remember the vital role Olive Schreiner played in her country's history. Her fame is due not only to her writing but also to her courageous behavior during the Boer War, which gained her much sympathy but aroused the hatred of the English government. As a result, she was banished to an unhealthy and inhospitable part of the country and forced to live as a virtual prisoner, a situation that had a disastrous effect on her health.

Her train was expected at the station in Amsterdam between 10 and 11 P.M. Instead, it arrived at one in the morning and my guest was so distraught that I had to wonder whether she was suffering a nervous breakdown. It turned out that in Creisau [Silesia], where she had been staying with Count and Countess von Moltke, people talked constantly of the impending war. At the home of her host, who was the nephew and heir of Germany's most important field marshal, everyone was obsessed with the dreadful events, which seemed inevitable. The train to Holland had been repeatedly delayed by mobilization, a state of affairs that vividly reminded my friend of all the horrors she had so recently experienced in South Africa.

Amsterdam and the relaxing atmosphere of my home gradually restored Olive Schreiner's spirits, until July 31, 1914, when the evening papers announced that the Dutch army was to be mobilized as well. She immediately decided to leave for London, fearing that otherwise she would never see her homeland again. Early the next morning, I took her to the station to catch the train for Vlissingen. Normally the station would have been virtually deserted at that hour, but it was bustling with men who had completed their military service years before, husbands and fathers who had responded to the government's call to enlist and were leaving their homes to head for our borders. Gravely, they bade farewell to families who were more often than not being left to fend for themselves.

Once the train had vanished from sight, I tried to comfort some of the women who stood there, in tears. As soon as they realized that I was genuinely concerned about their welfare, they began to bombard me with questions. In many cases, their husbands, the fathers of their children, had taken the wages they had received the previous evening, in the belief that the government would provide for their families. And, completely in good faith, these women were now asking me where to go to collect the promised money. Others were wondering whether the baker, the butcher, the milkman, or the grocer would extend credit to them while they were waiting for their payments from the government. I realized that comfort was not enough, that means had to be found to provide the basic essentials for these women.

Deeply impressed by what I had seen and heard that morning, I returned home to convene an emergency meeting of the board of the Association for Woman Suffrage. I described what I had seen just a few hours previously and everyone agreed that we should try to provide some form of direct assistance. We knew in advance that, even if preparatory measures were taken immediately, it would still be some time before government aid was made available.

Our first action was to send a letter to the executive committees of the various branches of the Association for Woman Suffrage. The letters urged that it was our duty to relieve as much as possible the suffering that had arisen here as a result of the hostilities in Europe. We proposed setting aside our suffrage work for the time being in order to provide needed support. We also included suggested actions for committee members. Even though it was a Sunday, we succeeded in getting our letter copied and sent out right away.

The next day we had a leaflet printed and immediately distributed in working-class districts by Boy Scouts and Girl Scouts. It carried an announcement aimed at women facing financial difficulties because the family breadwinner had enlisted. We informed these women that they could approach us for advice and support, and that we were even willing to help out with money.

In the same day's newspapers, we announced that many women and children urgently needed assistance until the government could organize some regular form of welfare. We asked for donations to help provide this support. Bakers, grocers, milkmen, and people who ran soup kitchens and similar establishments were asked to accept receipts signed by us in lieu of cash with the understanding that we would subsequently settle these debts.

We worked late into the night. The next morning, just as we were about resume our tasks, a group of women involved with work similar to our own approached us to discuss a possible merger, which, of course, we immediately agreed to. For some months, I devoted all my energy to that large women's committee, and although I cannot deny that it helped alleviate suffering, I am not really a supporter of long-term philanthropic work. "By helping relieve the consequences of war, are we not also contributing to its continuation, to all the horror and degradation it causes?" I wondered in desperation. Then I thought of the ancient cathedrals, of art treasures and of priceless libraries that had been destroyed in all the madness. And I thought still more of the dead and the maimed, of the thousands of families that had been divided, of the children and wives whose fathers and husbands had been sacrificed to the pride of those who governed them. More and more clearly I realized that, while the men who enlisted had helped make this tragedy possible, we women could have quite possibly ended the slaughter by collectively refusing to meet the needs caused by war and by ignoring the pressure to keep society going. If women had *not* agreed to take over wherever needed, if they had *not* been willing to perform the work of men, then the governments would have been forced to abandon the whole disastrous venture.

I wanted to call on women from every nation to protest together against the horrors of war. Perhaps we could even find a way to end the hostilities. Living as I did in a country that was only indirectly affected, I was nonetheless acutely aware of the terror experienced by women in those lands that were more immediately involved. How much worse, I wondered, must it be to have to endure everything at first hand?

While I was thinking about this problem and about how to realize my plan, I received a letter from Berlin, in late October 1914, which stated that under the circumstances the German women had decided to abandon their plans to hold an International Woman Suffrage Alliance conference in Berlin in June 1915.

I was informed of this in my capacity as president of the Association for Woman Suffrage, and, as such, I decided to call an emergency meeting of our foreign affairs committee. Referring to my Berlin letter, I emphasized the need for women from various nations to meet on neutral territory. After some discussion, the committee eventually came around to my way of thinking. As a result, an appeal was sent out at the beginning of November to the board of the International Woman Suffrage Alliance and to the presidents of the affiliated associations. The final paragraph read,

> "In these times of burgeoning hate and war among nations, we women must show that we at least can maintain solidarity and mutual friendship.
>
> Although it appears impossible to hold our congress in Berlin as planned, we nonetheless suggest that a meeting of the alliance should still take place in a neutral country. The plan would be to discuss alliance matters during the day but to provide additional opportunities in the evening to air the female perspective on the current situation in Europe. As Holland is probably one of the easiest countries to reach, we would like to invite the alliance to hold its conference in our country. We are, of course, prepared to make all the necessary arrangements."

One of the alliance's secretaries, Miss Chrystal Macmillan from London, supported our suggestions in a private note that accompanied this official letter.[15] She also proposed that all the international women's organizations be kept informed of our plans and be invited to attend the conference, which would include discussion of the peace plans devised by the various peace associations. These letters and announcements were published in the December 1914 issue of *Jus Suffragii* (The Right to Suffrage), the monthly magazine of the International Woman Suffrage Alliance.[16]

The answers I received over the next few months were hardly encouraging. Most of the alliance board members regarded my suggestion to meet as something of a political blunder. Others felt that it was a pointless idea. "Wait until after the war," I kept hearing. With the exception of Miss Macmillan, I received little support, even from the boards of affiliated associations, because, as more than one member wrote, "Personally I think it's a good idea but my organization just doesn't want to hear about it."

But the *Jus Suffragii* invitation also brought me many messages of sympathy, even from women in countries directly involved in the war. Consequently, I realized that I would achieve my aim more quickly and effectively if the conference were organized by a number of individual women rather than by a specific organization. This kind of gathering could concentrate on the antiwar campaign, whereas in the alliance, dedicated to the interests of woman suffrage, protesting against the war would be considered merely an additional task. But no matter how clearly I explained it, the central committee of the Dutch Association for Woman Suffrage felt unable to support me, although a number of individual members sympathized with my aims.

But by now I was no longer alone. Dr. Mia Boissevain and Rosa Manus, both of whom had been invaluable in organizing the impressive "Woman 1813–1913" exhibition in Amsterdam, had by now also offered to help.[17] We decided to invite a number of women known to be sympathetic to our cause from the nearest neutral or warring countries. They were asked to attend a preparatory meeting in Amsterdam on February 12–13, 1915. Three Belgian, four German, and five English women responded to this invitation.[18] In addition, we received many messages of solidarity from Scandinavia. And so we embarked on preparing our plans with our foreign guests and a number of other Dutch women. From all the support that came from organizations both at home and abroad, and from all the offers of help from women in neighboring countries, it soon became clear that we were absolutely right to think that the conference had a real chance of succeeding. Consequently, we decided to organize it as soon as possible in The Hague. Dr. Anita Augspurg and Lyda Gustava Heymann, two prominent figures in the German woman's movement, and Chrystal Macmillan and Kate Courtney from England had decided that, personal circumstance permitting, they would leave for Holland as soon as possible to help with preparations.[19] Of our compatriots, we were particularly indebted to Jeanne van Lanschot Hubrecht, Cor Ramondt-Hirschmann, and Hanna van Biema-Heymans.[20] It was largely due to these energetic and talented women that, despite all the difficulties, the delays in the mail, the lost, censored, and confiscated letters, we still managed to organize an international conference in just two months that was to be attended by a great many women from twelve different countries.[21]

It was a time of extremes, and along with the messages of support there were also, inevitably, feelings of suspicion that we had been paid by one of the warring nations: by Germany, to be precise. Yet, like their German sisters, the English and Dutch women had agreed to support the conference financially except where these costs would be covered by voluntary donations. But despite that, the rumor circulated that we were supported by the German government. Once it became apparent that we intended to ignore this kind of insinuation, our plans started to be regularly attacked and ridiculed. But nothing could dampen our hopes or quench our fervor. Our secretaries worked solidly from early in the morning until late at night. Piles of letters and telegrams arrived and were dispatched each day and a constant stream of invitations were sent out all over the world. Even our opponents were impressed with the news that the conference would be led by a woman of world repute, none other than Jane Addams, the founder of Hull House in Chicago, a well-known pacifist who would be accompanied by a large group of American women.[22]

Some countries obviously feared the potential influence of our conference, as was demonstrated when the English government halted all ferry service to Holland just eight days before the first meeting in The Hague, forcing 180 English women to abandon their plans to participate. This move also thwarted the plans of the French women, who would have had to travel to the Netherlands via England.[23] When the Holland-America Line's *Noordam* was detained in England with forty-plus members of the American delegation on board, we began in earnest to fear that all our work had been in vain, but fortunately these women managed to reach The Hague just in time for the opening of the conference. And despite England's opposition, it was represented not only by Chrystal Macmillan and Kate Courtney, who had both worked hard on arrangements for the conference, but also by Mrs. Pethick-Lawrence, who had sailed from America.[24] Naturally everyone who attended was well aware of her sacred duty to do everything she could to stop the slaughter and destruction of war. Although bloodlust and jingoism dominated the outside world, at the conference they were notable by their absence. Women from enemy nations reached out to each other in sisterhood and worked together in an atmosphere of complete harmony.

We decided to create a special commission, whose members included myself, to compile a list of resolutions to be brought before the conference. The resolution calling for an end to hostilities and a start to peace talks based on the principle of justice for all nations was particularly dear to my heart, as was the plan to form a committee of delegates from neutral countries that could negotiate between the enemy forces. We subsequently discovered that many of the resolutions adopted by our conference that focused on the idea of a just peace were included in President Wilson's famous "Fourteen Points."

At the end of the conference, it was decided that a women's deputation would present our resolutions both to the neutral countries and to those at war.[25] Miss Jane Addams and I agreed to assume responsibility for most of the work involved. We were asked first to visit the Dutch premier and minister of foreign affairs and then to inform the governments of England, Germany, Austria-Hungary, Switzerland, Italy, France, and Belgium in person of the plans and proposals adopted by the women's conference in The Hague. As I was still feeling somewhat weak from a bout of flu, I gratefully accepted the offer of Mrs. F. W. van Wulfften Palthe-Broese van Groenou, with whom I had stayed during the conference, to look after me during our travels.[26] Dr. Alice Hamilton, professor of social hygiene at Harvard, agreed to act as the companion of Miss Jane Addams.[27]

On May 5, 1915, we were received by the Dutch premier, Cort van der Linden, and the minister of foreign affairs, Jonkheer Loudon. Miss Addams explained the reason for our visit. She particularly emphasized the fact that it was the neutral countries' duty to offer to mediate between the hostile nations. During our interview, it became increasingly obvious that Premier van der Linden was himself a committed pacifist. This venerable old man clearly felt that a cease-fire should be declared as soon as possible. Thinking back, I can still hear him asking somewhat irritably, "But aren't the women in these countries just as warmongering as their male counterparts?" To which Miss Addams replied, "Women can't vote in any of the countries involved in the war, so it's rather difficult to get one's views heard. What you read in the newspapers are the opinions of only a handful of female writers."

We were received on May 13, 1915, by the English foreign secretary, Sir Edward Grey. He was particularly impressed by the number of German women present at the conference. He was also interested in the fact that the German government had done nothing to prevent these delegates from attending. I explained to him that in Germany it is the local authorities that have the power to issue passports, with the result that some women were able to travel to the Netherlands while others were forced to remain in Germany. I added that I greatly admired the German delegation because they were certain to have a difficult time once they returned home. Sir Edward Grey, now Viscount Grey, told us that in his opinion President Wilson of the United States would play an important role in any future peace talks.

The next day, Miss Addams met with Mr. Asquith, the prime minister, and I spoke at a women's meeting about the conference and the proposals it had adopted. On May 15, we left for the Netherlands. On the boat, we saw yet more evidence of the misery caused by war. Our fellow passengers included a great many young women, some with babies in their arms, some with children of three, four, or five years of age, and some of them in advanced stages of pregnancy. Although none of them spoke any language but English or had ever set foot outside of Britain, as the wives of German nationals they were now regarded as the subjects of a hostile nation and had been exiled from their native country. Their husbands had either enlisted in the German army or had been sent to internment camps by the English government. I should, however, point out that Britain was not the only warring nation to implement such measures against its own women. But this particular example clearly shows the tyranny of a system that robs a woman of her nationality if she marries a foreigner or if her husband changes nationality during their marriage. A number of governments have since recognized the injustice of this law and have attempted to introduce reforms at an international level.

We resumed our journey on May 19, setting off for Berlin. On arrival, I immediately contacted our ambassador and presented him with my letters of introduction. Meanwhile my traveling companion visited the American Embassy. Thanks to the efforts of our respective diplomats, we were received the following day by the minister of foreign affairs, Herr von Jagow. Like Sir Edward Grey, he expressed his hope for peace in the near future and his conviction that this initiative should be taken by the neutral countries under the leadership of President Wilson. But the minister also admitted his own pessimism and predicted that, although the present generation would never again think of waging war, man's militant nature would eventually prevail and lead him to resort to violence.

"By then," I commented, "women will probably have the power to help run governments alongside men."

Herr von Jagow agreed that here indeed lay hope for the future, "If women can influence governments with their superior feelings, then the world will be a better place."

The next day, Saturday, May 22, my companion was received by the minister of internal affairs, Herr von Bethmann-Hollweg. I could not accompany her because my ambassador had been unable to go through the necessary formalities. Bethmann-Hollweg emphasized the importance of an honorable peace for all nations and again hoped for the intervention of the neutral countries.

The previous evening, while Miss Addams was addressing the German Women's Council, I had made a call on that good and honest Social Democrat Eduard Bernstein.[28] I was also welcomed by his large family. Finally I was able to meet a German who regarded the whole situation without the slightest taint of prejudice and in terms of an international perspective.

We left for Vienna on May 23, the very same day that Italy declared war on Austria-Hungary. Needless to say, the city was in a state of high excitement.

The next day, despite the fact that it was Whit-Monday, we visited our respective ambassadors, who promised to arrange for us to meet the ministers of foreign and internal affairs: Count von Stuergkh and Baron Burian. We were eventually granted appointments for later that week. Both ministers seemed deeply affected by Italy's declaration of war. In contrast to statesmen such as Von Jagow and Sir Edward Grey, they felt that President Wilson was unfamiliar with Old World politics and thus not the right man to intervene. Rather, they argued, this was the task of the neutral countries of Europe. Count von Stuergkh found it hard to believe that the world could stand by and do nothing while Europe was destroying itself. He thanked us for our visit and said, "This is the first time in eight months that someone's talked sense in this office."

That evening we left for Salzburg and Innsbruck en route to Bern. But first we addressed a women's club of fifty Austrian women who listened to the story of our pacifist crusade with rapt attention.

In the Swiss capital, Dr. Gertrud Woker, who was a well-known figure in academic circles, arranged for us to meet both the minister of foreign affairs, Herr Hoffmann, and the president, Herr Motta.[29] The president turned out to be a highly intelligent and amiable man with whom we had a long and extremely useful meeting. At one point he said, "How is it possible that women from those countries involved in the war haven't simply rebelled against the fact that their male compatriots are being slaughtered and mutilated by the thousands!"

As we left him, President Motta promised that he would speak to the pope on our behalf. "Benedict XV is a good friend of mine," he said. "I know him and I'm sure he'd like to meet you."

Although it was forbidden in Switzerland to promote peace publicly, we requested permission to address an open meeting for women on the subject of "die Frauen und der Krieg" (women and the war). We were not only granted permission but were even given the use of the town hall, where we drew a large crowd on this occasion.

We left Bern for Rome on the morning of June 13. No sooner had we crossed the Swiss border than all the train windows were boarded up so that we could see nothing of the landscape though which we were traveling. Whenever we stopped at a station we were aware of a great bustle and commotion. Young men were singing and cheering as they went off to war. Italy's war had just begun, so its people had not yet experienced pain and suffering. Those who remained behind were clearly disappointed. For us, having seen the carnage that war had inflicted on Germany and Austria, it was dreadful to see how excited these young people were as they set off for their appointments with death or injury.

The next day an overfull train finally brought us to the Eternal City. We had been traveling for more than twenty-four hours. Nonetheless, we set out the same morning to meet our respective ambassadors, who had arranged for us to visit the ministers of foreign and internal affairs: Signori Salandra and Sonnino. But this meeting was less than satisfactory, since both statesmen were intoxicated with the glamour of battle, not yet aware of the full horror of war. What a state of high excitement reigned throughout the city! The streets were filled with hundreds of thousands of people possessed by the spirit of war.

Caricatures of Minister Giolitti, the one man who had the moral courage to oppose Italy's involvement, were on sale everywhere. We even saw a cheering crowd parade a wooden dummy of the statesman, which was subsequently strung up from a gallows. This stay in Rome taught us how easy it is to sway public opinion and also that it is simply irresponsible to allow an exclusively male parliament to make the decision to declare war.

"It took just two days," we were told, "for the public to come around to the idea of war." In fact, all that was needed were a few dishonest newspaper stories that spread lies about the enemy nations, a couple of reports about the outrages tolerated in those countries, plus a few articles to instill the fear that Italy would suffer the same fate as had befallen others unless the government acted immediately. The result: people believed that, were they to stand by and do nothing, their fatherland would be plunged into chaos and disaster. So strong was this message that the vast majority of members of parliament failed to escape its influence. Needless to say, none of the Italian women were receptive to our message of peace.

But we were more successful with the pope. His Holiness granted an audience at the Vatican not only to Jane Addams and myself but also to our two companions. In this meeting, which lasted more than one and a half hours, Benedict XV proved to be an extremely civilized and educated man. But it was also clear that, although he had dedicated his life to the pursuit of knowledge, he was not always a sound judge of society in all its complexities. The pope assured us in all sincerity that every attempt to secure peace was certain of his backing and that he was willing to consider all ideas on the subject. In terms of women and their role in society, this Prince of the Church felt that in general they should exert more influence on the rearing of children and that they should have a greater say in education.

But when Mrs. van Wulfften Palthe asked His Holiness whether this influence should be extended to the level of national government, the pope was suddenly unable to provide us with an answer.

In two nights and a day, we journeyed from Rome to Paris, where we called on the Dutch and American ambassadors to arrange our meetings with the highest of government officials. That we eventually met both the president and the minister of foreign affairs was, however, thanks to Monsieur Longuet, a member of parliament and the grandson of Karl Marx, the world-famous father of socialism.[30] Longuet knew the most effective way for us to meet with both Viviani and Delcassé. The latter declared to us that, even after months of war, France would never agree to a cease-fire, no matter how favorable the terms: "We have resolved to destroy Germany's power and will do whatever necessary to achieve that aim." All our reasoning power could not penetrate his wall of hate and revenge.

Our second visit was with Monsieur Viviani who appeared calmer and more dispassionate. Although he was apparently predisposed toward pacifism and feminism, Viviani thought that the time was not yet ripe for France to adopt the peace ideal in any permanent form.

Was it any wonder that we were deeply disappointed by these representatives of the French people? And there was worse to come! Blinded by circumstances, the president and vice president of the French Women's Council had signed and published an article in the newspapers of Paris that attempted to discredit both Miss Jane Addams and myself in the most scandalous fashion. This article was based on false reports in the French press of our conference in The Hague which neither Madame Siegfried nor Madame Avril de Sainte-Croix, the two signatories, had actually attended. Monsieur Otlet, a Belgian who had been present at the conference, had tried to interest the Paris newspapers in his experience, which clearly refuted these women's erroneous claims. But the French newspapers obstinately refused to publish his point of view.

When we complained to the central committee of the French Women's Council about the way in which we had been treated, Madame de Witt Schlumberger, the president of the French Woman Suffrage Association, invited both us and Mesdames Siegfried and Avril de Sainte-Croix to have tea at her house. Madame Avril de Sainte-Croix was apparently unavailable, but Madame Siegfried did appear, in the company of a coterie of women as chauvinist as she.

We were asked to describe the conference, but there was no way of convincing our opponents that they had misinterpreted its events. Basically, they argued that they were first and foremost French women supporting their country in its hour of need. In their opinion, thwarting their government's plans was tantamount to treason. They had been deeply disappointed to find that we disagreed and therefore failed to sing their praises in our press. Hence, they refused to retract a single word of what they had published in the French press. Meanwhile, we soon discovered that not *all* French women shared their views. The following afternoon we were invited to visit Madame Duchêne. At her home we met pacifist women who had had the courage to disapprove openly of the French government's actions.[31]

From Paris, we traveled to Le Havre, which at that time was the seat of the Belgian government. Although our papers were perfectly in order, the authorities were determined to make trouble. When we arrived, first the French and then the English police insisted on going through first our documents and then our luggage. Of course, they found nothing untoward, but we were still carted off to face the police commissioner, who subjected us to a thorough interrogation. We had no wish to hide the reason for our visit and immediately produced the address of our hotel. We had sent a telegram from Paris to book rooms there and had received notification of our reservations at once. However, no one wanted to assign a room to us when we finally arrived. After a lot of fuss, we were eventually allowed to eat in a small, out-of-the-way room. Soon after we had finished our meal, it was made clear to us that our departure would be appreciated. Of course, we guessed that the police must have had a word with the owner. But why? Were they scared that pacifists were planning to corrupt the ideals of the English soldiers stationed there? There was no chance of that! Given the mentality of multitudes of people in the warring nations, we knew well that not only would this be a useless exercise, it would also land us in a great deal of trouble.

The police commissioner pointedly informed us that "the Paris train leaves at 5 P.M." Although we had no wish to remain in Le Havre a moment longer than necessary, we nevertheless tried to arrange appointments with Ministers d'Avignon and Broqueville. Broqueville had left for the front, but d'Avignon agreed to meet us that afternoon. He assured us that Belgium would welcome a swift conclusion to hostilities: "but unfortunately it's not up to us to take the initiative as we are too closely associated with France and England."

Later that evening, totally exhausted, we arrived in Paris. After wasting yet another day having our passports checked, we finally left for London on June 18 in the hope of returning to Holland the following morning. However, unbeknownst to us, England was forcing foreigners traveling from France to stay for a week before permitting them to continue their journey to any of the nonallied countries. Thanks to the influence of a few friends in high places, we had to stay only for five days, time we spent discussing ways of promoting peace with a number of like-minded men and women.

I must now backtrack to the conference in The Hague, where we had decided to form an association of conference delegates whose aim it would be to attempt to achieve the pacifist ideal. It was to be called the "International Committee of Women for Permanent Peace," a name later changed at the 1919 Zurich conference to the Women's International League for Peace and Freedom. For the duration of the war, Rosa Manus and I were asked to coordinate among members in different countries. We were invited to join the committee as vice president and first secretary and were made primarily responsible for organizing the printing and mailing of the conference report.

Miss MacMillan worked with us during the first few months, and we were later assisted by Miss Emily Hobhouse from England, who is known in Holland for her humanitarian work in South Africa during the Boer War.[32] Apart from that, Rosa Manus and I were solely responsible for the time-consuming work of replying to a deluge of letters from throughout the world, often containing information that we had to pass on to women in other countries. We also received reports of the work of pacifists in many lands, which we summarized and published in a monthly bulletin sent to all our members. Through this kind of work, we maintained contact with pacifist women from every corner of the globe so that soon after the war they were able to work together effectively.

In August 1915, Miss MacMillan arrived from London with the important message that the English statesman Lord Crewe had decided the time was right to form a union of neutral countries to work toward the establishment of peace talks. Miss MacMillan had also succeeded in getting this statement confirmed in writing. The same afternoon, we met with the Dutch premier to inform him of these plans. Premier Cort van der Linden was extremely interested although he felt unable to pursue Lord Crewe's proposals before the American government responded about its possible role as mediator. During our talks, he commented, "I have to know as soon as possible what President Wilson thinks of all this."

I immediately offered to leave the next day on the *Nieuw Amsterdam* for America so I could speak with the president of the United States in person and sound out his opinion of these proposals. A ship's cabin was reserved at once by wire. The same evening I was issued my passport and the necessary letters of introduction. In great haste I bought a few things for the journey and spent the remaining time with Miss MacMillan composing a list of questions I was to present to President Wilson. The questions:

1. With the advent of mediation between the enemy nations, would America insist on acting alone and without the collaborative efforts of the major neutral countries in Europe? Does President Wilson consider this to be the most effective approach?
2. Or would President Wilson prefer to collaborate with the major neutral countries in Europe?
3. If so, would President Wilson want to assume leadership and to invite the collaborative participation of other countries?
4. If President Wilson considers that the neutral countries of Europe should assume the functions of mediators, would America be prepared to participate through the presence of one or more delegates?
5. Or does President Wilson feel that a single neutral nation in Europe should act as mediator? If so, is he prepared to assist if invited by that nation to do so?
6. If President Wilson agrees with the view expressed in point 5, which European nation does he feel to be the best suited to become mediator?
7. Would the presence of American delegates involve the stipulation of any particular conditions? If so, what would these conditions be?

Early on the morning of August 25, 1915, I was welcomed to New York by Miss Heyde, the private secretary of Mrs. Chapman Catt. Miss Heyde brought me to Mrs. Catt's house, where I was to enjoy a most relaxing and hospitable stay.

As soon as I arrived, I learned to my acute disappointment that President Wilson was refusing to accept any more visits about peace talks. To make things worse, the Dutch ambassador had left for San Francisco and his deputy was also away. This was all extremely depressing, but, while trying to work things out, I was visited by Miss Balch, a well-known pacifist from Boston, who not only had participated in the conference at The Hague but also had been one of a group of delegates to meet with the governments of Scandinavia and Russia about our plans and proposals.[33] Miss Balch had come to New York with no other goal than to provide me with as much support as she could. She had freed herself from all her obligations in Boston so she could be completely at my disposal. Of course, I accepted this unexpected offer wholeheartedly.

Our first task was to write a letter to President Wilson requesting a meeting at his convenience and briefly stating our purpose. We had to wait several days to hear that President Wilson would not agree to a White House meeting, since he wished to avoid publicity. Therefore, he suggested that we speak with Secretary of State Lansing or with Colonel House. They would then be able to inform the president of our talks. We wired Mr. Lansing for an appointment and received an immediate reply that he would expect us the following morning. So, after lunching with Norman Angell, the author of *The Great Illusion*, Miss Balch and I took the next train to Washington.[34]

Our meeting with Mr. Lansing was disappointing. He talked so much that I hardly had a chance to ask our questions. Clearly it became vital to see Colonel House, also a good friend of the president, and that same day we sent a telegram to his estate in Manchester, Massachusetts.

"See you tomorrow afternoon" was the reply, which meant that we had to leave Washington at five-thirty that evening. We arrived in Boston at 11 A.M. and, after having quickly freshened up, we continued our journey. Our meeting with Colonel House was much more promising. He gave me ample opportunity to describe the reasons for our visit. And afterward, he said that he felt I should talk with President Wilson directly and that he would try to arrange an interview for me.

While I waited for my invitation to the White House, Miss Balch and I stayed with Miss Jane Addams on Mt. Desert Island, a beautiful place where many wealthy Americans spend their summers.[35] After some time, I received a reply from President Wilson stating that he expected me on Wednesday, September 15, but that I was to come alone, since he could not receive guests from any of the countries involved in the war.

This visit also proved disappointing. No matter what I asked, the president replied that America was going through difficult times and that he was therefore unable to be definitive. Because the situation could change at any time, he had to have the freedom to act spontaneously. Even the most superficial or informal of statements would involve some level of commitment, which had to be avoided at all costs. He said, "I have to be able to act immediately in the most appropriate and effective way possible." In addition, he believed that the neutral countries in Europe were capable of taking the initiative independently and he would not regard such a development as hostile to the United States.

My impression during this visit was that Woodrow Wilson was a man of high ideals, but that he lacked the power to realize them. He seemed unaware that his potential power to help end the war was hampered by the fact that he had never visited Europe and that, as a consequence, he frequently misjudged the situation there.

Before meeting with the president, I had avoided publicity and refused to give lectures or interviews. But afterward I could see no real objection to a few speaking engagements in Chicago. For each of the five days I spent there as the guest of Mrs. Wilmarth, I gave one or more lectures not only on war and peace but also on woman suffrage.[36]

After our meeting, the president sent a friendly note to Miss Addams, which she thoughtfully passed on to me, knowing that it could be of use back in the Netherlands should anyone cast doubt on our talk. I have always kept that letter, not for the reason I mentioned above but as a token of the president's kindness,

THE WHITE HOUSE
WASHINGTON   September 23, 1915

My dear Miss Addams,
    I warmly appreciate your kind letter about Dr. Aletta Jacobs. You may be sure that it gave me great pleasure to meet so interesting a woman.
                     Cordially and sincerely yours
                          (w.g.) Woodrow Wilson

Miss Jane Addams
Hulls Cove, Maine

The same *Nieuw Amsterdam* of the Holland-America Line, on which I had arrived in New York on August 13, now brought me back to Holland on October 5. Apart from receiving precise instructions about what to do should the ship unexpectedly strike a mine, we proceeded without undue incident until we dropped anchor at Falmouth. For some obscure reason, the English authorities insisted that we remain there for a week, and the boat was repeatedly searched from deep in the engine room to the farthest outreaches of the rigging; the stocks of coal were turned upside down; every corner of the lounge was also searched; and of course our papers were checked exhaustively, down to the last comma.

After seven long days of being anchored at some distance from the quay and not being allowed to step ashore, we finally heard the signal to sail. Fortunately we reached Rotterdam without further incident. In fact, we arrived so early in the morning that I was even able to report on the very same day to our ministers for internal and foreign affairs on my trip to America and my visit to President Wilson. I spent the remainder of the war years collaborating with Rosa Manus on the work entailed in maintaining the International Committee of Women for Permanent Peace.

No sooner was there a cease-fire than everyone suddenly insisted that we must arrange a women's conference. Although personally I felt it would not be possible to organize a well-attended event as soon as was wished, I helped in whatever way I could to prepare for the conference, which was to take place in Zurich starting on May 5, 1919. A week before this date, I left with Mrs. C. Ramondt Hirschmann and Mrs. F. W. van Wulfften Palthe-Broese van Groenou for Switzerland.

At that time, German train service was still extremely irregular. Strikes and disturbances were common. Hence, we decided to reserve seats from Arnhem to Switzerland on the special train organized for the annual fair in Basel. We left Arnhem at 6 A.M. A compartment had been reserved for the three of us in the middle of a crowded train packed with male passengers. We were counting on reaching Switzerland the next morning but soon heard from our fellow travelers that there was a fresh outbreak of strikes in Germany particularly affecting the area around Frankfurt.

At the border station of Elten we were told that the situation was so bad that the Dutch train would be turning back. We were given the choice of either returning home or continuing at our own risk. Without knowing what awaited us, we three were the first to insist on proceeding. Some of the men agreed to accompany us, but the vast majority took the first train back to Arnhem.

Our group decreased at each station, and finally we arrived in Frankfurt with only three of our original companions. It had been a tortuous journey. Repeatedly we waited on cold platforms until a train materialized to take us a stage further. No one could provide us with definite information. Everything depended on the railway people. It took five days to reach Zurich, where we arrived at five in the afternoon to be welcomed by our American friend, Miss Balch, and a group of local women. They told us that because of the present difficulties, which had also completely disrupted the mail, the conference had been postponed for a week. I devoted all my energy both to the preparations and to the conference itself.[37] When the central office was later transferred from Amsterdam to Geneva, where the League of Nations was housed, Rosa Manus and I, having already indicated that we no longer wished to take a leading role, considered our work completed.

Meanwhile I had moved from Amsterdam to The Hague. I was hardly back from Zurich when I received a semiofficial invitation to tour Germany with two traveling companions of my choice so that I could see for myself the disastrous effects the continuing blockade was having on the population's health. In fact, I was offered so much help, including all my expenses, that I hesitated at first because I obviously had to maintain a certain independence to be able to judge the situation objectively.

While I was still considering the best way of acquiring accurate information in order to implement relief measures, Miss Jane Addams asked if I would like to join a commission that consisted of herself, Dr. Alice Hamilton, and Miss Carolina Wood from America. The group's aim was to gather data on the current German food shortage. These three women intended to visit Germany along with a commission of four members selected by the English Society of Friends. It was an offer I gladly accepted.

We arrived in Berlin on July 7 to be met by Dr. Elisabeth Rotten, the German representative of the Society of Friends, who had agreed to act as our guide and adviser. Our tour lasted three weeks. The people were in such a state of misery and despair that I felt I simply could not also visit Austria and Hungary as had been originally planned. It would require more strength than I possessed. Instead I decided to return home to publish an account of my experiences. My aim was to rouse public sympathies for providing extensive aid to these starving people.

Although I stuck strictly to the facts, I found that to be accepted for publication, I still had to minimize some of what I had seen. No one was willing to believe the sheer scale of suffering in Germany. I was most struck by the ways in which the health of younger people had been undermined. What was to become of these sickly children? What future was there for a nation where 40 percent of the population was suffering from tuberculosis?

In Germany, apart from encountering affliction at every turn, I became well aware of the fact that half a million prisoners of war were still being held in Siberia. Nothing had been heard of many of them for months or even years. Wives and parents often did not even know whether their loved ones were still alive. I had seen so much on my tour that it was some time before I realized fully the plight of the prisoners of war. But months later, as winter approached and I became increasingly obsessed with the state of the world, I suddenly remembered those poor wretches attempting to survive in the cold inhospitable wastes of Siberia.

In November 1913, when I had traveled from Japan to Germany, my route had taken me through Siberia where I had seen a convoy of political prisoners at one of the train stations. Their fate was now shared by thousands and thousands of young men, the victims of war. I knew that something had to be done for these people. I was eventually approached by a group of women who suggested that we launch a campaign on behalf of the prisoners of war to facilitate their repatriation. I agreed to run this committee and right from the beginning I was greatly helped and supported by Baroness W. van Lijnden-von Schmidt auf Altenstadt and Mrs. L. Eschauzier-Pabst. At first it was difficult to convince people that a year after armistice there were still at least a half million

Germans, Austrians, Hungarians, Czechoslovaks, and Turks exiled in the Siberian wilderness. It was something about which virtually no one had heard and the newspapers had even rejected our announcements because no one could believe we were telling the truth.

By this time, I had received official information from Germany and Austria and was being sent regular weekly updates. Our first task was to contact various women's organizations around the world so that they might launch their own national campaigns to help repatriate prisoners of war. Many foreign associations responded to our appeal; others wrote to say that they were already involved with this issue. Our committee organized public meetings, published the information we received from abroad, and collected money to be used for warm clothing and for the prisoners' return journeys.

After we had repeatedly requested its help, the International Bureau of the Red Cross finally took up this cause. Fridtjof Nansen, the great Norwegian who was later to help the victims of the Russian famine, agreed to work toward reuniting the Siberian prisoners of war with their families.[38] We now realized that we had completed our task and arranged to donate the money we had collected to the Red Cross.

Although I had chosen these duties of my own free will, once they were completed I decided not to continue with this kind of work. The years were taking their toll and my energy and stamina were gradually diminishing. I felt overwhelmed by the extreme emotions of the war years and more especially by the years that immediately followed. In my quiet study perhaps I could still produce something, but not in public life. Hence I decided to set down these "memories of my life and work." They would comfort me in my old age, and the younger generation might even benefit from my experiences.

But I have to admit that, after years of intense involvement, I could be easily distracted from my life of leisure. For example, I could not resist an invitation to participate in the conference of the International Council of Women held in Christiania in the summer of 1920. As this was to be the first council meeting since the outbreak of the war, many of my friends from all corners of the globe would be there. When I thought of all these people, I knew immediately that I had to go too. It would also give me the opportunity to spend a few days in Germany to review its economic progress and the health of its people.

I soon realized that this country, with a population of over sixty million, needed more than simple philanthropy to recover. The state both of the people and the land itself had deteriorated dramatically since my previous visit, despite the aid sent from throughout the world to alleviate the suffering caused by the war. All that well-intentioned charity was directly undermined by the Treaty of Versailles, which was based on hate and revenge. Without realizing that Germany's destruction would also signal the decline of their own land, the chauvinist French remained fixed in their absurd wish to ruin Germany in order to feel secure. In my view, the Treaty of Versailles had to be thoroughly overhauled if there was ever to be a lasting peace.

I thought that women's organizations in various countries should become involved. If they were to demand the treaty's revision, then other more powerful groups would perhaps wake up to what was going on. I sent a personal appeal to several prominent women and to all the women's organizations known to me. But I soon discovered that the most I could expect was the support of individual women, since the organizations would not risk involvement. Nonetheless, I remained convinced that my campaign had a real chance of success. Had I been a few years younger and richer, I would have taken on all the work myself. As it was, I eventually had to abandon this cause, with the hope that the 1921 Vienna conference of the Women's International League for Peace and Freedom would include my ideas as a point of discussion.

My suggestions were not accepted as proposals of the Dutch Committee for Permanent Peace for the conference. So I decided to go to Vienna to see what I could achieve personally. Fortunately, at one of the preparatory meetings, the president, Miss Jane Addams, asked me to address the conference on ways of preventing war. This was an ideal opportunity to explain my ideas in a relatively short speech in which I could also describe the existing peace treaties as active threats to the continuation of peace. I emphasized also that peace organizations should make strong efforts to urge the revision of these treaties, even if such actions meant abandoning all other activities.

I said, "Let us spend a year campaigning in all those countries directly involved and then we can hold an international conference at which the organizations that share our views will be able to discuss this issue." My proposal was enthusiastically adopted in Vienna, but that was as far as the matter went. Nowhere, not even in Holland, was my plan put into action. And, regrettably, my own infirmities prevented me from putting my shoulder to the wheel.

Meanwhile, the situation in Central Europe was becoming more perilous each day. Respected politicians and prominent newspapers openly predicted that Europe was on the brink of destruction. And they cited the peace treaty as the main reason for this impending catastrophe.

It was at about that time that the board of the Women's International League for Peace and Freedom was due to hold its annual meeting in Freiburg. The president of the Dutch branch, who was also a member of the board, was asked to contact other committee members to stress the importance of holding an international conference in the near future. The agenda would consist of just one subject: the proposed revision of the peace treaties. There was an overwhelming response to Mrs. Ramondt-Hirschmann's appeal. After some discussion, it was decided that a conference concentrating on achieving a "new peace" rather than attempting to patch up the existing treaties would be organized, and held in The Hague.

From December 7 to 10, 1922, delegates debated the possibility of creating a lasting peace based on demands other than those included in the Treaty of Versailles.[39] Despite the fact that it was hardly the time of year to travel by sea, Miss Jane Addams agreed to direct the conference in person. Accompanied by a large number of American delegates, she made the crossing in such good time that she was also able to take over some of the conference preparations.

As for me, I could do little more than support the whole event in spirit as I was unable to undertake more than a fraction of the work involved. I was all too aware that I had reached a point at which I had to put strict limits on my continuing involvement in public life.

So, having briefly described my work for the pacifist cause, I would like to conclude this chapter by stating that as far as I know, I acquired not one single enemy during my involvement with this cause, only a large number of loving male and female friends with whom I have shared many moments of great joy.

I am still frequently reminded of the enduring gratitude of the many women and girls who were stranded here at the beginning of the war. They were forced to appeal to me for help because their papers were not in order or they had no money to continue their journey or even because the Vlissingen boats were full to capacity. Many of them knew my name from the international woman's movement, some of them bore letters of introduction, and others had called at the suggestion of mutual friends.

Thanks to the many relationships I have been able to develop over the years, it was surprisingly easy to help these stranded women. My modest home became a busy shelter for girls and women of different nationalities who had never previously met and who found themselves sharing a room or even sleeping in the same bed (although usually we managed to resolve each situation after a couple of days). I have often been deeply moved by the gratitude expressed not only by the women themselves but also by their families.

It would be going too far and getting rather too personal if I were to start quoting from all the letters I have received, but I would like to include a poem written in 1923 by one of my wartime friends on the occasion of my birthday.

> With fresh belief, your Life's Ship sails,
> Your hand held firmly on the helm,
> Your gaze the lofty night sky hails,
> To search for Peace's distant realm.
>
> Beset by human grief and pain,
> Yet weakness you will never show,
> For we'll be freed from Nightmare's chains
> Sure as God's dawn, that much you know.

Alone but strong, you sense a breeze,
Enfolding you gently and with ease.
It is a sign for our unhappy breed
That Love and Justice is what we need.

No more children will we propagate
To be devoured by war, death, and hate.

For Dr. Aletta Jacobs with respect and gratitude
February 9, 1923
Franz Wegner

NINE

PROSTITUTION

My Concern Meets with Opposition; Respectable Women Do Not Get Involved with This Kind of Thing • Conflict with a Professor • My Experiences in London via Dr. Drysdale and Through My Own Practice in Amsterdam • My First Articles on This Subject • My First Lecture on Prostitution in Rotterdam in 1897 and How It Was Received • The 1909 Congress in Budapest • Adventurous Journeys • Traveling to Sarajevo and What We Found There • Lectures on This Subject in South Africa • "An Open Letter to the Women of South Africa" • Further Involvement with This Issue

R eaders will remember how, while I was still a young student, I was so abruptly confronted with the fact of prostitution and the misery it causes. I was deeply affected by that young woman in the Groningen hospital who was universally shunned and who awaited her death as a form of deliverance. For me, meeting her was a true revelation. She made me confront the tragedy of prostitution and I have always felt intense sympathy for its victims the world over, particularly in terms of the humiliating way in which governments control these women's bodies.

But I was not yet fully aware of how the nation's health is also adversely affected by prostitution. As I was a simple village girl, all this was simply beyond me, although I did intuitively feel that here was an issue involving not only the interests of the women themselves but also those of society at large. My experiences in Groningen made me determined to find out more about this subject, although those people who could help me were less than willing to do so and often made it perfectly clear that respectable women do not concern themselves with such matters.

Prostitution was not a word mentioned in polite society. Even educated women made it quite plain that this subject was definitely beyond the pale. And on the few occasions a man was prepared to discuss this issue seriously, I was invariably confronted with his expert opinion that "prostitution is a necessary evil. It's existed since time immemorial and there's no way it will ever be eradicated."

In my view, evil, necessary or otherwise, simply had no right to exist. My sense of justice was outraged by the theory that society was in some way obliged "to try to provide healthy women" so that men might indulge their carnal desires.

Many was the time I tried in vain to break down that wall of blind prejudice! For instance, I remember a particular debate with one of my professors. He declared openly that, as everyone knew, man's physical well-being depended on fulfilling his sexual urges and that society was therefore obliged to ensure that these needs were catered to with the minimum of risk to his health.

"Well, if that's what you think," I replied, "you'd better make sure that your daughters are made available for this purpose."

Unfortunately I was unable to pursue this line of thought as the professor abruptly stormed out of the room after informing me that I had no right to discuss subjects I knew nothing about. This struck me as ironic, for my one desire was to find out as much as I could about this issue, yet, as this instance demonstrated, all my efforts seemed doomed to failure. I was constantly being put off with vague generalities, and whenever I requested specific authors and titles on this subject at the Leesmuseum, my request was invariably greeted with either suspicion or apparent incomprehension.

The first person who was prepared to talk to me honestly about prostitution was the eminent doctor Charles Drysdale, whom I met, as I mentioned before, in London after I had completed my training in the Netherlands. Thanks to his practical experience and theoretical research, he was able to answer my questions fully and meticulously. Dr. Drysdale also took me to visit one of the London institutions where prostitutes, or women suspected of prostitution, were subjected to medical examination.

Just as in Groningen, I felt physically revolted by the experience. I simply could not understand how a doctor could put himself in the position of judging whether these social outcasts should be allowed to continue their grim profession. I was able to speak with some of these unfortunate women. Almost invariably they came from working-class backgrounds. They had been forced to fend for themselves from an early age without sufficient guidance or protection, with the result that once they had strayed from the straight and narrow, often through no fault of their own, their lives rapidly deteriorated.

When I returned to Holland, I soon became aware of the Reverend H. Pierson's campaign against brothels and the official regulation of prostitution.[1] I read everything I could on both sides of this argument and my opinions, which coincided with those of the Reverend Pierson, were regularly published in the newspapers and magazines of the day. Being a doctor had shown me the dire consequences of the evil of prostitution. My clinics were frequently attended by young women whose symptoms were the result of transmitted infection.

I have seen much misery caused by marriages involving young men who did not realize that they were still suffering from a venereal disease when they wed the woman of their dreams. In addition, as the only woman doctor in the Netherlands, I was consulted by prostitutes about diseases that I never even knew existed. This is not the place to go into any detail. Suffice it to say that, after ten years of medical practice, I was well aware of most of the forms of prostitution and of the victims it left in its wake.

I soon realized that, although many women are ignorant of just what is for sale in this world and end up by paying with their health, a great many young men also fall victim to what is viewed as merely a tradition. And ignorance often leads to disaster. Increasingly I began to recognize the need for education. Despite my respect for those who campaigned against the regulation of prostitution and my sympathy for Mrs. De Klerk-van Hogendorp's recently founded Women's Association for Moral Advancement, I believed that information had to be freely available.[2] I felt that young men and women should not be let loose in society without first being educated about the secret risks that threaten them from all sides. The Association for Moral Advancement seemed to have little to offer in this respect. It was a vehemently religious organization interested in only one category of membership.

Whenever there was a chance of publishing, I jumped at the opportunity to express my opinions on this vital subject. And I often received mail from mothers and spouses who clearly shared my views. The gifted writer Hélène Mercier (1839–1910), who was responsible for the founding of Ons Huis (Our House) in Amsterdam, wrote to me in 1895 about one of my articles that had been published in *de Amsterdammer, Weekblad voor Nederland* (The Amsterdammer, Weekly of the Netherlands),

> No, speaking the truth is never threatening when it involves some high moral aim. And I feel that it is a real boon that a subject which used to be treated as men's dirty secret or as material for literary realism can finally be approached with *complete* moral integrity by *women* themselves. It is ridiculous that women have always dissociated themselves from an area that directly involves them as *wives* and *mothers*.

I was thrilled to receive the approval of a woman whose work for society I so greatly admired. Hélène Mercier's encouragement also helped me to laugh about the insulting letters I had received from people who were too cowardly even to sign their spiteful missives with their own names.

"You must be truly depraved," wrote one of my anonymous correspondents, "to enjoy dishing up all this dirt."

Another unknown writer wanted to know if there were other supposedly respectable women in Holland who knew as much about this subject as I.

Some months after I published my article in *de Amsterdammer*, I received a letter from Mrs. Rutgers-Hoitsema, the president of the Society for the Advancement of Women's Interests, asking me to speak about prostitution at a public meeting in her home town of Rotterdam.[3] This issue had never been discussed there at an event that was open to both men and women. Bearing in mind the nasty letters I had been sent as a result of my rather restrained article in *de Amsterdammer*, my husband and a number of well-meaning friends strongly advised me not to agree to this lecture.

"You never know what can happen at a public meeting," my husband said, "You could end up being the target of the most dreadful insults."

I was well aware that this could happen, and, since I had always disliked public speaking, I had every reason to refuse this invitation. But each time I decided to write to Mrs. Rutgers to make my excuses, I began to wonder whether I could allow myself to evade this responsibility. Did I really have the right to avoid informing the wives and mothers of Holland about the presence of the most appalling dangers just because I was frightened of a little unpleasantness? Was this not the perfect opportunity to expose an evil that had always been either ignored or glossed over completely? After much hesitation and indecision, I wrote to Rotterdam to accept the society's invitation. I carefully prepared my lecture and meticulously cross-checked details and ideas against the views and judgments of other writers in this field.

The meeting was held in November 1897. The *Nieuwe Rotterdamsche Courant* included a businesslike but detailed report of my lecture. It said, "This gathering was attended by a large audience of ladies and gentlemen. In her introduction, Mrs. Rutgers-Hoitsema, the president of the Society for the Advancement of Women's Interests, expressed her pleasure that a woman had agreed to address other women on a subject of this nature in public." Once I had finished, the president announced that I would now be available to respond to questions relating to my lecture. All the reactions were extremely matter-of-fact and not in the least improper.

My lecture was published some weeks later. I still have the clipping, but can no longer trace its source, in which an Amsterdam newspaper describes how its editorial board, after reading my pamphlet, was struck by the dignity with which the author had tackled such a delicate subject, "We had to admire the sheer courage it took to expose such a contentious issue."

But that was just one opinion. Others, including the right-wing press, went to great lengths to insult and undermine a woman who had dared discuss such "filth" in the company of ladies. By now I was quite used to such insinuations. For I had taken that first step, which, as everyone knows, is always the hardest. And whenever I have subsequently been asked to speak publicly on the issue of prostitution, I have gladly accepted the opportunity of focusing on a realm urgently in need of reform.

Fortunately, since the beginning of this century, university students have grown increasingly interested in this issue, obviously of particular relevance to them. I try to read everything published in the Netherlands on this subject. Hence I came across an article written by a senior student for *Minerva*, the weekly newspaper of one of the Dutch student organizations. "Men and Women: The Mythical Double Standard" was the title of this extraordinarily perfidious and cynical piece. The writer, whose name I will omit from mention as he now no doubt deeply regrets the abominable theories of his student years, was in no way aware of the responsibility he had assumed by writing this text. However, his views were expressed with a certain virtuosity, and appeared in a periodical read by the majority of Dutch students. I felt that there was a real danger that the article could influence recent high school graduates eager to adopt the attitudes and opinions of an older student.

Of course *Minerva* received many protests and I was repeatedly asked to join the debate. Mothers of students, teachers, and the students themselves stressed that it was essential that this student paper should also include my views on sex and prostitution. And I agreed to their request. Anyone who peruses the March 20, 1902, issue of *Minerva* will see how I tried, as a woman doctor, to explain to these students the social consequences of sex in its various forms. For instance, I emphasized the fact that no illness has ever been caused by an unfulfilled libido. With a healthy lifestyle and a little willpower, any young person, male or female, is quite capable of practicing a little sexual abstinence. I also attempted to disprove the assumption that men are less socially reprehensible because of their misdeeds than their female partners. Although both may have acted incorrectly, I argued that a man who evaded fatherhood's responsibilities and depended on the immoral laws of the day that forbade the determining of paternity was far more guilty in the eyes of his child and of society at large than was the mother who had brought that baby into the world.[4] Finally I mentioned the fact that syphilis and its consequences have cost society more lives, more money, and more tears than the grand total of all other diseases put together.

My endeavors met with considerable success. As a result of this article, I received many messages of thanks and letters from young men asking for advice and information concerning sexual problems, real and imaginary. In some cases I advised a young man to discuss the matter with his mother, and it came as something of a disappointment to hear, "No, there's no way I can talk with her. Mother knows nothing about this."

In 1909 an international medical conference was being planned for Budapest at which the issue of prostitution was to be included as a subject for discussion.[5] I registered myself as a participant but, as I was feeling a little overworked, I decided to leave for the peace of Tatra Lomnics, in Hungary, a few weeks before the event was due to begin. In my mind's eye, I can still see myself standing at the station of this health resort, which at that time was virtually unknown in the Netherlands. I had been traveling for thirty-six hours nonstop and, as I wanted to retreat to my hotel as quickly as possible, I kept an eye out for the carriage that was to be sent to pick me up. Fortunately, I immediately ran into a coachman who had indeed just come from my hotel. But he began to protest vehemently when I tried to board his carriage. He had been told that he was to pick up a doctor from the station, and there was no way that a woman could be a doctor. No matter how much I reasoned with him, he remained absolutely adamant. I had to muster all my patience until, once it become evident that a male doctor was nowhere to be found, he finally relented and brought me to the hotel, which was located high up in the mountains.

There history repeated itself once again. A male doctor had been expected and the best room had been reserved for him in the hope of gaining his endorsement. It seemed such a pity to waste all that luxury on a mere woman. But in the end I managed to engineer a successful invasion. Much to my surprise, I entered my beautiful room to be greeted by a large vase of roses that had been sent "from some friends, to welcome Dr. Jacobs." How on earth had anyone managed to uncover my secret vacation plans? After a few discreet inquiries, I soon managed to unravel the mystery. My arrival had been ceremoniously announced in the newspaper published for Tatra Lomnics's foreign residents. A woman from Budapest, whom I had met several times during my suffrage tours, had read it and had been kind enough to organize this surprise on behalf of herself and her family. And the flowers were only the beginning. Thanks to her concern, I was anything but lonely in this distant spa town. She introduced me to a number of families she knew I would enjoy meeting. Among my new acquaintances, I met a charming old lady who smoked large and aromatic cigars morning, noon, and night and was also extremely interested in the current campaign for women to be granted the same political and economic rights enjoyed by many male citizens.[6]

She even let me stay in her large and luxurious house while I was attending the medical conference in Budapest. The servants had already been instructed to attend to my every whim, a carriage waited for me whenever I needed it. So I attended the conference in style! There I was most interested in the meetings that dealt with the treatment and prevention of the consequences of prostitution. Almost all the doctors who spoke were defending one or another of the systems of regulation. No one went so far as to suggest that prostitution should be eliminated altogether. When it was my turn to speak and I commented that it would be far easier and more effective to prevent prostitution rather than to have to deal with its consequences, I was audibly dismissed as just another hysterical woman.

One of the speakers at these meetings was a doctor from Sarajevo. He described, with much ado, measures taken by the Austrian government to prevent the spread of infection through prostitutes. By coincidence, after attending the International Medical Congress in Berlin a few years previously, I had been invited to work in Sarajevo on behalf on the Austro-Hungarian government. This city was to achieve world fame in the spring of 1914 when the assassination of the heir to the Austrian throne provided the necessary pretext for launching the last war. Had I taken the job, my work would have consisted of caring for Turkish women forbidden by the Koran to be treated by a male doctor.[7] Although I had never seriously considered accepting this offer, since then I have always had a soft spot for Sarajevo. When I heard that a group of doctors was planning an excursion to that city, I immediately signed up with their party. The doctor who had described the Sarajevo hygiene measures was kind enough to inform the authorities of my visit. No sooner had I arrived at my hotel than I was greeted by a shady-looking individual who announced that he had been sent by the government to accompany me to the district where prostitution was officially sanctioned.

Without going into too much detail about what I saw, I will say only that 80 percent of the girls I met had been brought in from elsewhere with the promise of lucrative jobs that naturally had failed to materialize. Most of them had come from the mountainous regions of Hungary, some of them scarcely more than children. My question about what was being done to help sick prostitutes received a short but cynical answer, "They're sent to a hospital. And if they don't get better we dump them on the other side of the Italian border!"

Deeply impressed by what I had seen and heard in Sarajevo, I made a full report of my experiences, which I sent to my friends and associates in Budapest. I asked them to inform the Hungarian government of the terrible fate awaiting their innocent female subjects in this neighboring land. Bearing in mind the local attitudes toward sexual morality, I doubt that my efforts met with success. But perhaps the situation has improved in Sarajevo since it has been under Serbian rule.

For some time I had been planning a world trip with Mrs. Chapman Catt, the well-known leader of both the International Woman Suffrage Alliance and the woman suffrage movement of the United States. Shortly after returning from Hungary—probably in early 1910—I received an urgent request from the women of South Africa, and particularly from the Boer women, to help them organize a campaign for woman suffrage. Mrs. Catt had received an identical invitation on behalf of the English-speaking women of South Africa. The International Congress of the International Woman Suffrage Alliance was to be held the following year in Stockholm from June 15 to 22, 1911. We decided that after this event had ended we would travel directly to South Africa as the first stop on our world tour. We wanted to gather information about the countries and peoples we visited and about the social and legal position of women. In addition, we intended to put this experience to practical use by persuading and helping women to launch their own campaigns for political rights.

Once I reached Cape Town, I became convinced that it was essential to extend my program's scope. A number of women had asked me to help in their crusade against brothels and the regulation of prostitution. Their campaign was also directed against other women who actually believed that it was in the interests of "respectable" women that government bordellos should be opened wherever such facilities were not as yet available. These women were actually in the process of trying to convince the government to adopt their plans.

I was urged to provide some form of guidance on this issue because, as my invitation stated, "Public ignorance or the ignorance of those whose duty it is to pass or enforce laws is the greatest enemy of all individuals who oppose regulated vice."

I decided to look into the current laws and investigate the prevailing situation so that I could provide the most effective help and advice possible. Mrs. Solly from Cape Town, who led the antiprostitution movement of South Africa, gave me a great many useful addresses and contacts.[8] Needless to say, what I encountered defied description. As usual, there was never any question of considering the women's interests. No one stopped to think about the plight of the prostitute or of those infected, often through no fault of their own, with a venereal disease. The existing regulations were designed with the sole purpose of protecting men; women's needs were treated as entirely irrelevant.

I addressed women's meetings on the issue of prostitution in Cape Town, Port Elizabeth, Bloemfontein, Kimberley, Pretoria, and Johannesburg. And wherever I went I received a great many messages of gratitude. When I arrived in a town, I would find that everything had already been arranged and that women would have come from far and wide to hear my lectures. Sometimes vast distances and lack of transportation would prevent many of my potential audience from attending, and I would be asked to publish my ideas and opinions in the local newspapers or magazines. I did so in my "Open Letter to the Women of South Africa." Thousands of copies of this straightforward article were printed in both Dutch and English and sent to women living in even the most distant farmsteads.

In this letter, I described the inherent dangers both of official brothels and of the regulation of prostitution. I explained to these women that prostitution is not a "necessary evil"; rather, it is simply the evil that undermines society more than any other and causes the most dreadful diseases among both men and women, guilty and innocent alike. I tried to demonstrate how little point there is in subjecting prostitutes to medical checkups because a woman who may be healthy at the time of examination can still be infected immediately afterward.

My statement ended with the following words, "Those who wish to prevent the spread of disease as a result of prostitution or who would even attempt to eliminate the very existence of this social cancer must begin by educating our sons from an early age about the dangers involved. Once they have been warned by their parents, their teachers, and their doctors that, no matter whether she lives in a brothel or works on her own, no prostitute can be trusted to be free of disease; once they realize the consequences of infection and are no longer legally and morally encouraged to indulge in this evil, then we will see the advent of a society that consists of decent men and decent women with no place for those diseases that are the disgrace of any civilized nation.

"However, the dawn of this era will in no way be accelerated by the licensing of brothels and the existence of a 'Contagious Diseases Prevention Act.' Hence, it is the duty of all women to campaign for the repeal of these measures, which were adopted at a time when people were still ignorant of the way in which venereal diseases are spread."

After South Africa, I visited East Africa and Asia. Wherever I went, I tried to find out as much as I could about the prevailing situation in sexual and moral terms. I encountered a great deal of suffering, but unfortunately it is impossible to help work for improvement when one is only passing through.

In June 1913, the International Woman Suffrage Alliance held a conference in Budapest. The fact that the entire event was dominated by the campaign against prostitution was due to what Mrs. Catt and I had experienced during our world tour.[9]

Unfortunately the beginning of the last war meant that the plans discussed at the conference ultimately were not realized. With the world in flames, many of our number felt—and in my view quite correctly—that we had to dedicate all our energies to the peace movement, because what was the point of instilling high moral and sexual values in our younger generation if they risked being slaughtered in a war or losing all sense of morality?

Finally, I should add that L. J. Veen of Amsterdam published my book, *Women's Issues*, in 1899. In it I discuss three topical issues, the second of which is "The Legal Regulation of Prostitution." The two other articles are devoted to "Woman's Economic and Political Independence" and to "Family Planning."

TEN

MY UNION WITH
CAREL VICTOR GERRITSEN

A Brief Outline of the Life of C. V. Gerritsen • How I Met Him • Our Life and Marriage • Bicycle Trips • Scottish Hospitality • The Conference of the International Council of Women in London • How Gerritsen's Public Life Influenced My Own • His Campaign to Reorganize Poor Relief • My Twenty-Fifth Anniversary as a Doctor of Medicine • We Visit America • His Death

I have mentioned the name of C. V. Gerritsen so frequently in the previous chapters that I would now like to devote the following pages to our mutual friendship, love affair, and marriage. I also want to stress the profound influence he has had on every aspect of my life. Let me begin with a brief outline of his life.[1]

Carel Victor Gerritsen (born February 2, 1850) was the eldest of the six children of Henri Gerritsen and Elisabeth Brasser Rijs of Amersfoort. His father was a wholesaler in the grain and feed trade. Carel did well in primary school and subsequently lodged with a teacher, Mr. Van Otterloo, in Amsterdam so that he could attend the local business-preparatory high school. Whenever he later spoke about that period, his fondest memories were of his classes with Mr. N. G. Pierson (who later became a professor, the president of the Nederlandsche Bank, and finally a government minister). Pierson had the ability to stimulate his students' enthusiasm both for economics and for social issues. Once Carel had successfully graduated from high school, his one desire was to take the university entrance exam so that he could continue his education. But this proved impossible. His father needed him to help out with the company. He was forced to return to Amersfoort, live at home, and work for the family business.

This arrangement was bound to present difficulties. Both his parents were strict old-fashioned Protestants. Every Sunday they attended church; Carel's father was also a member of the parish council. In the afternoon, the minister would come by for tea. Of course, the children were also obliged to attend church and, during the minister's Sunday afternoon visits, they were expected to listen attentively to his lectures and admonitions. Of course, each child in turn was duly prepared for confirmation.

Carel had no wish to be subjected to all this. He refused to go to church, to say grace before meals, and to stay at home for the minister's Sunday visits. He also had no intention of getting himself "confirmed." This led to a spate of quarrels in which it soon became obvious that neither side was willing to budge an inch. Carel eventually left for London where he soon found an administrative post in a merchant's office.

It was at that time that the freethinker Charles Bradlaugh refused to take the oath in Parliament.[2] There ensued a tremendous fight between him and the attendants in Parliament which, despite his enormous strength, ended with Bradlaugh being physically ejected, his clothes torn to shreds. This was but the first of a number of similar scenes. Nonetheless the voters in his constituency kept faithfully electing him. Finally, in spite of his courage and perseverance, Bradlaugh was forced to abandon this unequal struggle.

Gerritsen soon came into the contact with Bradlaugh's associates and defenders and through them he met Annie Besant, Dr. Charles Drysdale, and various other English social reformers. He ended up becoming firm friends with most of these people. As I have already mentioned, without his ever having met me in person, Gerritsen sent me letters of introduction to these friends, and it is thanks to him that I met with them during my stay in London.

After living for a number of years in London, Carel suddenly received news from Amersfoort that his father, suffering from a serious eye ailment, would probably be left partially or completely blind. Carel would therefore have to return home as soon as possible so that he could help run the family business with his younger brother, David. But he decided not to live at home, preferring instead a space above the office. Through a network of foreign contacts, Carel even managed to expand the business. He spent his evenings studying and strove to promote new ideas in this narrow-minded and predominantly anti-revolutionary city by giving lectures and writing articles that he paid to have printed and distributed among the local population.[3] As I mentioned in chapter 2, he managed to create quite a reputation for himself, particularly when he made no secret of his friendship with Multatuli, who even stayed with Carel when he came to give a lecture in Amersfoort! He also maintained his English contacts, and, business permitting, he regularly visited London for short breaks.

Several years later, he started a weekly newspaper in Amersfoort called *Ons Blad* (Our Paper) in which he generally also wrote the lead article. In 1881, he was elected to the Amersfoort Town Council where he constantly clashed with the extreme right-wing local administration. A major element in this conflict was Carel's opposition to the regulation of prostitution. He wrote a pamphlet on this subject, which included both the social and moral aspects and additional medical information that I provided. He also campaigned against the use of child labor in factories and other places, lobbied for better education and for the admission of girls to boys' schools, and advocated pensions for council workers. Outside of the council, he campaigned for a number of causes such as schooling for bargemen's children.

In May 1886, Gerritsen moved to Amsterdam where, the following autumn, he entered the university so that he could attend the lectures of Professors Quack and Pierson. He received his intermediate teaching diploma in political economy. His influential paper on the Nederlandsche Bank, in which he argued for its transformation into a state bank, was published in 1887.

In early 1888, he was one of the initiators of a campaign against the high-handed actions of the governing body of the "Civil Duty" electoral association, with particular attention to influential members who regularly decided among themselves who was to join the town council and who would represent Amsterdam in Parliament. This conflict led to the resignation of a number of members dubbed "radical" and, following the example of the Geuzen, to the founding of a new and radical electoral association called "Amsterdam."[4] Gerritsen was one of the leaders of this organization, which aimed at representing all the local citizens so that minorities would also have a fair say in council meetings. The result was an antiliberal coalition of radicals and church groups, which won a landslide victory in the 1888 autumn elections. The old guard was overthrown and among the new members was the first Radical, none other than C. V. Gerritsen. At first his sole ally was one of the older members, Mr. W. Heineken, yet he fought tirelessly against monopolies and concessions, against police behavior, and against whatever in his view was in any way oppressive. Later he gained support from a new member of the council, Mr. M. W. F. Treub, and also from *de Amsterdammer* journalist J. de Koo, whose acerbic articles greatly influenced public opinion. Along with Treub, Gerritsen successfully campaigned for badly needed reform of the labor act. It is thanks to these two men that almost the entire country was to follow Amsterdam's example and impose maximum working hours and a minimum wage.

In February 1893, Gerritsen became the first Radical member of parliament when he was elected to represent the district of Leeuwarden. Needless to say, he had no intention of renouncing his beliefs just because he had entered Parliament. Doubtless inspired by Bradlaugh's example, he introduced a private member's bill proposing a free choice between taking a Christian oath or swearing a simple pledge, a procedure that would also apply to regional and local councils. Much to his pleasure, this bill was passed and its principles entered the statute books. He remained a member of parliament until September

1897 when he was replaced in Leeuwarden by a Social Democrat. In 1901, he was offered a new candidacy but turned it down since he was by then devoting all his energy to the Amsterdam City Council. On September 5, 1899, he had succeeded Mr. Schölvinck as the alderman for commerce and poor relief, in which capacity he managed to produce much fruitful and lasting work. I should also add that his initiative and intrepid courage were responsible for the establishment of the council medical service, despite the opposition of Amsterdam general practitioners.

Apart from Treub, Gerritsen was also supported by such council members as Hugo Muller, Kouveld, and Den Hertog. Outside the council, his views were reflected in papers such as *de Amsterdammer, Weekblad voor Nederland,* which was edited with great insight by that extraordinary journalist, J. de Koo. (In time the Dutch Radical Union was formed; when it merged in 1901 with the Liberal Democratic Union, the word *radical* was abandoned.) Sometimes Gerritsen found himself opposed by his former supporters. This was one of the reasons he decided to resign as an alderman in 1902. He held to this decision even when the town council named him as alderman again the following September, although he continued to work as a regular council member.

Wherever he served—which included being a member of the Provincial Estates for several years—Gerritsen fought for equal rights for men and women, for better conditions for the working classes, and for improved hygiene (in their homes, for their children at school, and so forth). On the Amsterdam City Council, he championed the development of public services, and it is thanks to him that monopolies were eliminated and businesses such as the Amsterdam Omnibus Company, the (English) Gas Company, and Bell Telephone were eventually taken over by the city and converted into publicly owned companies.

And this concludes a brief outline of his working life, which achieved much for the society in which he lived.

As I already have mentioned, Gerritsen and I had begun corresponding after my first examinations. When I contracted typhus, he repeatedly came by, although he never gave his name. He was in the audience when I defended my dissertation and before my departure for London he sent me letters of introduction to many of his good friends there. Despite all this, it was some months after I had set up my Amsterdam practice that I finally got to meet him in person.

He had actually visited my parents some time before and had asked my father's permission to be able to visit me. I burst out laughing when Father told me this. To be honest, my impression was that he was an old-fashioned and rather diffident young man, although this was in no way suggested by his letters. As far as I was concerned, that interview with my father had killed any notion of romance, and I felt not in the least excited about his impending visit.

On January 20, 1880, I received a neatly written letter in which Gerritsen informed me that he had met some of our mutual friends in London who had asked him to convey their greetings. He wanted to relay these messages in person and asked if he could call the following Sunday afternoon at teatime.

My reaction was quite simply, "He only dares to show up because he has the excuse of a few messages from London."

My youngest sister, Frederika, who was at that time teaching math and accounting at the girls' college in The Hague, was present when Gerritsen finally appeared. We had already made tea. Both of us were diligently doing our needlework. I was embroidering flowers on dark blue silk and my sister was making fine lace. The needlework broke the ice at once. The expression on Gerritsen's face made it quite clear that he was astounded to find us occupied with anything as domestic as handicrafts! I asked him jokingly exactly how he had imagined this woman with whom he had up to now exchanged only a series of serious and rather formal letters? Did he really think that I spent my entire life with my nose stuck in a book? To show him that my embroidery was more than a passing fancy, I produced further examples from my work basket. My sister and I told him that we had also made the dresses we were wearing, although I added that, as soon as I could afford it, I would happily consign this task to more expert hands.

From then on we talked as if we were old friends. We immediately began to discuss the lives of women whose biographies had been published, and Gerritsen told us that he owned an extensive library that included several of these books.[5] By the time he got up to leave, he had stayed far longer than was normal for an initial visit. He apologized, but my sister and I said that it was all our fault because we had kept him talking for such a long time. He left with the promise that he would lend us the books we had discussed.

Although this visit had been a great success, some time passed before it was repeated. He sent the books and received a brief thank you note, and that was all for the time being. Then came March 8, the first anniversary of my doctorate in medicine. I had completely forgotten this date, and would have done nothing to celebrate it, had I not come down to breakfast and discovered a vase of flowers with a card from C. V. Gerritsen. He had written, "Do the women of Holland realize the deep significance of March 8, 1879?"

He was the one person who had remembered that special day. Along with his sister and brother-in-law, Mr. Hengeveld, he called that same afternoon to congratulate me and was amazed to find that there were no other celebrations. They asked me to have dinner with them at the Amstel Hotel and also invited my brother Eduard, who was garrisoned as an infantry officer in Amsterdam and by chance had dropped by to see me. We both accepted this invitation, and in this way I also got to know Gerritsen's closest relatives.

In 1880, we exchanged a few insignificant letters and Gerritsen occasionally visited me to deliver books that I had asked to borrow, but beyond that our contact remained limited. In March 1881, Gerritsen came by one evening a few weeks after the death of my much-loved father. He was well aware that I was devastated by my loss and it really helped to hear him speak admiringly of my father and express his pleasure at having known him.

I began to tell him how my father had also been a good friend and adviser to me. For his time, my father had extremely progressive views on politics and social issues, although during our discussions he took care to suppress any radical tendencies as he was worried that I would go too far and find myself in difficult circumstances. My father held mature and well thought-out opinions on a great many social issues. I felt I could discuss anything with him and he always had time to listen to me and to exchange ideas. Despite our frequent disagreements, he helped me achieve greater insight and a more considered point of view.

I told Gerritsen that I felt as if I had lost my only friend and knew that I would never find another like him. When I had finished, he asked me very shyly whether perhaps he could prove himself as a friend worthy of listening to everything I found important. He admitted that medical matters were a bit beyond him, but since we shared the same principles in terms of social concerns, in that respect we could certainly help and support each other.

We established an initial bond of friendship that evening. It was as yet an informal relationship, and I found it hard to imagine how I could discuss each day's problems and share opinions with a man I hardly knew. Was it not wiser to save all those issues for friends like Hélène Mercier, Cornélie Huygens, or Elise Haighton? At first our friendship consisted of exchanging a few more letters and seeing each other more frequently. Gerritsen regularly spent Monday afternoons at the Corn Market in Amsterdam, after which he would stop by between 3 and 4 P.M. when my office hours were ending. Then we would talk about subjects we had recently read about in newspapers or magazines. Sometimes we were still deep in conversation when he had to leave to catch his train for Amersfoort, and I would accompany him to the station so we could conclude our discussions.

It was a politically turbulent time. The clashes between the supporters and opponents of the proposed constitutional reforms to allow greater male enfranchisement gave us much to discuss. Gerritsen knew so much more about this realm than I. I grew increasingly aware of how much I was gaining from his friendship and guidance.

But I was also able to help Gerritsen when he became a member of the Amersfoort Municipal Council. He often dropped by unannounced to ask my opinion of some subject that was currently under discussion. For instance, we talked about the issue of whether girls' schools should be set up in Amersfoort. This was an idea I definitely opposed. I suggested that the council should simply allow girls to attend the various boys' schools. Gerritsen feared that the people of Amersfoort were not yet ready to accept so radical a measure and that waiting for them to come around to the idea would have an adverse effect on girls' education. I maintained that their eventual admission was better than opening separate girls-only schools.

Gerritsen also wrote a brochure to launch his council campaign for the abolition of the regulation of prostitution. I provided him with the necessary medical details, and together we discussed all the various social and moral arguments that could be used against this regulation. Whenever he was too busy or lacked inspiration, I would often write the main article for his weekly newspaper, *Ons Blad*. This allowed me to air my opinions on subjects such as "Raising Girls" or "Legal and Social Discrimination Against Women."

Gerritsen supported me strongly when I began to campaign openly for family planning in 1882 and also when I launched the crusade for woman suffrage early in 1883. We were gradually learning to trust each other's opinions. I would never publish a piece without first sending it to Amersfoort for approval and Gerritsen always consulted my opinion whenever his articles involved an issue that particularly concerned me.

When I reread the letters we wrote during the years 1881, 1882, and 1883, it seems to me that we were two young idealists with burning ambitions to reform the entire world! We discussed all kinds of problems. When I failed to reply promptly, I would receive a curt message demanding, "So what's up, why have I heard nothing more about (a particular letter), which you must have received by now?" Sometimes his note would end with a caustic comment, "I do hope you're not wasting your time on more needlework!"

During those years of collaboration, we dealt frankly with every issue we encountered, including that of sexual relations. Gradually we realized that we were two young people in the prime of mental and physical health, involved in a friendship that had acquired a deeper meaning. Our collaborative work had led to an inner understanding, a *Seelenharmonie,* or spiritual alliance. Marriage would have in no way disturbed all this, had we not both been convinced that no woman with a modicum of self-respect would subject herself to the current wedding vows. An additional problem was that Gerritsen lived in Amersfoort, and I had no intention of giving up my practice in Amsterdam.

We both considered and discussed the situation until we came to the conclusion that it would be better not to see each other in the foreseeable future and to write only if it became absolutely necessary. The months passed and we heard only indirectly what had become of each other.

In May 1884, I once again received a letter. Gerritsen wrote to say that he was spending some weeks in London because he was thoroughly fed up with life in Amersfoort. He had hoped to find a suitable job in London, but soon began to feel as miserable as he had in the Netherlands, and was now thinking of embarking on a major journey in the hope that a little diversion would improve his spirits.

In a few words, I encouraged him to pursue his plans. But, I wondered, how did I really feel about our separation? Despite my busy practice, which took up almost all my time, I felt that something was missing in my life. A busy job, work that involves love and dedication, should be a great comfort in times of adversity, yet somehow it never quite fulfills the needs of normal young people. I was clearly unhappy. Once you fall in love these feelings refuse to be sublimated into work, even the kind that is performed with love. I felt a sense of unease that was disturbing my emotional equilibrium. But I had no intention of giving in because I wanted to remain free and independent so that I could fulfill my chosen task to the best of my ability. For that reason, I decided to fight my inner feelings by convincing myself that marriage would in no way solve my problems.

In the spring of 1884, I had been caring for two young girls of twelve and fourteen. The children of a rich mercantile family in Amsterdam, they had become firm friends of mine. Their father had also been ill and was advised by his physician to leave with his wife for the waters of Kissingen. The idea was that I would take care of the children, accompany them to Lucerne at the beginning of August to join their parents, and then stay on as a guest of the family. I accepted the invitation, but with some conditions. I would happily take the girls to Lucerne and stay with them for a couple of weeks. After that I wanted to be free to travel around Switzerland as I pleased.

During the second week of my stay in Lucerne, I met three English people, a brother and two sisters, who were planning a walking holiday through one particular part of the country. It was soon agreed that I should accompany them. Shortly afterward, I was walking back and forth along Lake Lucerne at sunset when I saw a small steamship approaching with a number of men on board, including none other than Gerritsen! And he had seen me too. In fact it was no coincidence that he turned up in Lucerne because he had managed while in Amsterdam to discover my whereabouts. When I told him about the three English people and the walking holiday, he asked if there would be any objection to his joining the party. Everything was soon arranged, and the five of us left a few days later. We had agreed not to be too ambitious but to give ourselves time to wander down side roads or to pause at some beautiful spot where we could think and talk to our hearts' content. We also wanted to be able to skip the dull parts by taking a boat or some other form of transport. The plan was to walk from Lucerne via the Brünig to Meiringen and Brienz, and from there to continue to Spiez and Kandersteg before crossing the Gemmi to reach Leuk. We would then follow the Rhône to Martigny and from there we would set off to Chamonix.

When we had finally traversed the Gemmi and arrived in Leukerbad (Loèche-les-Bains) where we intended to find lodgings for just one night, I found myself hesitant to leave so soon. I was particularly interested in the methods used in this health resort and had decided to accept an invitation from a local doctor. I would have to stay behind for two days and take the train in order to catch up with the others on the second evening. Everything went according to plan, but when I arrived at the station, only Gerritsen was there to meet me. He told me that our English friends had gone on to Martigny from where they planned to head home via Paris.

What were we to do? Should we continue our journey as planned and face the consequences? We decided to come to a decision the following day.

We both agreed that a legal marriage was out of the question. On the other hand, the only disadvantage to a marriage of "free individuals," in which both of us maintained our full freedom and economic independence—even continuing to live apart—would be the offense to conventional attitudes. As two completely independent people, we would be able to live, for better or worse, according to our own beliefs. Our union was based on mutual respect and a shared philosophy of life.

All the objections were easily outweighed by the happiness our union would bring. Eventually we decided to spend our vacations together, but to continue our lives as before. Never for one moment did I doubt that the way in which we had chosen to live was anything other than highly moral. On the contrary, we were both convinced that future marriages would be based on such conditions, which would also increase the chance of lasting happiness.

In late 1885 and early 1886, Gerritsen began to feel that he wanted to leave Amersfoort and move to Amsterdam. This wish was made all the more intense because he wanted to give up business so that he could resume his education.

We looked for suitable accommodation for him in Amsterdam. I hired some staff, and the house was furnished according to our mutual taste. And, of course, we also discussed the question of whether we should live together. However, I was afraid that if we flouted public opinion, my practice would suffer and I would risk losing my economic independence. So we decided not to take that final step, but inevitably our lives became more intimate now that we were living so close to one another. Hardly a day passed when we did not exchange at least a note.

During the first two years he lived in Amsterdam, Gerritsen attended university lectures in constitutional law and economics, and I could always rely on him to keep me informed about new developments. In turn, my influence was quite obvious when in 1888 he and a number of other progressive men founded the Radical Union, the first political party to include woman suffrage in its manifesto. It was also the first party to grant membership to women on the same conditions as to men.

In the spring of 1890, Gerritsen left to spend three months in Paris with the twin aims of attending lectures in political economics and finance and of improving his knowledge of French. Rereading his letters from that period, which describe everything he saw and encountered, I am particularly struck by one story that now seems strangely odd and naive in this era of the internal combustion engine. In a letter of June 19, 1890, I read the following, "Yesterday, among all the hundreds of carriages on the Champs Elysées, I actually saw one without a horse! And would you believe me if I told you that this extraordinary vehicle was moving just as fast as its neighbors, with their elegantly trotting ponies? It was like a large Tilbury coach and is called a 'charette.' It had two male passengers, one of whom was steering it with a long rudder attached to a front wheel. This 'charette' was powered by steam, with a little engine located beneath the vehicle that made no smoke or noise. What an extraordinary invention! Who knows what further miracles of this kind may one day be generated by electricity!"

Shortly after Gerritsen returned from Paris, I began to prepare to leave for Berlin where I was to participate in an international medical conference. I was particularly excited about this trip because there was a real chance that I would meet my old physician friends from England and also a great many celebrities of various nationalities. Everything lived up to my expectations and I still remember this conference with great pleasure.

Because of his stay in Paris and my trip to Berlin, Gerritsen and I saw virtually nothing of each other for several months, although we kept in constant touch by letter. Gerritsen was also going through a difficult period with his staff. And I was becoming increasingly aware of my desire to have a child. All this eventually brought us to a point, in the winter of 1890 to 1891, when we realized that we would have to organize our lives in some other way. The question was how. Once again we considered the possibility of living together without first getting married. But would I then dare have a child in the full knowledge that he or she would suffer as a result of our battle against conventional morality? And would Gerritsen, who by now wanted to enter politics, encounter all manner of difficulties because he was not legally married? Of course, these problems seem quite trivial nowadays! Why not simply keep your head held high and live out your principles with pride?

We decided to take a long holiday together in the summer of 1891 so we could come to some final agreement. Our travels took us via Paris and Saint-Malo to Jersey and Guernsey before we finally returned home by way of London. Walking the length and breadth of these delightful and temperate islands gave us ample opportunity to plan for the future. We weighed the pros and cons of marriage and those of simply living together until we finally came up with a solution. We would live together and get married, but beyond that we would remain free and independent of each other. I would use my own surname; I would continue with my practice and retain possession of my capital and earnings. We would live in the same house, but maintain separate apartments with the exception of a shared dining room and parlor. We would each furnish our apartments ourselves, and at the end of every year household expenses would be added up and divided by two. Each of us would pay for our own clothes, books, and other personal expenses. We would also work out all the domestic arrangements as carefully as possible. In this way, we felt that we could ensure each other's freedom within the marriage.

Once we had agreed on these conditions, we decided to go ahead with our plans as quickly as possible. As soon as we returned to Amsterdam, we set about looking for suitable accommodation. However, it turned out to be extremely difficult to find something that fulfilled all our requirements. We were making little headway, so finally we decided to purchase a house and have it remodeled. We eventually found a suitable building on the Tesselschadestraat that later also became the corner of the Roemer Visscherstraat. We lived together in that house until Gerritsen's death, and I stayed on there alone until 1911.

All the alterations and organizing took far longer than expected, and only in April 1892 were we finally able to move into our home. To avoid any outside interference, we spent the days between the announcement of our marriage and the wedding itself with friends in London.

Although the councilman who officiated at our wedding gave a speech that attempted to reconcile two such radical elements as ourselves with the legal proceedings at hand, his efforts did nothing to prevent my look of total indignation when I had to swear publicly that I would "obey." Since then, I have spoken, written, and done whatever I can to get that vow of obedience removed from the civil marriage vows. It is wildly out of date and casts a suspicious light both on the men who sign the marriage register, and, more especially, on those who continue to enforce it. For, in fact, even in the most conservative families, no one honestly expects "obedience" of a wife. Of course, as everybody knows, those men who imagine that they are at all times obeyed are the ones most likely to be duped. Nonetheless, since many people consider their wedding to be the most important day of their lives, why should they be forced to take a vow that they have no intention of keeping?

In September 1893, we realized that we were expecting our first child and looked forward to the great event with a sense of profound happiness. Even as late as the beginning of the seventh month, I performed an exhausting forceps delivery. And I maintained my practice up until my last day of pregnancy, yet still found the time to make the baby's layette myself.

In January 1893, Gerritsen was nominated as a parliamentary candidate for Leeuwarden. He was to be the first candidate fielded by the still youthful Radical Union and was up against the well-known Friesland liberal, Mr. J. Troelstra, whose son, P. J. Troelstra, the current leader of the Social Democrats, was at that time attending the University of Groningen.[6] It was a difficult election campaign that involved all the Radical Union speakers. Meetings were held night after night across the entire district. But no matter how late Gerritsen returned to Leeuwarden from these meetings and how many hours he had spent traveling, he still found the time to write me about the day's events before finally retiring to bed. No wonder that, with the help of his young and idealistic supporters, he was eventually elected to represent Friesland and entered Parliament as its first Radical member.

Despite all the pressures of the election, every single letter Gerritsen sent me reveals how delighted we both were with impending parenthood and how this event was constantly on our minds.

But the baby we had wanted so badly was to live for only a single day. A mistake made by the midwife cut short its life and I simply cannot describe how devastated we felt. It took me years to recover from my grief. But looking back, despite all the sorrow I still count myself lucky that I know how it feels to be a mother, that I have held my child in my arms, even though it was for but one day.

Life went on as before and we both returned to our appointed tasks. Work permitting, we took our meals together but saw little of each other for the rest of the day. If the weather was good and I could finish work by half past three, I would accompany Gerritsen on one of his many tours of the harbor establishments for which he worked so enthusiastically and where he had managed to introduce a great many improvements. On other occasions, I joined him on an inspection of the many council organizations for poor relief. We walked the length and breadth of many new neighborhoods and backstreet districts, so that Gerritsen, who was not an Amsterdamer by birth, could prove in meetings that he knew the city through and through and was well aware of everything that was going on.

Every vacation or brief holiday was spent traveling. At first we mainly went on walking trips but in 1894 we started taking our bicycles so that we could get to know more about life both at home and abroad. We also kept notes on our travels, which we later developed and published as our "Travel Letters."[7] We often took them along as information with which to compare the social situation, laws, and practices of the Netherlands with those of other nations. We rarely visited a country or district merely for the beauty of its landscapes; we were more concerned with broadening our knowledge of the country and its people. When visiting a village or city, we would make a point of talking to the inhabitants, which often produced much interesting information and many useful contacts. The briefest of meetings frequently led to a lengthy correspondence and even friendship.

When we first took to our bikes, we decided to join the international cyclists' association. That decision helped us enormously with introductions and information because we always looked up the association's representative in every place we visited. As a rule, these men were friendly and educated people who were only too happy to help us.

We would set out early in order to arrive at our destination before midday. This meant that we had time to visit a factory, school or college, or a museum or some other institution. If it was somewhere especially important, we would stay overnight, otherwise we would leave the same afternoon. Then we would take care to reach our lodgings before dusk, so that, were we not too tired, we would have time enough to write up the day's events. We divided this work so that

Gerritsen described one part of the day and I the other. We became so adept at coordinating the two halves that, when these reports appeared in print, no one realized that they were the result of a collaborative effort.

In this fashion, we visited Denmark, Norway, and Sweden. Through a number of trips, we got to know almost all of Germany and also large parts of France, England and Scotland, Switzerland, northern Italy, Austria, and Hungary. I would now like to describe a few of these journeys in greater detail.

On one occasion, we took the train to Dresden, where we stayed for several days to visit the neighboring districts by bicycle. We then set off on an ambitious tour of the Saxon district of Switzerland. Our baggage, which consisted of a solitary suitcase, had been sent ahead to Prague, while we took a few basic essentials with us on our bicycles. After Prague, we quickly headed for the Bohemian Woods and Linz, which is located on the Danube, and from there we took a boat to Vienna. We stayed there for a week before leaving for Steiermark [Styria] and Innsbruck via the Salzkammergut. Then we took the Brenner Pass to Franzenfeste where we managed to get lost, spending two days struggling with bumpy tracks and primitive lodgings until we finally reached Belluno where we took the train to Venice. From here we left for Padua and Verona, continued to Lake Garda, and took the boat to Riva. After that, we headed via Trento to Bolzano where we made a brief detour to Merano and then again took the Brenner Pass, to Innsbruck. The few days we still had left were devoted to cycling through the Mittelwald to Munich before taking the train back to Amsterdam. In all, this journey took us approximately nine weeks.

In the same way, we set off another year for Antwerp and cycled to Ghent, Kortrijk, and Boulogne, spending a day and a night at all the well-known resorts along the coast until we reached Le Havre. From here we proceeded to Honfleur and followed the Seine via Rouen to Paris. In Rouen, we met a friendly representative from the cyclists' association who was both a lawyer and a cycling fanatic. He provided us with so much interesting information about Rouen and its beautiful surroundings that we decided to stay on in order to take a few day trips with him and his wife. When we returned to the city from these trips, the couple told us much about the daily lives of the inhabitants of Rouen. This meeting led to a friendship and correspondence that lasted for many years. After Paris, we made a major detour, which took us via Nancy and Metz, through Luxemburg to Liège and Maastricht until we headed back home.

I would like briefly to describe one other journey, not simply because it was one of our most ambitious but also for the many happy memories associated with it. It was in the summer of 1898. After three days of cycling, we arrived in Vlissingen where we boarded a boat to England and then took a train to London. After touring for a few days, we decided to accept an invitation from an old friend, Dr. G. B. Clark, to stay at his beautiful estate in Surrey.[8]

This host, too, was an avid cyclist. Each morning and afternoon he took us on magnificent tours of the area and accompanied us on the first part of a major trip to Scotland. We left Surrey for Windsor and followed the Thames to Oxford and Stratford-on-Avon, which is known the world over as the birthplace of the greatest of English playwrights. We stayed in the Shakespeare Hotel where the rooms were not numbered—each was named after one of Shakespeare's plays. Then we left for Birmingham where we stayed for several days to investigate workers' conditions in this center of English industry. Subsequently we rode a train to avoid some particularly monotonous landscapes, but took to our bicycles again in Carnforth, which is on the edge of the Lake District of Cumberland and Westmoreland. That day we reached Windermere, where Londoners often came to spend long weekends. Because of a bank holiday Monday, we could stay only for one night since all the Windermere hotels were fully booked. The next morning, therefore, we left for Keswick where we spent some time making day trips. Our plan was to reach Glasgow in a day but we ran into a downpour in Ecclefechan and had to stay put. We knew that town as the birthplace of Thomas Carlyle and as his final resting place—in the rather unimpressive local graveyard. Out of respect for his memory, we decided with some trepidation to stay at the local pub, which was primitive but clean. Since the next day was also rainy, we decided to take the train to Glasgow. There was so much to see and to learn that we stayed for a week making day trips. On one of these we discovered the town of Lanark with its many spinning mills. I was particularly interested in this place because it was here that Robert Owen had introduced his socialist experiments.

One evening in our hotel in Glasgow, we met a representative of William Beard and Co., a mining concern from Bothwell. When he realized that we were interested in seeing a coal mine, he invited us to accompany him. Bothwell was a half-hour train ride from Glasgow. To prepare us for our visit, we were shown drawings of the mine's many shafts and tunnels. Then we were supplied with miners' outfits. I was given boys' clothes, but still had to roll up my sleeves and trouser legs to move freely. My hair was covered with a cap and I felt well protected. We were accompanied by a good-natured overseer who did his best to give us a guided tour. Descending into the shaft sent shivers up my spine, for it seemed to take forever to reach the required depth of six hundred meters. After waiting under a sort of bell jar so that we might become accustomed to the air pressure, we set out on the tour, which took hours and which I will not describe in any detail. Much has already been written about coal mines, which tend to be the same the world over: a wretched combination of ominous darkness, difficult access, and inhuman, extremely burdensome, and badly paid work. In short, this is the world that Zola so graphically depicted in *Germinal*. This long and exhausting journey, much of which was made bent over or even on all fours, left a deep impression on both of us. I felt great compassion for the toiling miners and for their unfortunate ponies who are doomed to spend their lives in the dark without ever seeing the sunlight again. To be honest, toward the end of our tour I was covered with sweat from the heat, and all my exertions, and I was also feeling increasingly exhausted. But we were to be spared nothing because one of the miners suddenly said to our guide, "There's something wrong!" Apparently an electrical cable had broken, causing the coal trucks to be held up in one part of the mine. At the same time, the elevator that had brought us into the mine had also broken down and we were forced to walk some distance to the next shaft.

I have never been happier to see daylight than at the moment we finally surfaced after spending many long hours underground! And I can hardly describe the grubby state in which we emerged, our noses, mouths, ears, and eyes full of coal dust. Fortunately, there were hot baths waiting for us at the home of our hosts, where I discovered, when I removed the protective cap, that my hair was stiff with dirt. We were reasonably presentable after an hour's ablutions, but for days afterward I felt as if my mucous membranes were still covered with dust.

Nowadays, a visit to a coal mine is not an uncommon occurrence even in our country, as we have a large state-owned company in South Limburg. But when we descended into that pit in Bothwell, it was considered extremely unusual for a woman to agree to such an undertaking and not be put off by a lot of well-intentioned warnings. I have never regretted my visit because it left me with an indelible impression of miners' lives.

After spending a fruitful week in Glasgow, we took to our bicycles again and headed for Oban via Inveraray. We had planned to spend a few days there but, since it was full of seaside visitors, we decided to take the boat to Fort William and to cycle on to Inverness. We then continued to Gairloch and the Isle of Skye, which was much in the news at that time because of the crofters' revolt against the landowners. Famous for its stunning landscapes, Skye is visited by a great many English and Scottish families.

It took some days to cycle from Inverness to Gairloch. On the second day, we were frequently caught in downpours and had to take shelter repeatedly. Finally we decided to cycle on at full speed and stop at the first hotel we saw. Unfortunately, the heavens opened at seven o'clock in the evening, with not a house in sight, only one small church. We decided that the best plan was to ask if there was a train station somewhere in the vicinity. When we knocked at the presbytery door, we were welcomed in by a bachelor parson and his house-keeper. He said that we could stay there if I would help his housekeeper organize a room for us, and if we would care to join them in a simple supper. Of course, we accepted. During the meal, I noticed a chess set on a small table. The parson was a great chess enthusiast, so while Gerritsen browsed around the presbytery library, I engaged this elderly vicar in a game that lasted until well past midnight. Early the next morning we were ready to resume our travels, but the housekeeper informed us that we had to stay a little longer; the reverend had gone out at the crack of dawn to catch a couple of rabbits for a meal, and we simply could not leave until he had returned! When he came back, he literally begged us to stay on for a few more days. He was so well-meaning that we eventually agreed to stay for another day, and in this way we managed to get a glimpse of the life of an English village parson. It did not seem a very enviable lot.

Once we had returned from Skye to Gairloch, we decided to take a different route to Inverness. We then headed toward Aberdeen and followed the Dee to Braemar. In Balleter, we visited the Ballaterach farm where Byron grew up and fell in love for the first time, with Mary Robertson, the farmer's daughter. This idyll provided the inspiration for a number of beautiful poems, although since they were written the farm had changed beyond all recognition.

Braemar, Queen Victoria's summer residence, was also worth a visit. From there, we had to negotiate two difficult mountain passes in order to reach our next destination. We left Braemar early in the morning. The weather was peerless until we reached the first mountain top where we were suddenly engulfed in thick mist, our visibility cut down to less than a yard. This mist was so cold and wet that our clothes were soon sodden. What were we to do? On our way up, we had spotted a run-down cottage, the only sign of human habitation. We managed to trace our way back to the cottage, home to two sisters in their seventies who welcomed us warmly. They stoked a log fire so that we could dry our clothes. These women were two well-born ladies who had definitely seen better days. When they were no longer able to support themselves, their family had found them this bargain of a hut in the middle of nowhere. After a couple of hours, even with the mist as thick as ever, we felt impelled to leave such oppressive poverty. We asked if there was an inn in the neighborhood or some other house where we could stay the night. One of the old women directed us to the gamekeeper's lodge located behind their home. We left our bicycles behind. The gamekeeper was not at home, but we were received by his sister who, in true Scots fashion, was curt and rather gruff. This manner was something we recognized, and we were not in least put off; people usually turned out to be much more friendly than they initially sounded. "Come in," said the sister, "I'll put the kettle on. Let's hope the weather clears up and you can soon be on your way." In no time, there was English tea with bread, cheese, and eggs. The wood fire blazed, and we were joined by our host, Betsy Wallace, who talked to us as if we had known each other for years.

Her brother returned a little later. He was a big, warm-hearted man who immediately said that it was a good thing we had knocked at their door because there were no other houses nearby and, in addition, there was a dangerous bend a little further up the road.

The mist cleared at around five o'clock. We asked the gamekeeper whether it was safe to resume our journey or to return to Braemar. He went outside to check on the conditions and came back with the verdict that we should stay put. The weather was unpredictable; wherever we might head we could end up in an accident. They prepared a camp bed in the "good room" and shared their meal of stewed potatoes and weak coffee. The gamekeeper, we discovered, was an excellent conversationalist. He spent the whole evening relating anecdotes about Scottish farming life. The next morning the weather was clear and sunny, and when we set out to leave we discovered that our bicycles had been decorated with flowering white heather. Betsy had gone out early to pick a few bunches, which she said would bring us good luck. Neither brother nor sister would consider any form of payment for their generous hospitality, and, when I finally asked if there was some other way of expressing our gratitude, they said that they would appreciate it if we would write to them occasionally, to show that we had not forgotten them. And that, of course, is what I did. For a great many years, I sent Betsy and her brother a small Christmas present that I thought they would like. This would be answered with a brusque thank you note, an arrange-ment that continued until my parcel was eventually returned "undeliverable."

After this adventure, we visited the Trossacks and from there we made day trips to and across various lakes. We then cycled by way of Stirling to Edinburgh where we spent several days. Originally we had planned to cycle the whole way to London, but we realized that this would take far too much time. So we ended our tour in Edinburgh and returned to Amsterdam via London by train and boat.

In July 1899, the great International Conference of Women, the first in Europe, was to take place in London. It would be the second conference of the International Council of Women, which had been set up in North America in 1893. For months I had been looking forward to meeting many of the women from distant lands with whom I had been corresponding for years. Each time I received a letter asking, "Will I be seeing you in London?" my heart skipped a beat, and I was delighted to reply that yes, indeed, I would be attending. My joy at seeing, in one place, all these women who, like me, were campaigning for women's social, political, and economic interests, was all the greater for know-ing that Gerritsen was also planning to attend. I should add that he was one of the very few men who gave a lecture at the conference.

Many London families opened their doors to the foreign participants, and in such a generous way that it was impossible to say no. Mrs. Herbert Samuel invited me and my husband to stay for the entire event. The man who picked us up from Liverpool Street Station looked so youthful that we thought he was our hosts' son. Yet he was none other than Sir Herbert Samuel himself, who was to play such an important role in politics and become the first high commissioner of Palestine, a post he retains to this day. (I have already mentioned our acquaintance with the Samuels in chapter 6).

I soon met women such as the eighty-year-old Miss Susan B. Anthony from America, the minister Anna Howard Shaw, Mrs. Emmeline Wells (the widow of one of the first Mormons, who was also the governor of Utah for many years), the Baroness Alexandra von Gripenberg from Finland, the two Russians Madame

Anna de Filosofova and Dr. Kozakevitch Stefanofsky, and various women from Canada, Australia, and New Zealand.[9] Their initial reaction was invariably the same: amazement that I was still young. By this time I was a good forty-five years old, but, as the elderly Miss Anthony said, hugging and kissing me, "How can it be that you are the same woman of whom I have heard for so many, many years already!" I was to receive the same response from a great many of the women I was meeting for the first time in person.

At one of the first large dinners for conference participants, I was seated between Beatrice Harraden, the well-known English author of *Ships That Pass in the Night,* and the American writer Mrs. Charlotte Perkins Stetson. The latter had just completed her major work, *Women and Economics,* for which the Fabian Society in London had offered her an honorary membership. Some years previously, she had received an award in California for an essay on the workers' movement. Before the dinner was even over, Mrs. Perkins Stetson asked me if I would like to translate her latest work into Dutch. I said I would, and the very same evening I received a letter of confirmation from her. One year later, in July 1900, I completed the book by Charlotte Perkins Gilman (she had since divorced Mr. Stetson and married a Mr. Gilman). In Dutch, it was called *De Economische toestand der vrouw* (Woman's Economic Situation) and was published by Tjeenk Willink in Haarlem. But despite the extremely positive reactions of many newspapers and magazines, this book failed to make much of an impression. Yet "it touches on an issue vital to today's society" (*Algemeen Handelsblad,* December 23, 1900) because it is a powerful argument in favor of women's economic independence in marriage—from a moral, economic, and eugenic viewpoint.

I translated one other book some ten years later. It was called *Woman and Labor* and was written by the brilliant and charming Olive Schreiner. Academically, it would be hard to compare this book with Mrs. Perkins Gilman's, yet it deals with the same subject in sociological and ethical terms and can therefore be regarded as a supplement to *Women and Economics.*

Among the many festivities connected with this unparalleled conference, I particularly remember the evening at Stafford House where the guests were received by the Duchess of Sutherland and Lady Aberdeen. I also recall a splendid garden party in Gunnersbury Park given by the ladies de Rothschild. Trains were provided for the guests as well as special carriages to and from the station. I was also fortunate enough to be one of the twelve guests invited by Sir Richard Temple to spend two consecutive weekends at The Nash, his magnificent country estate in Worcestershire. I will not attempt to describe any of the other social events. Suffice it to say that they were so plentiful that life was a constant whirl of lunches, dinners, and even breakfast parties. However, I would like to point out that my invitations always included "and husband" or "and Mr. Gerritsen" after my name and that my husband was usually eager to take advantage of his inclusion.

When we returned to Amsterdam and spoke with friends and acquaintances about the conference, Gerritsen commented that this event had made him realize how a proud woman must feel spending her life regarded not as herself but as a mere appendage of her husband. For in London he was seen exclusively as Dr. Aletta H. Jacobs's husband. He said that this lesson is something every man should experience in order to understand the importance of women's struggle for independence. However, that week in London was apparently not dreadful enough to dissuade him from accompanying me to the next conference of the International Council of Women, held in Berlin in 1904. Here I will limit myself to commenting that this conference marked the consolidation of the International Woman Suffrage Alliance. It was also especially important for me, since here I first met Mrs. Carrie Chapman Catt, who was to become a close friend. In addition, I got to know the minister Anna Howard Shaw more intimately, and we too remained close friends until her death.

I would now like to illustrate the way in which Gerritsen and I related to one another as man and woman.

Naturally I took advantage of the opportunity provided by the Radical Union, and later also by the Liberal Democratic Union, for women to join on the same conditions as men and with equal rights. Not only did I believe in the party's principles; I was convinced that here people would be receptive to my campaign for improved conditions for women. So I became an active member.

Gerritsen was one of the party's leaders and hence I always knew what was going on. Not long after the Radical Union was merged into the Liberal Democratic Union, guidelines were developed for party members who were elected to office. A commission with Gerritsen as its chairman was formed to discuss a draft party platform. I was passionately interested in this plan and privately I was extremely critical of some of the points, which I felt did not go far enough. I also felt that there had been some unfortunate omissions. I tried to convince Gerritsen to ensure the inclusion of, first, the principle that gender would in no way influence the selection of officials and candidates were to be assessed solely on the basis of their competence and suitability; and, second, that if a woman were appointed, she would receive "equal pay for equal work."

Some time later Gerritsen told me that the party platform had been decided upon and that the commission had rejected my suggestions. "And what about you?" I asked. With an impassive expression, he replied, "I am just one member and I have already told you the commission's decision." And he refused to discuss this subject further.

A meeting was due to be held in Amsterdam to review the party platform and to debate the possible inclusion of additional amendments. I considered the options open to me to get my two points accepted in the program. This time, Gerritsen was definitely not the right person to advise me, since during the meeting he would have to defend the program in its unaltered form. He felt unable to help me find the best way to tackle this problem because doing so would make his own task all the more difficult. When I asked why the commission had rejected my points, he simply said that he was not allowed to divulge what had been discussed in a commission meeting. Perhaps I attached too much significance to the inclusion of these two points, but they obsessed me, and my husband's attitude irritated me to the point of rebellion. On the evening before the meeting, I asked him if there was still time to submit amendments. He replied that of course there was so long as they were delivered to the committee table before the meeting began.

As we set out the following day, I showed Gerritsen an envelope and said, "Here are the amendments I am going to hand in." He said, "I hope you know what you are doing. Because I'm going to oppose you as best I can!" That sounded ominous, but I was not going to be put off.

At the time there were very few female members of the Liberal Democratic Union, and at that meeting I was the only one present. When my amendments came up for discussion, the chairman asked me, with extreme formality, "Does Dr. Jacobs wish to expound upon her amendments?" I replied that the points in question were completely in accordance with our principles and as such could not be omitted from the manifesto. Hence, I felt that further explanations were unnecessary, but if there were any objections I would happily elucidate my point of view. There were indeed objections, first from the audience and then from the commission itself. And it was Gerritsen, the chairman, who opposed the inclusion of these two points with all his considerable intelligence. I feared that I was fighting a losing battle, but, because I was convinced that I was right, I did my best to disprove these arguments. Much to my delight, my amendments were accepted by a small majority.

After the meeting, Gerritsen came up to me, put his arm around my shoulder, and said, laughing, "I must congratulate you on your success!" The men who witnessed this scene were amazed, and one of the more prominent party members announced, "I am astonished that such a difference of opinion can be resolved like this!" Apparently everyone expected me to be thoroughly reprimanded for publicly disagreeing with my husband. How little these people knew us! The following morning, a report of the meeting in one of the Amsterdam newspapers criticized the whole event and used it as a pretext to attack woman suffrage. This was what happened when women began to meddle in politics: it led to public conflict between husbands and wives!

As I previously mentioned, Gerritsen served on the Amsterdam City Council up until his death and was a member of the Dutch parliament from 1893 to 1897. He was also a member of the Provincial Estates of North Holland until his death, and from 1899 to 1902 he was the Amsterdam alderman for commerce and poor relief. Because of his dedication to his work and our deep involvement with each other, I must have been one of the few women to receive a thorough education in both legal and practical aspects of many social issues. My situation also gave me the opportunity to exert influence whenever the interests of girls or women were under discussion. Of course, it is impossible to know precisely what influence I had, if any, but at least I had the satisfaction of involvement.

I was particularly pleased that, when Gerritsen became an alderman, he was asked to be in charge of Poor Relief, which included the city's hospitals, orphanages, and old people's homes. I was able to work indirectly for their improvement and for the abolition of various abuses I had encountered over the years at these institutions. Above all, the way in which poor patients were treated convinced us of the need for reform. "With energy and enthusiasm, with determination and courage," as one of the Amsterdam papers described his approach after his death, Gerritsen began to reorganize those antediluvian institutions so that they could provide more reasonable and humane forms of welfare. In this transformation, he was able to rely on the wealth of knowledge concerning modern attitudes toward such establishments we had compiled during our many trips abroad. Fortunately, by now these views were also shared by many people here in the Netherlands. But it took great courage and perseverance to pursue some reforms because inevitably the directors of these institutions and other interested parties opposed such measures purely out of conservatism or self-interest. No matter how much opposition he encountered, Gerritsen never for one moment wavered. On the contrary, he was inspired to make renewed efforts to achieve his goals.

It was particularly galling to see how Amsterdam doctors opposed Gerritsen's reforms of the medical services provided through Poor Relief. One wondered why they should resist the improvement of a situation that was unworthy of the City of Amsterdam and of council doctors employed to run these clinics for the poor. The only possible explanation for their attitude was that they were ashamed that some of their number had recently demanded an end to the inhumane treatment of poor people. It required a medical layman to take the initiative to reorganize these services along more humanitarian lines, and Gerritsen spared no one his all-too-obvious disapproval.

The unfair way in which Amsterdam doctors voiced their opposition had a disastrous effect on Gerritsen's health, which already gave cause for concern. When his proposals were passed by the council and he began looking for a physician to carry out his reforms, the doctors took their revenge by exerting such pressure that no one dared apply for the post for fear of repercussions within the medical establishment. This boycott threatened to undermine the reforms, which could easily have come to nothing had not Dr. Menno Huizinga finally come forward in defiance of the doctors of Amsterdam and agreed to become the medical service's director.

When Gerritsen died some years later, all the papers praised his "reform of Poor Relief medical services, which was a godsend to all poor patients" as being one of his most important achievements. My explanation that the Amsterdam doctors' behavior was due to a sense of shame was later borne out by what the physicians themselves published about the Poor Relief medical services. While Gerritsen is described as the prime mover of the reorganization, not a word appears about the prevailing attitude of the doctors themselves. Fortunately, in a book published on September 21, 1923 to mark the seventy-fifth anniversary of the Amsterdam Medical Circle, Dr. L. Heijermans, director of the medical service, describes his department's development and fully acknowledges the impact of Alderman Gerritsen's 1901 initiative.

At the start of 1904, Gerritsen began to suffer from strange and worrisome symptoms. Yet, when he consulted a doctor, nothing untoward was discovered. He decided that the symptoms were due to too much hard work. He suggested that I give up my practice entirely so that we could both take an extended holiday; then he would return in a much better frame of mind and an improved state of health.

I was extremely tempted by this suggestion, especially since we were planning to spend some time in North America to learn about the prevailing social conditions there. In order to meet with the American authorities and acquire the necessary contacts, we decided to start by attending the meeting of the Interparliamentary Union, which was to be held in St. Louis in August 1904.

Our plans began to take shape, but before I retired from my practice Gerritsen wanted me to celebrate the twenty-fifth anniversary of my doctorate in medicine. The day in question was March 8, 1904 (although, due to a mistake by the organizing committee, the festivities were actually held on March 18). Gerritsen also helped with the preparations but made sure that I knew nothing of what lay in store. A women's committee was formed to ensure that March 8, 1904, would be a day I would never forget. This committee consisted of the following ladies: Th. P. B. Haver, J. van Buuren-Huys, Martina Kramers, W. Drucker, Schöffer-Bunge, Van Loenen-de Bordes, and E. Kerlen.[10]

In a constant stream that began first thing in the morning, flowers, telegrams, letters, newspapers, and magazines from home and abroad were delivered to our house. They celebrated an event that was apparently important not only for myself but for a great many others as well. Many former patients took the opportunity to present me with tangible proof of their gratitude. In addition, the central committees of a number of organizations, which I was glad to see included workers' groups, sent messages of appreciation and friendship in letters, verse, and telegrams. All the national and local papers in Holland published shorter or longer versions of my life story, sometimes accompanied by personal memories and impressions. I would like to include a number of these pieces here.

In the *Sociaal Weekblad,* Cornélie Huygens wrote,

It soon became obvious that there was a considerable demand for female practitioners. Her practice was successful from the very start and grew daily. Considering the prejudice that existed against a "woman doctor," this achievement probably caused considerable astonishment, particularly in a country whose cautious attitude to the strange or new is positively proverbial. However, the reason for her popularity was immediately apparent to all those who met Dr. Aletta Jacobs in person.

For those who noticed this young girl's natural composure and observed her thorough and unflinching treatment of patients were convinced that she had found her true vocation, that as a doctor she had entered a field that would fully use her very considerable talents.

This tremendous strength of mind, *une grâce d'état* for any doctor, is obvious for all to see. Even in the most difficult of moments, her bedside manner remains clear-sighted, her hands firm, her voice gentle and encouraging, her influence calming. The writer of this article has had ample opportunity to admire how in these moments her innate femininity is combined with a masculine willpower. And here I would like to draw particular attention to the unique qualities of our first woman doctor that can normally only be appreciated by her patients and their families.

Total femininity is at the root of her entire being and reveals itself in all manner of details. The care with which she runs her home and her choice of hobbies eloquently attest to the fact that the interests of science need not weaken the aura of womanhood.

De Telegraaf ran an article written by a certain J. C. The following is an extract,

Whenever she speaks of unpleasant experiences, her calm and friendly face creases into an engaging laugh, although such incidents must have caused her considerable pain when they occurred. Nonetheless she has always fought her way through. This spirit was typical of her student days and is something she has always maintained, along with an absolute decisiveness.

She has clearly formulated opinions on various social issues. She is an activist, and also, whenever possible, writes about her ideas, addressing the public directly in a style that is simple and to the point.

Her medical practice has almost always been restricted to women, a group that had been consistently underserved; hence she has been consulted by ever increasing numbers of patients. This gave her the opportunity to thoroughly study the needs of people in general and women in particular and has provided her with the insight to understand how and where improvements could be introduced.

With this insight, she has always spoken out in support of measures that would lead to these improvements.

Often this involved considerable moral courage, as was demonstrated by her 1883 attempt to register as a voter, which she knew would be met with derision and slander.

Courageous is also the only word to describe her struggle against that most ancient of social ills: prostitution.

She has always been quick to help women whenever necessary. During her twenty-five years of medical practice she has had the satisfaction of seeing various of her initiatives become law, such as the measures now being introduced to improve salesgirls' working conditions, especially with regard to the time they must spend on their feet.

Even if she had done nothing further with her life, her achievements as a seventeen-year-old girl would have earned her the admiration of many. For devoting her next twenty-five years to the reform of major social abuses, for doing all in her power to help bring about women's economic and political independence, she deserves the respect of all concerned about the world's suffering, all who share even a twinge of that powerful feeling called altruism.

And when she stood waiting to receive me in loose, dark clothing that blended with the soft shadows of her room, she seemed, despite all her decisiveness and strength, the ideal of gentle, sensitive womanliness.

The Sunday edition of *de Echo* also included an article about me that concluded with the following:

I would like to add a few words of appreciation that may also serve to remind women that the fact they are now generally considered to be men's intellectual equals, and publicly respected as such, is largely due to the campaigns and personal example of Dr. Aletta Jacobs.

Over the years, the woman's movement has been blighted by the involvement of alien elements that have unwisely meddled in affairs that do not concern them, are beyond their understanding, and are being incorrectly exploited with disastrous results. There has been an unfortunate misunderstanding of the essential inner difference that incontrovertibly exists—though not with regard to intellectual equality—between men and women.

This is in no way the fault of women such as Dr. Aletta Jacobs, and it is disheartening to see how the glory of her life's work is soiled in such a clumsy, ignorant fashion.

When seeking to identify the commendable and the sublime in movements such as that for women's emancipation, one must always focus on the most intelligent and sensitive of leaders.

Dr. Aletta Jacobs is one such example, par excellence.

The women of Holland owe much to her.

And for the monthly magazine of the Dutch Association for Woman Suffrage, Miss W. Drucker wrote an article that opens with the following lines,

> Ten years ago, Mr. Louis Frank, the well-known feminist, remarked to me that it is a sad but undeniable fact that women who earn degrees tend now to be pedantic and arrogant. Whoever this may apply to, it is clearly of no relevance to the woman who celebrated twenty-five years of medical practice on March 18, the first woman to be awarded a degree in Holland, Dr. Aletta H. Jacobs. At first, no one would suspect that this cheerful and vivacious person is also a highly educated woman. Neither in meetings nor *en petit comité* [informally] does she employ the authoritarian tactics of the university graduate. She is a doctor to her patients, but not in daily life, and, as such, an example her male colleagues would benefit from emulating.

I have been writing this chapter with a pile of magazines beside me that come from the United States, Canada, England, Scandinavia, Germany, Austria, and Hungary. All of them include articles about my anniversary and my work. However, fact has been so frequently mixed with fiction that I will desist from quoting from them.

The committee organizing this day of celebrations laid a wreath that morning on Thorbecke's statue to honor the man who first permitted a woman to attend a university in 1871. That afternoon, a reception was held at the Unity building for all those who wished to congratulate me in person. Gerritsen accompanied me to this event, which attracted many guests.

Mrs. Haver gave a speech on behalf of the committee and many of the women of Holland, and presented me with a statue called "La Victoire." The base was inscribed with the words, "To Dr. Aletta H. Jacobs, 1879-1904, the first woman doctor of the Netherlands." Mrs. Haver also made a point of praising Gerritsen as being one of the first men in our country to appreciate a woman on her own terms and to support her constantly in her struggle for emancipation.

Without my knowing about it, Gerritsen had also invited the committee and a number of good friends to a festive dinner that evening.

Once the celebrations were over, I still wanted to attend the June 1904 conference of the International Council of Women in Berlin before we embarked on our trip to the States. In addition, there was much to be arranged before leaving the country for so long a time. The Child Welfare Conference was to be held in The Hague from April 7 to 9. This organization had developed out of the National Women's Council of which I was vice president. Since the president was abroad, I had to take her place at this event, so once again I found myself caught up in all the commotion involved in preparing a conference. Hence, we decided to complete this work and to make reservations on the Holland-America line for a late-July/early-August sailing from Rotterdam to New York.

During the last few days of our stay in Berlin, Gerritsen again developed the symptoms from which he had previously suffered. I began to dread undertaking an ambitious journey, but took comfort in the fact that nothing abnormal had been found in the many medical tests he had undergone. Probably, I hoped, the symptoms were due to a bad case of nerves. I felt considerably reassured when he was soon back to himself after a couple of days of rest. I hoped that the combination of a long journey and a new environment would improve his health.

After reading the latest books about North America, we felt prepared for anything we might encounter. But reality bore little relation to the books. We had both agreed to mail occasional articles to two Amsterdam newspapers. Gerritsen would write for the *Algemeen Handelsblad* and I would work for *de Telegraaf*.[11] We had been issued press cards, which were to prove invaluable in America. We discovered on this journey that journalists abroad enjoy many privileges denied to the regular tourist. In America, our press cards often proved more effective than even the most prestigious introductions.

When we arrived in New York, for the first time ever we encountered problems because of our different surnames. While America was always portrayed as a free and democratic society, we caused a positive uproar when we attempted to register at a fashionable hotel by signing our individual names. At Holland House, we were given the choice of either taking two rooms or signing for one under a single name. We opted for the latter. It was at my husband's insistence that *I* signed the visitor's book. We had to stick to this arrangement throughout our stay in New York and the rest of America.

Since we had arrived in New York well ahead of the start of the Interparliamentary Union meeting, we used the opportunity to meet many of the people with whom we had either already corresponded about social issues or to whom we had letters of introduction. Also, we were able to see more of the city than would have been possible otherwise. In addition, we benefited from much good advice concerning the planning of our journey through America and were able to collect all the information we needed to visit a number of important institutions in different states.

Here is one example of this process. Mr. Samuel Barrows, who was a member of Congress and a prominent expert on the American prison system, provided me with an official permit to visit any prison or reformatory.[12] I used it as often as I could, and along with the oppressive old-style prisons I was able to discover the admirable system that had been recently introduced into various reformatories and was as yet unknown in Holland. I wrote a detailed report for *de Telegraaf* about one of these visits, to the Sherborn Reformatory in Massachusetts, a women's prison. Not long after I returned to the Netherlands, something happened that made this article especially worthwhile. The director of the special women's prison in Gorinchem wrote to me that "reading your article has led to a extremely positive development. The chairman has presented our one inmate with a rose bush she can look after in her cell, with which she is absolutely delighted." What more could I have wished from my travel letters than that a little sunshine was brought into the inhuman existence to which we condemn so many of our convicts?

The letters that Gerritsen sent to the *Handelsblad* reveal that in all the states we visited, he gravitated toward studying labor conditions, in particular the relationships between employer and employee and the laws that influence them. He carefully studied education, libraries, and banking, and he kept detailed notes even on those subjects that were omitted from his travel letters and that he planned to write about at greater length in the future.

Apart from visiting a great many prisons, I was also extremely interested in the hospital system and the legal and social position of nursing staff. Wherever I went, I sought contact with the leaders of the woman suffrage associations in order to learn more about how this campaign was being waged in America and about the reactions of the various states.

On September 6, 1904, we left New York with three hundred congress delegates for St. Louis. The American government had provided two special trains, consisting exclusively of Pullman cars, and was also paying both for the journey and for our luxurious stay in St. Louis. En route we first visited Philadelphia, where we were received by city representatives who showed us the most noteworthy sights. Similarly, in Pittsburgh an excellent guide showed us around Carnegie's factories.

When the St. Louis meeting was over, the visitors were to be transported back to New York, once again in special trains. On the return journey, we first went to Kansas City and although we had only a few hours, we still managed to see much of the town because many private citizens offered to drive us around in their cars. The next day we arrived in Colorado. Another train, waiting for us in Colorado Springs, took us ten thousand feet above sea level to Cripple Creek where we visited a gold mine and a mine workers' camp. Had I been familiar with the books of Upton Sinclair, I doubtless would have viewed the miners' lives in a different light.

When we arrived in Denver, Carel and I decided to bid our companions farewell and stay on for a few days before heading west. I was glad that Gerritsen agreed to this plan because the commotion of the previous few days had obviously tired him and taxed his nerves. After several days' rest, he felt strong enough to resume our journey to Wyoming, where we wanted to visit Yellowstone Park. Next we headed for Salt Lake City in Utah. I had some good friends living there whom I had alerted to our imminent arrival. During our stay, we got to know far more about the Mormons and their beliefs than we had been able to discover from travelers' tales and newspaper articles. We both came to the conclusion that, like any faith, the Mormon religion is a mixture of good and bad that is in turn reflected among its followers. Since then I have often been able to argue against and disprove many erroneous ideas concerning the Mormons.

This book is not the place for a more elaborate description of our journey through North America. But I would like to mention briefly that we traveled from Utah to California, from San Francisco to Los Angeles, and from there to Arizona, New Mexico, Illinois, and then back again to New York. We had many opportunities to see the wonders of North America, including the Yosemite Valley in California, the Grand Canyon, and the cliff dwellings in Arizona, and, of course, Niagara Falls in upstate New York. Wherever we went, we tried to learn as much as we could about the land and its people, particularly its primitive peoples. I was fascinated by the lives of various Indian tribes and of the Negroes and, as far as was possible for an outsider, I attempted to communicate with them so that I could learn more about their world.

As the year drew to a close, I began to long for home, particularly since Gerritsen's symptoms were returning more frequently and he had visibly lost weight.

We arrived in Amsterdam in January 1905. All the political parties were busily preparing for a general election in June. We were hardly back home before Gerritsen was immediately asked to stand for Parliament in two constituencies. He had felt ill during the voyage and had scarcely ventured out of bed. He was now losing more and more weight. I feared that electioneering would seriously aggravate his condition, which I could not as yet name or evaluate. I used all my powers of persuasion to convince him not to stand as a candidate and to work for his party only insofar as his health would permit.

It made no difference. The election was a matter of national importance. The right-wing cabinet had to be thrown out at all costs. Personal concerns were to be put aside and there was no choice but to work with all one's powers toward this one vital goal. And as he pointed out, "You'd be the last to back out for reasons like that!"

Gerritsen accepted both candidacies, which meant that he was constantly shuttling back and forth between Schoterland and Den Helder to give speeches or to debate with opponents. And each time he returned home, I realized that he was looking progressively more unhealthy. I begged him to give up the election, to allow others to take his place. But he simply would not listen to me. Finally, when one day he discovered that he was unable to get out of bed, he asked me to call a physician who was also a friend of his. Although this doctor was clearly concerned by what he saw, he would not as yet risk a diagnosis.

It was on Election Day itself, just after Gerritsen had been cheered by the news of his victory in Den Helder, that, after consulting other doctors involved, Professor Pel broke the news to me that there was nothing they could do and Gerritsen was not expected to survive for long. In a relatively short time, his previously sturdy constitution was ravaged by stomach and liver cancer.

Gerritsen remained lucid up to the last day and was delighted that the left-wing parties had won the election. He talked about the new cabinet's formation with friends who came to visit and I had to relate or read aloud everything that appeared in the papers on that subject. He was unaware that the end was near, and I made sure he never realized just how ill he was.

He went quietly to sleep on July 5, 1905.

All the papers marked his passing with appreciative articles about Gerritsen's life and works. I would like to include a few extracts because they describe him so accurately.

From *de Telegraaf* of July 5, 1905,

It was as early as 1888 that Amsterdam voters first sent C. V. Gerritsen to City Hall and there, both as a Town Council member and as an alderman, he gave his best to public life. Of the small group of Radicals, he was always one of the most passionate, guaranteed to leave his opponents in a state of high fury.

His speeches certainly outraged a great many people, but despite this, and because of his energy, diligence, and dedication, he became an alderman in 1898 and was made responsible for Poor Relief and Commerce. Amsterdam owes much to him. As a new alderman, he immediately set about reforming the appalling state of welfare services and will be particularly remembered for the conflict that his medical service measures provoked among many of the city's doctors. He refused to give in and ultimately triumphed. Despite its recent introduction, this new service has already achieved wonders and is a godsend to all poor people in this city. This achievement undoubtedly represents Gerritsen's finest hour as an alderman.

And as the July 5, 1905 issue of the workers' newspaper *de Echo* attests,

There were certain characteristic similarities about all Gerritsen's achievements for this city: a common spirit and identity pervaded them all because each plan was conceived and developed by a man whose sole intent was to break with the past. He took on the task of sweeping away all that was faulty and pernicious and that proliferated in an era in which the work of the city fathers was still shrouded in secrecy, far from public scrutiny.

There is ample reason for us to regret Mr. Gerritsen's retirement from his post as Amsterdam alderman. To this day, we lack the knowledge, talent, extraordinary energy, and far-sighted policies of a man such as Gerritsen.

Death seldom comes at the right point in time; in this case it deals a particularly heavy blow.

For after a lifetime of work and sacrifice for the common good, this man has been struck down at the very moment that his life's ambition was about to be achieved.

Once again, I had lost my life's supporter and companion, and the future seemed dark and lonely without him.

ELEVEN

FROM 1905 TO 1911

The Prospects for Woman Suffrage under the Borgesius Government • Presenting Our Requests to H. M. the Queen During the Constitutional Reform • The Advent of English Suffragettes • The Copenhagen Conference and the Decision to Hold the Next Congress in the Netherlands in 1908 • Interviews with Members of Various Parliamentary Groups • Preparations for the 1908 Congress • In the High Tatras and Sarajevo • Convalescence in Zurich • Travel Plans with Mrs. Catt

After Gerritsen's death, it was a long time before I could resume work. I was well aware that he would not have wanted me to succumb to grief, and yet I found it very difficult to continue my life as before. Sorrow and lack of sleep had left my nerves in a terrible state. I felt even worse when the gray days of winter set in. A change of air seemed called for, and I decided to go to St. Moritz, which had not as yet become a vacation spot for foreigners seeking sports and leisure. Daily sunbathing improved my health enormously. What is more, as a stranger there, I met many people who were also trying to come to terms with grief, and hearing their stories helped me to get past my own sorrow.

When I returned to Amsterdam at the beginning of 1906, I launched wholeheartedly into my work for the Association for Woman Suffrage. The Borgesius-Rink government, which had assumed office in 1905, was preparing constitutional reforms in which Clause 80, the clause that defined the conditions of suffrage, would be left blank. "A blank Clause 80" had been the rallying cry of the parliamentary majority and had enabled the Borgesius government to come to power.

The constitutional reform commission had already been chosen by the time I returned from St. Moritz. Also, all the left-wing groups had formulated their own demands. But I felt that our association should be involved, not only with regard to this particular clause but also with regard to all aspects of the constitution that directly affected the lives of women. Anna Polak, W. Drucker, and M. W. H. Rutgers-Hoitsema assumed responsibility for this work.[1]

During the queen's visit to Amsterdam on May 3, 1906, Mrs. Rutgers-Hoitsema and I presented Her Majesty with a document that had been approved by the association. Clause 80 was formulated as follows: "The Law determines which men and women are entitled to vote and eligible to run for office." We also proposed the revision of all clauses that affected a woman's right to self-determination. The next day we presented a copy of this document to Mr. Rink, the minister for internal affairs, with whom we freely discussed the chances for constitutional reform.

We were not so foolish as to imagine that our demands would be immediately granted, but we believed that this approach would best acquaint both the highest authorities and the Dutch people with our demand that women vote under the same conditions that applied or would soon apply to men. Since we believed that this was the cheapest and most effective way of campaigning, we also sent copies of our document to every minister and member of parliament, to the council of state, and to all the newspapers. By the next morning, our demands had been seen by thousands of people. According to their political persuasion, the newspapers either endorsed or dismissed our work. That week's issue of *de Amsterdammer, Weekblad voor Nederland* included an illustration of the queen mother talking to the queen. The caption read, "Justice, my daughter, is something that brings greatness to a small country."

At that time, our association consisted of no more than two thousand members. For that reason, I made a point of visiting remote areas each week to speak about woman suffrage and to explore the possibility of establishing new chapters. We were always short of cash and were more than happy to accept the offers of local innkeepers to use their meeting rooms for little or no money provided we purchased our refreshments from them. I was usually accompanied by a younger association member in training as a speaker. I particularly remember my trips with Mrs. C. S. Groot, our incomparable "Marijtje," who later won the hearts of those who saw her in traditional rural costume North Holland.[2] Together we covered the entire area north of the IJssel River. She was always surrounded by a cheerful group of young women who acted as her entourage. They were invariably sensible but naive village girls who were thrilled to sleep in a real hotel.

I also visited a part of the province of Groningen with Mrs. Bakker-Nort, who was still studying law and had yet to imagine becoming a member of parliament.[3] We will never forget our extraordinary adventures on the trip to Veendam, Stadskanaal, and Winschoten, and they certainly deserve a place in this book. We held our first meeting in Veendam, and awoke the following morning full of high spirits because we had succeeded in attracting a number of new members who had immediately formed their own chapter complete with a governing committee. So we had certainly carried out our task in Veendam. The weather was good and in a couple of hours we were due to catch the horse-drawn tram to Stadskanaal, where we hoped to set up another chapter that same evening. We decided not to wait for the tram but to walk until it caught up with us. At first we followed the street, which petered out into sand once we left the built-up area. Until then the weather had been bright, but suddenly it began to rain heavily. Unfortunately, we were totally unprepared and were soon soaked to the skin, wading through mud in town shoes. We decided to take shelter at the first house we might pass, which turned out to be a small emporium. The bell rang loudly as we entered, but there was not a soul in sight. We looked around, but the place was apparently deserted. We felt it could be dangerous to wait so we resumed our trek through the mud and puddles. After several kilometers, we reached a small house and saw three women sitting inside. The youngest of the three invited us in. We did not have to introduce ourselves because they knew who we were. They knew we were the only nonlocal women likely to pass by since they had read in the newspaper that we had spoken on woman suffrage the previous evening in Veendam and were to speak the next evening in Stadskanaal. They let us dry our clothes by a blazing log fire and brought us cups of cinnamon coffee, which is considered a treat of the region but that we found virtually undrinkable. Meanwhile the women chatted in their dialect about woman suffrage and we soon realized that they were on our side. In fact they even provided us with a few new arguments!

The tram arrived at last and we said goodbye to our charming hosts. At about 6 P.M. we finally reached the inn at Stadskanaal where we were scheduled to speak, hoping to be greeted by a warm meal. Instead we discovered that the place was deserted, and without even any furniture. We heard from the local people that the innkeeper had gone bankrupt and disappeared. What were we to do? We knew no one we could ask to put us up for the night and were convinced that the meeting had been canceled altogether. After some discussion, we wired our Winschoten chapter, asking for a coach to be sent to fetch us and to bring us some food since we hadn't eaten since early that morning.

Meanwhile people were beginning to arrive for our meeting and, as always, we were happy to champion our cause. In the barn, we discovered a ladder, a number of empty barrels, and some rope. By placing the ladder over the barrels, we managed to provide adequate seating for the ladies, while the gentlemen—who were farmers—preferred to remain standing. We borrowed a few lanterns, which we strung up with the rope, and we had soon improvised the perfect atmosphere in which to convince our audience of the benefits of woman suffrage.

The coach arrived from Winschoten at about 11 P.M. and two of the committee members emerged with a large hamper full of the most delicious sandwiches and a bottle of good wine. The coachman did not want to return immediately as his horses needed at least an hour's rest. So we went back to the barn, sat down on our ladder bench, and used an empty barrel as a table for the sandwiches and wine. We finally left well after midnight and arrived in Winschoten between 3 and 4 A.M. I have never been quite sure whether our lightheartedness was due to the wine—and I must admit that I am not used to alcohol—or to the adventures of that day, but that long, dark journey in the dead of night through the middle of nowhere seemed to be over in a trice—so quickly that its memory still causes great amusement.

During this politically active period, there were many opportunities to publish newspaper articles about woman suffrage. We particularly welcomed any form of opposition because that automatically gave us the right of reply. For example, an article that appeared in *de Nederlander,* a newspaper edited by the excellent Mr. de Savornin Lohman, asked the question, "Will Woman Suffrage Influence the Course of History?" While the question was answered dismissively, the article also concluded that there were no reasonable grounds for denying independent unmarried women the right to vote. Obviously, here was a perfect opportunity to bring our demands to the attention of Christian-Historic women.[4] My approach argued that every reform, no matter how insignificant, has left its mark on world history, and therefore an important reform, such as the political equality of the sexes, would necessarily have a major influence on global events. In addition, I refuted all the objections of our otherwise likeable opponent. He responded to my comments, which meant that once again I had the right of reply.

We met with much opposition in the Roman Catholic press, but our counterarguments soon won us a great many new adherents in this camp. We certainly preferred this kind of opposition to that of the liberal papers, whose tactics were to ridicule our cause and then to ignore us.

Nineteen hundred and six proved to be a remarkable year for women's enfranchisement in a number of ways. After the International Woman Suffrage Association had been established at the 1904 Berlin conference, it was decided that the international activists would meet in Copenhagen in June 1906. All participating countries would be involved in the preparations. Holland was to be represented by twelve delegates led by myself as the association's president.

It was at the Copenhagen conference that we first heard an English suffragette describe her movement in terms of its national importance. She also revealed the truth behind newspaper reports that had been published throughout the world. From its inception, I had disliked this movement's militancy, but I had to admit that it had brought us closer to achieving our goal. Millions of people who had not heard or read of suffrage, and hence had never thought about it, were now being confronted with the subject almost every day, albeit most often in news reports full of half-truths and exaggerations. And many had come to the same conclusion as had the Bishop of London after sitting down to breakfast one day and discovering that a bomb had been placed under his chair. "If civilized women are driven to such extremes," reflected His Lordship, "they must attach great importance to the right to vote." As a result, he began to read statements published by moderate suffrage workers, and ultimately he publicly proclaimed his support for woman suffrage.

In Holland, we also profited from the struggle of these courageous militants. Many liberal newspapers now commended Dutch campaigners for their calm and moderate behavior; there was an obvious anxiety that we might choose to follow the suffragettes' example. Certainly their work helped us at least to the extent that we were no longer ignored and were sometimes even praised.

At the Copenhagen conference, it was decided that I should accompany alliance president Mrs. Carrie Chapman Catt to Austria-Hungary to help organize a local campaign. I have already described this trip in chapter 6. One other decision made at Copenhagen was of particular significance for us here in the Netherlands. Our delegation knew that the Dutch parliament would be debating the constitutional reform in either 1908 or 1909, so we decided to invite the alliance to hold their next conference in the Netherlands in June 1908. This invitation was gratefully accepted, and we returned home full of plans to ensure the success of "our" conference.

Nineteen hundred and six was also an important year for us as it marked the twelve-and-a-half-year anniversary of our founding.[5] We wanted to hold a day of celebration for our members, which would also create some useful publicity. This entailed a lot of extra work, but, needless to say, I always found many willing women for whom no task was too menial and no effort too great. They took on everything with love and dedication, whether it involved speaking engagements, helping a group of women to set up a new chapter, or simply working late into the night folding circulars, placing them in envelopes, and sticking on stamps. The Association for Woman Suffrage has always been able to count on committee members and volunteers to work selflessly and without expecting even the slightest token of appreciation. Because everyone was well aware of the importance of what we were doing, no sacrifice was considered too great to help further our cause.

Despite the seriousness with which we took our work, the general meetings, attended by all the local leaders, often seemed like parties and provided us with ample opportunity to encourage or console each other. This continued until 1906 when a small group of women attempted to replace the three members of the executive committee, including myself, who were up for reelection. The forthcoming 1908 alliance conference was also a factor in this whole situation.[6]

I was traveling with Mrs. Chapman Catt in Hungary during the election campaign but was delighted to hear that all three of us had won by an enormous majority. My pleasure came not simply from knowing that I could continue in the leadership but also because the association remained a strong and unified organization.

I continued to work throughout 1906, although it was always painful to return home to find that there was no one to share in my successes, to comfort me for each disappointment, and to consult on the most effective means of opposition. Most of all I missed the intellectual atmosphere I had enjoyed at home for so many years. Initially it was even difficult to send off articles without first showing them to a kindred spirit, as had been my custom with Gerritsen. Slowly I adjusted to the situation and regained my self-confidence.

Nineteen hundred and seven was also a busy year. Government circles were discussing married women's right to work, which had been scandalously curtailed by the Kuyper regime, but reinstated by the next cabinet, which included Mr. Rink as minister for internal affairs. Parliament was also debating the Children's Acts, and the Constitutional Reform bill had been submitted as well. These proposals directly involved women's interests and so our association soon had its hands full. We were very often involved in discussions with leaders of different political factions; we spoke with ministers and delivered requests to the government; we held public meetings and prepared information sheets. Our talks with these leaders often provided us with singular insights as to why these "peoples' delegates" opposed or supported particular proposals. The women we represented were always well informed about each subject that came up for debate. By contrast, some of the politicians had such a low opinion of female intelligence that they apparently considered it unnecessary to prepare for our discussions.

We were received by Messrs. de Savornin Lohman and van Idsinga and Count van Bylandt on behalf of the Christian-Historic group. I was asked to speak first and expressed the hope that these talks would lead to increased sympathy for our cause so that their group would advocate a revised constitution that included woman suffrage. Mr. van Idsinga reminded us that his party's members of parliament had agreed to meet with us so that we could inform them of any new developments concerning female enfranchisement. I pointed out that the situation was changing each day as women were becoming increasingly aware of the ways in which our country suffered as a result of their being unable to influence its laws. For instance, the new Children's Acts were about to be introduced. As pleased as we were that steps had been taken to provide for the legal protection of children, we nonetheless felt that it was absurd that these laws had been passed without the active participation of the women of Holland, who were, after all, the mothers of our next generation. Men had been solely responsible for these acts, which would radically affect the relationship between mother and child and introduce an element of government influence into an area previously considered to be a woman's domain. As if men were the ones who best understood the hearts and souls of children! These laws would have been very different had they been created by men and women working in collaboration.

I also spoke at length about still other laws, and about meetings and articles through which Christian-Historics who were not members of parliament had opposed woman suffrage. Mr. de Savornin Lohman then asked if we had ever considered that women might achieve just as much for society through their indirect influence as they would through more direct means. And if both men and women were able to vote, how would this affect family life? Johanna W. A. Naber replied, and Count van Bylandt then asked whether, if they were granted the franchise, women would also be prepared to fulfill military duties.[7] He said that in his mind's eye he could already see us marching along with our guns across our shoulders and, to make himself perfectly clear, he described the scene in graphic detail. We had just published an article on this very subject for the Roman Catholic newspaper *de Gelderlander,* so it was easy to refute his arguments. Finally Mr. Lohman commented in a friendly manner that his party had not yet considered any of this, and it needed to be thoroughly investigated before any decision could be reached.

We then met with a very different group. Association members M. G. Kramers and S. Tilma-Schaaff were received by Messrs. Troelstra and Ter Laan, the leaders of the Social Democratic Workers' Party. They flatly rejected any suggestion of woman suffrage. Although they felt that all men should be granted the franchise, they argued that women were not yet ready to vote. Mr. Troelstra added that he himself would oppose granting women immediate universal suffrage. It goes without saying that our representatives pointed out the inconsistencies of this argument. Moreover, they were parliamentary representatives of a political party that officially supported universal enfranchisement for both men and women.

I should add that we always mentioned in advance that we intended to publish a full report of all our talks.

Meeting these members of parliament made us realize how little they knew about this subject. Even those who supported our cause out of a sense of justice were, in general, unfamiliar with specific details. Hence, our association's executive committee decided to publish a small book containing all the various arguments used to support the introduction of woman suffrage and to send a copy to every member of parliament.

Apart from our suffrage campaign, we were also working day in and day out to prepare for the 1908 Amsterdam conference. We realized that we needed plenty of time to prepare because of our lack of experience, as this was the first international women's conference to be held in our country. We knew that we would need to plan everything thoroughly. The conference would be expensive and we were not certain that nonmembers would also be prepared to support us financially. We formed a steering committee led by myself with Miss W. Drucker as treasurer. She could call on as many members as she needed to help acquire the necessary funding. And although she was assisted by a great many other women, Miss Drucker was the only person who was directly answerable to the committee. As it turned out, her group was so successful that the money raised financed our campaign literature well after the conference had ended.

Mrs. Van Loenen-de Bordes assumed responsibility for all the organizational tasks, such as the hiring of suitable premises, finding lodgings for our guests, making name badges, cleaning the halls during the conference, and a thousand other similar items. Johanna W. A. Naber took care of press liaison and overseas communications. Mrs. van Buuren-Huys dealt with mail within the Netherlands and recorded the minutes of our numerous committee meetings. Mrs. Schöffer-Bunge and Mrs. Gomperts-Jitta worked to prepare the opening reception and all the other conference festivities.

I was not in charge of any one committee but coordinated all of them and tried to solve problems whenever they arose. The steering committee meetings were always held at my house. At first these took place monthly, later every two weeks, and finally once a week. Each member would report on her work and present ideas or suggestions. Then we would review the new plans and examine problems or mistakes. We soon managed to find a suitable location although it was at a price that seemed positively astronomical. For two thousand guilders, we were offered the whole of the Concertgebouw in Amsterdam.

Our president, Mrs. Chapman Catt, arrived two months before the conference was due to start. She was called "the uncrowned queen" by her many admirers because of her majestic demeanor, her natural authority, and her kindness. She and I were to work together on international business and on organizing the conference agenda. We also had to ensure that all the festivities and sight-seeing opportunities did not conflict with the conference itself.

The event was to take place from June 15 to 20. On Sunday, June 14, a recital was held in the main auditorium of the Concertgebouw. It lasted until midnight, when we were allowed to take over the building. Two women from the steering committee made sure that the entire place was cleaned that night. The cleaners were just leaving as the first visitors arrived at nine o'clock the next morning.

It would take an extended chapter to describe this event in any detail. But, in short, in my opinion the Amsterdam conference was never surpassed by any other meeting of the International Woman Suffrage Alliance and was perhaps only equalled by the 1911 Stockholm conference. The Dutch women certainly created quite a reputation for themselves as being excellent organizers.

I must not forget to mention that the reason we had originally invited the alliance to this 1908 conference was by December 1907 no longer relevant. The Borgesius cabinet had been forced to resign and was replaced by the Heemskerk government, which openly opposed our cause. Of course, we had hoped that the conference would help influence the constitutional reform debate. Although they were too limited in scope, we were nonetheless pleased with the proposed revisions. But now nothing would change for the time being and there was obviously no advantage to be gained from the conference in that respect.

On the other hand, it brought in hundreds of new members and marked an abrupt turnabout in public opinion. Many newspapers published detailed reports accompanied by illustrations both serious and humorous. *De Amsterdammer, Weekblad voor Nederland* was particularly notable for its visual material.

After the conference, I spent several weeks working with Mrs. Chapman Catt on the conference report, which was to be printed in Amsterdam. Our national committee also had business to complete and I was still busy with domestic duties as some of my five guests had decided to stay on after the conference. Once everything was back in order, I set off on a long and relaxing journey with Mrs. Catt. Our final destination was Geneva where the international board and committee members of the International Council of Women were due to meet in September. That still left us with plenty of time for our travels. My charming companion wanted to spend a couple of days in every German city we passed that she knew by name. In two weeks, we had traveled only as far as Freiberg, where we planned to spend some time. I mention these details as I have always felt that Mrs. Catt only feigned interest in the obscure towns because she was concerned that I should not tire myself out with too much traveling. Indeed, the conference and all its arrangements had completely exhausted me. But, after Freiberg, we still had a month in which to visit various places in Switzerland. During that time we also started to plan a world trip together.

Although my life was dedicated to work and did not allow for time to be wasted on fruitless pastimes, I still managed to indulge my wanderlust while investigating various aspects of life abroad. My initial visit to St. Moritz in the winter of 1905–1906 had proved so beneficial that I decided to spend a month each winter in this particularly beautiful part of Switzerland. Each time I reencountered a number of French and English people with whom I had become friends during that first winter. Every other summer, my travel plans were determined by the International Woman Suffrage Alliance conferences, after which I would embark on a major journey through the particular country in which the event had been held. In 1909, a year after Amsterdam, a conference took place in London that had mainly been arranged to allow for a thorough revision of the alliance's rules and regulations. I did not feel like staying on in England, which I had already visited on many occasions. Moreover, I had not yet recovered from all the hard work of the previous year. For these reasons, I resolved to enjoy a peaceful and extended summer holiday. Eventually I chose Tatra Lomnics in the High Tatras, which was at that time an unknown resort mainly frequented by the Hungarian nobility. I have already described my reception there in chapter 9. Although it may not have been peaceful, my holiday in the Tatras certainly did me good.

Countess Pejacevich, a committed feminist and campaigner for woman suffrage in Hungary, introduced me to many people of greater and lesser importance. I particularly remember Count Zichy, also well-known in Holland, who lost his right arm in an accident when he was thirteen years old. He often read parts of his autobiography to me from the original manuscript—his story was as yet to be published—and I was particularly interested in the feelings he experienced while his arm was being amputated. He refused to use any form of narcotic or local anaesthetic and described every sensation throughout the operation and especially his emotional reactions. He then resolved to master all the skills that people normally perform with two hands, and his achievements were quite staggering. He even performed as a one-handed pianist of great skill in our own Concertgebouw.

Another of the interesting people I met was Baroness Lipthay, who loaned me her horse and cart for long journeys. At her home I was introduced to a Hungarian government minister who told me wild stories of political intrigue and corruption, of nobility rule in a country rife with bribery and corruption.

The international medical conference began in Budapest in early September. Baroness Lipthay invited me to stay in her splendid home and to use her carriage whenever I needed it. Her servants had been alerted, and when I arrived at the train station in Budapest there was a coach waiting to pick me up. A whole suite of rooms had been prepared for me in her magnificently luxurious house so that I could work quietly or receive the many friends I had made during my previous visits to the city. These women formed a young and enthusiastic group of campaigners dedicated to woman suffrage and to the advancement of women in general. Despite their youth, they were certainly extremely well informed.

I have already described the medical conference and how I later accompanied a delegation of doctors to Sarajevo. On the first night of that trip, I met Frau Dr. Rosen, the wife of a Wiesbaden doctor, who like me was a woman traveling on her own. We shared a sleeping car and soon became firm friends as we had so much in common. She was also an experienced traveler and had many clever ways of making a long journey *gemütlich*.

Our first stop was at Sarajevo, the capital of Bosnia, which was still under Austrian rule. It was one of the strangest towns I have ever seen, half-Eastern and half-Western. The population consisted of seven ethnic groups, all of which were represented on the city council. I was particularly fascinated by the Turks and Spaniards, and it was here that I managed to visit a genuine harem.[8] When I notified the city authorities of my request, I was invited to visit a young Turk, one of the most distinguished in the city.

I arrived at his somewhat unsightly house in the company of two other women. We were received by a grubby maid-servant who showed us into a room where we were welcomed by the master of the house, who was sitting on a chair strewn with cushions. He was dressed in the Turkish style with a fez and baggy trousers. However, his behavior was Western, the result of having been raised in the house of a teacher in Leipzig. He removed the Turkish pipe from his mouth as we entered and asked us courteously whether we preferred to speak German or English. A few years previously, the father of this twenty-four year old had presented him with five wives. They were all beauties, he announced proudly, but they would be unable to talk to us as they only spoke their own language. However, he was prepared to act as interpreter. Before we visited the five wives, we first talked with the happy husband. I asked him whether, as a man of Western education, he did not find it intolerable for a woman to have to live in the Turkish fashion. If they loved him, they would be extremely jealous of each other. Alternatively, it was also possible that they did not love him because no one had consulted their opinions before the marriage took place or had stopped for one moment to imagine how bitter the whole event must have been for them.

He agreed with everything I said but pointed out that this was, after all, the Turkish custom and that a man's importance was judged by the size of his harem. I told him that in 1890 I had been asked by the Austrian government to work as a doctor in Sarajevo. In terms of my own safety, it was just as well that I had turned down this offer because otherwise I would have certainly incited the Turkish women to rebel against their inhuman situation.

After this introduction, we then left for the women's quarters, a nine-by-ten-meter room with a wooden floor. Five mattresses with colorful fabric on them were placed against the rough wooden wall. There were two high, slitlike openings with wrought iron lattices so that no one could escape or break in. These windows were located at such a height that the women were also unable to see outside. In this room they spent their days and nights together. In my opinion, their looks left much to be desired and their clothes were extremely shabby. All five rushed up to us to show off their babies, and we were careful not to favor any one of these tiny creatures more than the others. After seeing other parts of this run-down house, we returned to the master's room, which all five wives were now permitted to enter. Turkish coffee was served, and we tried to converse with these women, but once our host began to translate, it was patently clear that he was altering our questions and inventing his own replies. During this visit, we were seated on a sofa, the Turk was sitting on a chair, and the five women were gathered on the floor at his feet, despite the fact that there were other chairs in the room. However, I should add that I have seen very different harems in both Cairo and Jerusalem.

I was also particularly interested in the Spanish inhabitants of Sarajevo. These women certainly had more freedom than their Turkish counterparts. They were allowed to appear in public as long as they were completely enveloped from head to toe in a dark garment so voluminous that not even their hands could be seen. But direct contact eluded me because the introduction I had requested only arrived on the day I was leaving.

Frau Dr. Rosen and I said goodbye to the doctors in Ragusa [Dubrovnik] because we wanted to stay on to enjoy the panoramic landscape and temperate climate. This is not the place to describe the journey in detail, although I should warn other travelers about the ferries that took us from Ragusa to Montenegro and from there on to Fiume [Rijeka]. Not even during my subsequent journeys to the Orient have I seen such horrific scenes of beds, chairs, sofas, and upholstery literally crawling with vermin. Apparently the locals found all this quite normal. We spent several weeks touring this area before returning to Wiesbaden where we went our separate ways.

The 1909 elections in Holland had brought a right-wing victory, keeping the Heemskerk cabinet in power. Obviously there was no chance that woman suffrage would be introduced while that group was in office, so the association concentrated on campaigning and on increasing our membership. While we had eighty-one chapters with seventy-five hundred members, the committee was convinced that these figures would need to be trebled or quadrupled before we could be powerful enough to persuade the government to introduce female enfranchisement.

In late 1909, Mrs. Chapman Catt wrote me again about our world tour. But by now it was clear that she was seriously ill. I had repeatedly advised her to undergo an operation, but she had refused to listen to me. I also often felt unwell, and my Amsterdam doctors had determined that my complaints were due to overwork and advised me to take a complete break. Although she was extremely ill, Mrs. Catt wrote me, "Now about yourself. I expect if you were an American your malady would be called nervous prostration. You are overworked, I am sure. The trouble with us all is that, when we overdo, we do not take time enough to recover. If you want to escape from all the troubles, come over here and I shall be glad indeed to take you into my household at any time."[9] While we were both in this state, there was obviously no question of travel to Africa or Asia.

Shortly afterward, I was staying in London with Mrs. Adela Stanton Coit,[10] who told me that she had suffered from exactly the same symptoms a few years previously and that she had completely recovered after taking a cure at the Zurich sanatorium of Dr. Bircher-Benner, at that time still known for his sensible diets and not for being one of Freud's more fanatical supporters.[11] So I left for the sanatorium on the Züricherberg in June 1910 and, in contrast to all the advice about taking "a complete break," I soon found myself on my feet from dawn to dusk, climbing mountains, doing gymnastic exercises, being massaged, and following a diet consisting almost exclusively of fresh fruit. I lost a lot of weight and gained an enormous amount of energy. Much attention was also paid to maintaining a state of mental well-being. After three months, I was able to return to Amsterdam, completely cured.

Meanwhile Mrs. Catt had found that she could no longer avoid her operation, and, once she had recovered, she felt like a new person. Now we could finally begin to arrange our world tour, although we would first have to attend the 1911 International Woman Suffrage Alliance conference in Stockholm. We had to make definite plans because if Mrs. Catt were to leave America long before the conference, her affairs would have to be arranged meticulously, as she would be away from home for almost two years. The same applied to me, and so our travel plans had to be settled well in advance.

Of course, we were both inundated with warnings from well-meaning friends that it was most unwise for two women to travel alone through Asia and Africa. Unprotected travelers such as ourselves, I was told, risked all manner of danger.

In the Netherlands, for the next few years our work for woman suffrage would be restricted to public education, and I realized that my personal involvement was in no way vital to that process. I could leave the association to be run by an excellent committee under the leadership of Mrs. van Balen-Klaar. I could also rent out my house and put my furniture into storage. Once all that was done, and given that I had regained my health, I was determined to leave, all the more as another good friend from America, the Reverend Anna Howard Shaw, had written me to say, "If Mrs. Catt does not go around the world with you, why should we not go together? It would be an awfully good thing for us both if we only could forget suffrage for a time."

But Mrs. Catt did indeed go, and I will describe our journey in the next chapter.

In 1909 and 1910 the "overworked" diagnosis was not without reason. Apart from all the work I have mentioned here, I also wrote a booklet containing biographical sketches of six extraordinary women I had known and befriended. Only one of them was still alive.[12] I had had Gerritsen's and my travel letters from America brought out as a book and had translated and readied for publication Olive Schreiner's excellent *Women and Labor*. All this, plus numerous newspaper and magazine articles on a wide variety of subjects! I should also add that in 1898 I had written a text to accompany a volume of anatomical illustrations called *Woman, Her Structure and Internal Organs,* which is now being reprinted for a fifth time.[13] I compiled this book because at that time there was nothing available in Dutch for a lay audience about the female body, specifically on the position and function of the genital organs. Many of my patients had repeatedly asked for more information on this subject.

TWELVE

A WORLD TOUR

Preparations • Staying in Sweden and Norway • In South Africa • Around the East Coast of Africa • A Visit to Palestine and Syria • In Egypt • The Philippines • In China and Japan • I Return through Russia[1]

It is extremely difficult for two people to prepare for a major journey when one lives in New York and the other in Amsterdam. To make matters worse, we had been unable to agree on which countries we most wanted to visit and where our trip should begin. Mrs. Chapman Catt wanted to visit the Philippines, while I longed to explore Java and Sumatra. It took a lengthy correspondence to sort all this out and to determine how long we would be away. We soon came to an agreement: I would go with her to the American Philippines and she would accompany me to the Dutch East Indies. We had also agreed to depart immediately after the 1911 International Woman Suffrage Alliance conference to be held in Stockholm from June 12 to 17. The one issue we had been unable to resolve was whether, after the conference, we should leave directly from England or sail first for New York so that Mrs. Catt could arrange her affairs before we embarked on our travels.

With typical American efficiency, Mrs. Chapman Catt had already determined the price of a round-the-world ticket, how long we would stay in each country, and all the attendant pros and cons of traveling that way. However— and this perhaps reflects the freedom-loving nature of a Dutch woman—I found it hard to accept the idea that a travel agency would dictate exactly where I was to be for the next year and by what means I would be traveling. I wanted to leave it all to chance and to travel from one country to the next at our own convenience.

Eventually, we agreed to adopt my approach. But we still had to work out our first port of call. In the preceding few years, South African women had repeatedly written urging me to visit their country to help convince their Dutch-speaking sisters of the importance of woman suffrage. Mrs. Chapman Catt had received a similar request from the English-speaking women but was at first unwilling to accept this invitation. She suggested that I go to South Africa on my own and then return to England to begin our journey together. I had already corresponded with a number of South African women about these plans when I received a letter from New York dated March 11, 1911. It began,

"When we first talked about going to South Africa, I conceded that point to please you, for I thought you very much wanted to go there. In the meantime, I have become so much interested in going there myself that I would regard it as a disappointment if we should cut that country out of our itinerary. My reason for wishing to go there is that which first made you want to go, and that is that I believe we will be able to do a good deal of good there. . . . Now I wish very much to go to South Africa. If you do, let us consider that as settled, for it is manifestly the first country we must visit."

Finally, we agreed about the two most important points: we would visit South Africa and we would not buy round-the-world tickets, so our journey could be spontaneous. It was now simply a matter of finding the best way of getting to Cape Town and how much that would cost.

When almost everything had been arranged, we found ourselves bombarded with advice and dire warnings, which increased as the day of our departure drew near. Of course, we were bound to suffer from the most dreadful bouts of homesickness! But my companion, who had thought of everything, knew the remedy for this too: we had only to make sure that we did not get homesick on the same day so that one of us would always be able to comfort the other. Despite many other objections, by this point nothing could dissuade us. And, many people supported our plans, for, after all, we two needed a long relaxing journey so that we might return to the woman suffrage campaign with renewed vigor.

Before us still was the International Woman Suffrage conference in Stockholm. Mrs. Catt had arrived at the end of April so that she could, as usual, take over the final and most important preparations. I arrived in Stockholm with several of my compatriots at the beginning of June. It seemed almost criminal to be discussing subjects other than the conference with Mrs. Chapman Catt and I knew from experience that, as the opening approached, it would be almost impossible to distract her from international work. Once my two compatriots and I had had enough of Stockholm, we decided to visit Dalecarlia in the days leading up to the conference. This trip was inspired by Selma Lagerlöf's books about farming life.[2] We found the long journey from Stockholm to Rättvik quite exhausting, but were amply rewarded by the beautiful land-scapes, costumes, and farms of Dalecarlia.

Even when the conference had ended, Mrs. Catt was unable to leave imme-diately. As always, she first had to compile a report and complete other international work. She estimated that these duties would take at least a month, which indeed they did. I had anticipated this and had agreed to visit Lapland with one of my Dutch companions and, time permitting, to visit the North Cape as well. We reached Abisko, our first destination, after spending two nights and a day on an express train. Abisko is the site of the Swedish National Park, in the center of which is an excellent tourist hotel. At first the whole area looked like a wasteland, but the longer we stayed the more aware we became of its natural beauty, of the magnificent butterflies, the rare birds, strange insects, and numerous plants and flowers. The mountains of Lapland loomed up in fantastic shapes and in the evenings reindeer came down from the ridges in great herds. We tried to approach them, but they were so timid that they fled immediately. Of course, now that we were in Lapland, we also wanted to meet the Lapps. They lived high up in the mountains and we traveled for an entire day to reach even the nearest of their camps. Because of a nearby railroad, the inhabitants had had considerably more contact with civilization than some of the groups we would later meet. They were able to buy needed items in a store instead of having to make everything themselves from local materials and with home-made tools. They were also subject to Swedish law and were obliged to send their children to school.

After a few days, we left this strange world and crossed the northernmost border, which divides Sweden and Norway. We knew that if we were lucky with the boat schedule, we could visit the Lofoten Islands, my favorite part of Norway, and the North Cape. Fortunately, our luck held and on a peerless day we were able to see that famous phenomenon of the sun rising and setting in the same instant. During our travels toward the North Cape, we frequently came into contact with Laplanders who had lost few of their original customs and traditions.

On the way back to Stockholm, we spent a day in Kiruna, at that time still a relatively young city. It is surrounded by a vast sweep of iron-rich mountains. Most iron is extracted from mines deep underground, but these high moun-tains also provide iron ore, which is being removed by a number of English and Scottish companies. To that end they have laid a railway line from Kiruna to Narvik, from where the ore can be shipped. I had hoped to discover something of the workers' conditions there but unfortunately the opportunity eluded me.

Once we were back in Stockholm, I discovered that Mrs. Catt had left a few days previously for England. There was a letter waiting for me, which explained that she wanted to visit London as soon as possible to settle some affairs there. Although her plans were as yet uncertain, she hoped that she would be able to take the *Walmer Castle* to Madeira on July 15 and then catch the *Saxon* a week later so as to embark on our journey to Cape Town. Since, there was nothing left for us to do in Stockholm, we took the night train that very evening. After two nights and a day, we were back in Nijmegen so I could chair the summer meeting of the Association for Woman Suffrage and could personally say goodbye to all my many friends.

My Dutch companion had developed a taste for travel and asked whether she might accompany me to South Africa. I had no objections since Mrs. Catt was also taking a young American friend. On July 11, we both left for London where we found Mrs. Catt still deeply immersed in her work. It was clear that she would not make the July 15 sailing. We decided that the two Dutch women would go on to Madeira as planned and meet up a week later with the two Americans, so that we four could travel on together to Cape Town. I have never regretted the eight days I spent on Madeira; they made an indelible impression on me.

Despite the fact that the *Saxon* arrived in Cape Town early in the morning, we were met by a crowd of women who had come to greet us on behalf of a number of women's organizations. It soon became apparent that our visit was considered important not only with regard to woman suffrage but also because our help was needed on a number of other social issues. I was immediately asked to address women in every South African city on the dangers of prostitution. This was an extremely timely subject, since many women in South Africa actually wanted the government to set up brothels in those places where they did not as yet exist! I have already written a brief account of this in the chapter on prostitution. We stayed for two weeks in Cape Town, delivered several speeches a day, had discussions with women's clubs, and still managed a great deal of sight-seeing. We were inundated with all sorts of invitations.

After Cape Town, we decided to visit Port Elizabeth. Mrs. Catt left by boat with her American companion and I and my companion took the train. I chose this indirect route because it gave me the chance to visit that great South African woman, Olive Schreiner, with whom I had been corresponding for some time and whom I also knew through her books. After a twenty-four-hour train journey, we arrived early one morning and found Olive Schreiner waiting to meet us. Both she and I felt as if we had known each other for ages, as if we were old friends. She towered above me as a talented writer, yet we felt like soulmates, for each of us was completely dedicated to fulfilling our life's tasks. Every word she uttered attested to her great love for humankind. But, unlike me, she was not first and foremost a feminist; instead she invested all her energy in helping those who most needed her assistance and support. She was such a loving person that she could forgive the ruling class's treatment of the weak and helpless by attributing their errors to a lack of understanding. Her pen was her chosen means of helping the downtrodden; with it she attempted to educate society's more powerful members. Although her contemporaries failed to appreciate her, her compatriots misunderstood her, and the English government persecuted her for her courageous actions, nothing could undermine her fundamental belief in the human race. "Mankind is still in its infancy," she once wrote to me, "but there will be a better world one day." For me, the day we spent together bore witness to her ideals.

It would be doing Olive Schreiner an injustice not to include her in the ranks of feminists. Even though the women's movement was not her primary commitment, her book *Woman and Labor*, which I translated into Dutch, shows how clearly and ethically she understood it. She later wrote me to say that the day we spent together was a "red letter day" that she would never forget. For me, it was a revelation to find a woman in a far-flung corner of South Africa who, had she lived in the Netherlands, would have probably been my greatest helpmate and supporter.

Perhaps I am going into too much detail here. About our South African journey I will add only that I stayed with ex-President Steyn and his family; that I attended a meeting in Bloemfontein that revealed much about the people of the Orange Free State and at which General Herzog argued for retaining both English and Afrikaans as official languages; and that we were among the few travelers who journeyed through Rhodesia [Zimbabwe] to Victoria Falls and the Zambezi. Mrs. Catt and I were invited to spend a weekend on the farm of General Smuts, who was at that time the minister for internal affairs.[3] Unfortunately, we had run out of time but still managed to spend a full day with the general and his wife. Of course we also did plenty of sight-seeing and were particularly interested in exploring such local industries as the ostrich farms and the ostrich feather market in Port Elizabeth and in investigating workers' conditions in the gold and diamond mines. We realized that, with the possible exception of gold mining, these three major industries would soon lose their importance if women were to become less obsessed with adorning themselves with diamonds and feathers, or if they simply no longer had the money to buy these ornaments. Few suspected that, with the advent of the Great War, the latter possibility would in fact become reality.

Although our trip was intended as a break from suffrage work, there was hardly a day during our three months in South Africa when we did not speak at some meeting on female enfranchisement, on the women's movement in general, or on a subject that had some connection with prostitution. Our free days were spent traveling by train to particularly remote locations. In Cape Town, we were honored to receive a letter from the director of South African Rail that read, "A first-class carriage is to be reserved in the middle of the train for Dr. Aletta H. Jacobs and her companion, wherever they may be traveling in South Africa. They are to be treated with special care throughout their journey." Mrs. Catt received a similar letter. This official order helped us greatly during our travels in South Africa.

Our last meeting, in Durban at the end of October, was attended by both Boer and English women who had come from all parts of the country. It was here that Mrs. Catt set up the South African Alliance for Woman Suffrage, which in turn joined the International Woman Suffrage Alliance. We then left South Africa, well satisfied with our visit's success.

We found that four cabins had been prepared for us on the *Avondale Castle*, a cargo ship that was sailing along the east coast of Africa to Port Said. Our Boer friends were full of concern for our safety because it was an old and rickety vessel. However, we had purposely chosen this boat because it stopped at each port for anything between a few hours and a day or two, allowing us to get some idea of these extremely diverse harbor towns. The journey was full of contrasts and, after twenty-eight days without undue incident, we finally arrived at Port Said, our final destination.

Here we first realized how lucky we were not to have had our journey prescribed by a round-the-world ticket. During our four weeks on the little freighter, we had heard nothing of the outside world and did not know that the day after our arrival the king and queen of England were due to visit Port Said en route to India for the celebration of their coronation.

Our plan was to leave Port Said immediately for Cairo and to spend a couple of weeks in Egypt before leaving for India. But when we heard of the royal visit, we realized that we would arrive in India in the middle of the festivities and would have little opportunity of seeing the country in its natural state. So we decided to alter our itinerary.

When we arrived that evening at our hotel in Port Said, we discovered that it was possible to stay the night but that we would have to leave the next day, since all rooms had been booked long in advance because of the festivities. A boat would be leaving for Jaffa at 2 P.M. the following afternoon, and we were assured that it was still possible to make reservations. It was well after midnight when we finally decided to take that boat and to visit Jerusalem and its surrounding area for about ten days. We left early the next morning to collect our passports from our respective vice consuls. We then obtained cash with our letters of credit, which again involved visits to different offices, reserved places on the boat to Jaffa, and brought most of our baggage to Thomas Cook Travel after putting aside everything we needed for a ten-day journey. In addition, Mrs. Catt and I also had to reserve places on a *de Nederlander* boat that was due to sail from Port Said to Colombo in January. Of course, all this had to be done at high speed so we would be on time for the boat going to Jaffa.

How glad we were later that we had decided to go to Jerusalem! We managed to see both Palestine and Syria (which in fact we had no choice but to visit) while these countries were still unspoiled. From what I am told, they have now been completely modernized and can no longer be compared to their prewar state or, as Mrs. Catt put it, their state "before the world grew mad."

There was but one reasonable hotel in Jaffa. In Jerusalem, we had to find lodgings in the American-Swedish settlement that has been so romantically described by Selma Lagerlöf. In both Jaffa and Jerusalem, all the people looked like homely Sleeping Beauties who had been abruptly awakened after two thousand years of sleep and were still going about their business in their traditional clothes and according to their traditional customs. Now nothing is left of that era but the churches and a few other historical curiosities, around which a new city is being built, much as ancient Rome lies inside modern Rome.

Once we had seen all the sights of Jerusalem we decided to return to Port Said but discovered to our horror that there were no boats sailing from Jaffa because of an outbreak of smallpox that had claimed two lives in one week! We were advised to go through Syria to Beirut and, from there, to take a boat that did not stop at Jaffa but went straight on to Port Said. So, with our guide and plenty of provisions, we piled into two carts, each of which was drawn by three horses and fitted with rough wooden benches secured to iron bars. After several days of lurching along dirt tracks and through fields of stubble, we finally arrived in Tiberias. We crossed the Sea of Galilee in a row boat to reach a small railway station and then spent several hours in a primitive train to Damascus. All this has now been changed and modernized.

As this is not the place to go into any detail, I will outline only the most important aspects of our subsequent journey. When we reached Beirut from Damascus, we decided to take a ship we were certain would not call at Jaffa. We boarded the next boat, and as we sailed out of the harbor we realized what kind of vessel we were on. There were some twelve hundred emigrants and only a handful of first-class passengers. We steamed past Jaffa, but something else foiled all our efforts not to end up in quarantine. During the night before we were due to arrive, an old woman who was traveling to America with her children suddenly collapsed and died. As a result we had to drop anchor outside Port Said and no one was allowed to leave the ship. Eventually we were permitted to go on to Alexandria under the yellow-green warning flag. But when we arrived, we were forbidden to dock. After three days, we were informed, "It has been impossible to prove that the old woman did not die of cholera."

This medical chicanery resulted in our being sent to the Alexandria quarantine station where we were confined like prisoners for four days. We were then allowed to leave, but were obliged to inform the authorities of our destination and of the hotel at which we intended to stay. After paying extortionate bills for our lodgings, for the compulsory medical check-ups, and for a number of other services we had not requested, we discovered that our baggage had been marked with a red cross to show that we had just been released from quarantine and should be avoided. We ordered a car so that we could quickly board the next Cairo train. However, the driver carefully made sure that at Alexandria Station our tickets were marked with a cross so the Cairo authorities would know what kind of visitors they were dealing with. When we arrived in Cairo late that evening and were yet again forced to submit to a medical examination, I decided to make use of my medical title. I asked to speak with the senior physician and gave him my card. I assured him that both my companion and I were in perfect health. As a result we were allowed to proceed to our hotel and had no further dealings with the Egyptian government.

Our stay was an uneventful one. In Cairo, we found ourselves once again assuming our role as the enlighteners of women. Yet we had far more opportunity to learn about the lives of Turkish women than to exert any influence of our own. Nonetheless, the experience resulted in a series of new acquaintances, and, during the 1923 International Woman Suffrage Alliance conference in Rome, I encountered an Egyptian delegate whom I had originally met during this visit to Cairo.[4]

Early in 1912, Mrs. Catt and I said goodbye to Cairo and to our two traveling companions, and boarded the *Princess Juliana* to Ceylon [Sri Lanka]. The possibility that woman suffrage would soon be introduced in Holland probably explains why, after less than three days at sea, I was presented with a petition signed by thirty-six passengers requesting that I speak on this subject. I may be a committed campaigner but I must admit that there, somewhere in the middle of the Indian Ocean, it was rather too hot to be thinking about giving lectures . . . But it was a pity to waste an opportunity and so, with the captain's permission, the second-class dining room was turned into a conference room for the occasion. All the first- and second-class passengers were present when I began my speech at 4:30 that afternoon. There was so much interest that our debate was still in full swing when the hall had to be transformed back into a dining room at 6 P.M. The next day, Mrs. Catt was also asked to speak. In this way, the issue of woman suffrage became "the topic of the day," and we were often drawn into other passengers' discussions.

Our beautiful and extremely comfortable ship finally landed at Colombo on January 20. We spent several enjoyable weeks in Ceylon, including some days in the splendid city of Kandy where we caught up on our correspondence and saw the local botanical gardens. I was particularly intrigued by this visit because I wanted to know if these gardens were more impressive than 's Lands Plantentuin in Buitenzorg [in Java]. We arrived in Paradenya, where the gardens are located, at 7 A.M. one morning and found that they were completely deserted apart from a young student who offered to be our guide. While showing us the most important plants, he drew our attention to an exceptionally tall palm tree crowned with an immense crest of blossom. This was the Taliput palm. He told us that it flowers once in a hundred years and then dies. A little farther on he pointed to another tree that was called the Royal palm.

I will say no more about these magnificent gardens except to add that that day marked an end to my perfect *Seelenharmonie* with Mrs. Catt. For in Ceylon, India, Burma, Penang, Singapore, and Java, we saw many avenues of Royal palms and (in my opinion) we saw the Taliput palm on only one other occasion. After some time, Mrs. Catt began to mix up the two names so that each time we saw these trees I could not repress an "Oh look, some more Royal palms!" to which she would immediately reply, "You mean Taliputs!" This was inevitably followed by an altercation concerning the botanical differences between a Taliput and a Royal palm. Eventually we both began to tire of the subject and agreed to look the other way whenever we glimpsed these controversial trees. We managed to keep this up until we reached the 's Lands Plantentuin in Buitenzorg where we were given a tour by the director himself. And needless to say, he pointed out these very trees. Somewhat cheekily I asked him to explain which was the Royal palm and which the Taliput. He stared at me in astonishment but answered my question and proved that I had been right all along. For a second, Mrs. Catt and I glanced at each other, but said nothing.

Here I take a giant step forward both in my story and in time. Early one morning in Manila, I awoke to discover Mrs. Catt sitting on my bed and reading the following verses to me:

To Aletta

A year ago today, dear friend,
We started on a cruise
Around the world, we said we'd go
And would ourselves amuse.

Our friends and foes alike agreed,
We'd never come around,
We'd fight and quarrel sure as smoke
Our friendship run aground.

One ship, they said, would carry you,
And one would carry me
And should we meet another day
We'd never speak, you see!

But here we are together still
And better friends I'll say
Than when we on the Saxon sailed
A year ago to-day.

But then my dear, I'd have you know
It is a Taliput
That palm they call the Royal one
On that I'll stake my mut.

And if you will admit it is
With you the summer seas
I'll sail, till death shall part us two,
If not, I'll say adieu.

July 18, 1911–July 18, 1912

Quoting this simple but sensitive poem, I find myself at a loss for words to describe our life in this fascinating part of the world, which included a plethora of countries and peoples, customs, sights, and personalities. Anyone interested in discovering more should consult my *Reisbrieven uit Afrika en Azië* (Travel Letters from Africa and Asia), which have been published as a book and cover this period of my life in considerable detail. At the risk of stating the obvious, I would like to add that we always managed to combine work with play and never lost sight of our journey's aim: to study the legal and social position of women in every country we visited and, wherever possible, to help organize these women so that they could improve their lives.

We often met people by chance who were later to help us enormously. This was the case during our trip from Buitenzorg to Sindanglaya. We had borrowed an extremely primitive carriage, but the landscape was so stunning that we preferred to cover great distances on foot. A little way ahead was a carriage similar to our own with a passenger who, like us, got out and walked. He came up to us and introduced himself. His name was easy to remember: Del Pan. We quickly realized that he was a well-educated and sophisticated individual who had traveled extensively. He was as familiar with America as Mrs. Catt was and spoke to me about Holland with an understanding that would be the envy of many Dutch persons. Del Pan had been born in the Philippines of Spanish parents. He had studied law at the University of Madrid and was now working as a high-ranking government official. When we met him, he was traveling to Sindanglaya, where he intended to stay for several days. After we had visited Buitenzorg, Sumatra, and other parts of the Dutch East Indies and finally arrived in Manila some months later to begin our tour of the Philippines, our meeting with Del Pan proved to be particularly useful. The American authorities and even the governor went out of their way to help us, but Mr. Del Pan himself proved invaluable as an excellent and charming guide who introduced us to local people and customs. Because he was so well traveled and, like us, always had a specific purpose in mind, he knew exactly what would most interest us and organized our itinerary accordingly. I still have an official government document issued to Mrs. Catt and myself that declares us to be school inspectors permitted to visit and investigate any school on the islands. To this day, I still receive the government's annual report on the schools.

As I left the Philippines, I felt that country could gain much by following Java's example in terms of exploiting natural resources, but, conversely, Java could learn from the Philippines about education, hygiene, and the people's development.

On the day that we were to leave Manila, we were visited by the many friends we had made during our six-week stay who came to say goodbye and to present us with souvenirs. Where else but in America or in one of its colonies would the governor and his wife personally come to bid farewell to two unofficial visitors? We were even more surprised by their cordial gesture of a box of fresh roses for each of us, which we found in our cabins on board ship, a gesture that brightened up an otherwise difficult journey.

After the Philippines we visited China and Japan. We had been advised not to proceed beyond the coast of China; although the second revolution had ended, there was obviously a third in the offing. However, we had received so many dire warnings during our travels that we now tended to take them all with a grain of salt. In China, we learned much and met many extraordinary people. Moreover, our visit was vital in terms of the women's movement. The Chinese women's movement, such as it was, lacked any form of organization or unity of purpose, and it had appropriated the militant methods of the English suffragettes. When I asked these women why they had chosen such a radical approach, I was surprised to hear that, instead of reporting on feminism throughout the world, the Chinese press had reported on only the campaign tactics of the English suffragettes. No wonder that, when Chinese women began to demand their rights, their first action was to break all the windows of a parliament building.

Although both of us opposed the suffragettes' methods, this trip once again demonstrated that their actions had made women all over the world aware of their own disadvantaged positions and of the need for organized campaigns. Even in the most remote corners of Africa and Asia, we were confronted again and again by the influence of the suffragettes, mainly because newspapers eagerly seized on such sensational stories while ignoring more moderate efforts to achieve reforms. We were frequently forced to admit that radical action certainly makes the world sit up and take notice. On the other hand, our visit also influenced the women of China to adopt a calmer and better organized approach.

When we arrived in Yokohama, we each received so many letters urging us to return home that we decided to shorten our visit to Japan and to proceed no further. The original plan had been that either Mrs. Catt would accompany me back to the Netherlands via Russia or we would travel together to Honolulu and San Francisco and then slowly across America to New York, whence I would sail for Holland. Both plans were now out of the question. Eventually we decided that I would return through Russia to the Netherlands and Mrs. Catt would go home via Honolulu. We agreed that, soon after our separation, each would prepare a record of her travels she would then send to the other.[5]

The women we met in Japan were very different from those in China. None were prepared to fight for their rights in the way that their Chinese sisters were. But we met with a number of women's groups and urged them to begin organizing themselves. In 1923, I was delighted to be visited in The Hague by four Japanese women who asked my advice about forming a women's movement in Japan. They particularly wanted to know what kind of campaign would be the most effective in terms of achieving the right to vote and what further goals they should bear in mind.

During our world trip, we saw countless extraordinary sights and met many remarkable people. We greatly valued all we had learned, yet by the end of our journey our most powerful feeling was gratitude that we had been able to perform such useful work among the women of Africa and Asia.

I saw Mrs. Catt off at Yokohama as she embarked on her voyage to Honolulu. I had several days to wait for the train that would take me from Vladivostock to Berlin because the Trans-Siberian Railway left only once a week. I had been told that there were no good seats left on the next train but that I would be able to make a suitable reservation on the one after that. And that was precisely how it worked out. I spent several days wandering around Japan on my own, then sailed for two days on a Russian boat from Tsuruga to Vladivostock, where I found an excellent compartment just for me in the middle of the train. Although I was the only woman on the Russian ship, I had not imagined that there would be no other female passengers for the whole of the journey through Siberia. That was probably why I had been given a compartment to myself, but in any case there were few other travelers.

When we arrived in Harbin on the afternoon of the following day, we had to wait almost an hour for the Peking train. Our new passengers included Prince Heinrich of Prussia, the brother of the German Kaiser, and his vast retinue, which included two representatives of the Trans-Siberian Railway, several Russian generals, and a number of other officials. These fellow travelers provided at least a little diversion from the endless journey through an inhospitable landscape.

There were few first-class passengers apart from myself. Twice a day I took my meals in the spacious dining room alongside Prince Heinrich's entourage while His Imperial Highness and two of the Russian generals ate in a smaller dining room. I talked several times with these gentlemen about war and peace, and about women's rights. Occasionally there was a knock at my door and a high-ranking officer would enter for a neighborly chat about pacifism. All this took place in late November 1912. Had I known how close we were to war, I would have certainly spoken out—in a fashion that could well have endangered my life. In one of my discussions with a German general, I obstinately insisted that war could never break out in any of the civilized countries because their people were simply too highly developed. How wrong I was!

Sadly, I must now conclude this chapter because the scope of my book is too limited to be able to include everything I discovered traveling with my intelligent, experienced, and observant companion. During this trip, I wrote two newspaper articles a week that were later published in book form. However, it was not always possible to include what I found personally interesting. For it was a year in which, for the first time since my husband's death, I felt a sense of profound happiness. I spent each day surrounded by love and intelligence, in the company of someone I respected and whose views I shared. During the sixteen months we traveled together, I came to realize that Mrs. Chapman Catt is one of those few principled women who, in days gone by, would have been declared a saint.

THIRTEEN

FROM 1913 TO 1924

A Survey of the Last Ten Years • The Death of Mrs. Haver • The First Public Woman Suffrage Events in 1913 and the National Petition • An Interlude of War and Work for Pacifism • The Resumption in 1915 of the Suffrage Campaign and Its Consequences • Passive Suffrage Is Granted, Then Universal Suffrage in 1919 • I Move to The Hague • The 1921 Festivities to Mark the Fiftieth Anniversary of My Entering the University • My First Ballot • I Recover from a Serious Illness • Celebrating My Seventieth Birthday • Conclusion

I arrived home at midnight after traveling by train for more than two weeks. The next morning, the secretary of the Association for Woman Suffrage arrived while I was still in bed to break the sad news that Mrs. Th. P. B. Haver, one of our best and most efficient workers, had died a few days previously. She was to be cremated the next day and the executive committee was hoping that I would agree to speak at her funeral.

I was deeply shocked by Mrs. Haver's death. Although I was well aware that she had been incurably ill for some time, I had still hoped to be able to thank her for her invaluable work and to reassure her that we would continue the fight for women's advancement. She had visited me one evening shortly before I left on my world trip and had seemed particularly dejected about our rate of progress. What would happen if our most important campaigners were to fall sick or die? Perhaps she had had a premonition of the fatal illness that had slowly robbed her of her vitality. Because my heart and mind provided me with the right words for this sad occasion, I agreed to speak at her cremation.

Mrs. Haver's death was a serious although not unexpected loss for the woman's movement. The association's committee and members decided to postpone the reception that was to be held to celebrate my return as none of us felt in the mood for a party. It was eventually held some time later, and the warmth of my welcome convinced me that I was still greatly valued despite my prolonged absence.

The Heemskerk government was still in power. With a new general election coming up, the three left-wing parties—the Liberal Democratic Union, the Liberal Union, and the Free Liberals—decided in June 1913 to form an antigovernment coalition. As in 1905, constitutional reform was again under discussion. The left-wing coalition proposed revising Clause 80 and all relevant articles so that universal male suffrage would become a part of our constitution and all obstacles blocking the future introduction of female suffrage would also be removed. I protested to my own party because I felt that it should stick to its manifesto, which specifically advocated a constitutional revision granting universal suffrage to both men and women. However, I failed to attract any support and soon realized that all my efforts were bound to fail. But when I read the bill proposed by the antifeminist Christian parties in power, I knew that, in terms of suffrage, it was vital that we women join the campaign to bring down a government that offered us precisely nothing. Minister Heemskerk had had the gall to announce in Parliament that "the women of Holland simply do not want to vote!" That was reason enough to call on all our thousands of members and supporters to protest vehemently against this government.

During my travels with my wise and experienced companion, I came to realize that, where social reform is the goal, there is little point in attempting to convince government ministers if one has not already won over the voting public. Hence, I suggested to our committee that we should hold a demonstration in The Hague to prove that a great many Dutch women actively desired the right to vote. The demonstrators would then proceed to a large meeting where speeches would be made not only by women but also by representatives of various political parties. The committee's reaction to my proposal indicated that it was not yet ready to undertake public action. The plan sounded too much like the suffragettes! Eventually we agreed on a compromise proposal. A protest meeting would be held in The Hague. Those who attended from throughout the country would be free to choose whether or not to join the march from the train station to the hall. It would also be possible to make one's own way there.

This was to be our association's first public action. On Sunday, May 4, 1913, hundreds of members attended the event. We were forbidden to march past Minister Heemskerk's house and were led through various back streets to the Zoological Gardens, where the protest meeting was to be held. I was not in the least disappointed by this change of route because there was no point in demonstrating to Minister Heemskerk that his views were incorrect; he was well aware of women's desire to vote. Our job was to win public approval. And when the great day came, many of our members managed to overcome their personal reluctance and joined the march to publicize our principles on the streets of The Hague.

The protest meeting was also a great success. The large hall in the Zoological Gardens was filled to capacity and all the left-wing parties sent their best speakers. We received messages of sympathy from many important associations and prominent individuals. We had made an excellent start and, although unable to vote in the next election, we still managed to work as hard as even the most energetic and well-organized of the political parties.

On Election Day, in June 1913, like many other campaigners I was attending the International Woman Suffrage Alliance conference in Budapest. It was here that we received the good news that the Heemskerk government had been forced to resign. However, our joy was tempered by the fact that the socialists had refused to help form a left-wing government. All this eventually resulted in the creation of the minority cabinet led by Cort van der Linden. We were far from happy with this turn of events. We already knew the prime minister's views because, as a minister in a previous cabinet, he had shown himself to be an antifeminist who opposed all efforts to raise women out of their disenfranchised state. Nonetheless, we were convinced that this government would introduce constitutional reforms that would at least include the proposals put forward in the three parties' election manifesto. But, of course, that was not enough in itself. Our actions in The Hague proved that women could also campaign through holding public events, and these tactics were soon adopted by our various branches.

The following September, we were also encouraged by the contents of the queen's speech, which for the first time included the issue of woman suffrage. The queen announced that the government was to present a revision of the constitution that would grant the franchise to all men above a certain age and remove the legal obstacles to woman suffrage.

That was certainly a healthy sign and one that spurred us on to still greater efforts. In a his most recent speech, Prime Minister Cort van der Linden had expressed his wish to govern according to public opinion but had earlier stated that the introduction of woman suffrage was like taking a leap into the unknown. So we needed to refute both of these assertions directly. To disprove the first of his comments, we organized a national petition drive demanding constitutional equality between men and women. Within a few months, we had obtained a grand total of 165,000 signatures, at which point the war forced us to end this initiative. With regard to Van der Linden's second point, we wrote to the governments of all those countries where woman suffrage had already been granted in order to inquire how it had worked out in practice. Our letter was sent to the Australian parliament and all the individual states of Australia, to the governors of the various states in America in which women could vote, and also to the governments of Norway and Finland. We soon received the replies we needed, which we then printed and mailed to every member of the government and to the press.

In August 1913, at the opening of the Peace Palace and during the International Peace Congress in The Hague, we organized a series of public meetings in Amsterdam and The Hague with speeches by various foreign delegates. We greatly valued their involvement as the conference involved much hard work and several of these notable figures were in fact unwell. Most of those who accepted our invitation were personal friends of mine. They were Countess Bertha von Suttner from Austria; Monsignor Dr. Alexander Giesswein, the papal prelate of Hungary; Dr. Carl Lindhagen, the mayor of Stockholm; Mrs. Sewall, the American president of the International Council of Women; and Madame Jeanne Mélin from France.[1]

Apart from the main campaign, we also adopted other highly effective tactics. Each afternoon, large numbers of women with suffrage ribbons and flags would distribute pamphlets in working-class districts and speak to small groups of women. Some women also started hiring tents at the weekly markets in order to sell inexpensive knickknacks and make suffrage speeches to a steadily growing audience of marketgoers. As a result of all this hard work, we managed to attract hundreds of new association members each week.

Suddenly, all this work had to be abandoned with the outbreak of war in the summer of 1914. As a committed pacifist, I initially empathized with the women and children who had been left behind as I also did with the young men in the armed forces. I felt that it was my duty to alleviate suffering wherever possible, an aim to which I devoted all my time. But was this really women's most important wartime task and one that I too should be involved in? Certainly, from time immemorial, women have been regarded as the providers of comfort and the healers of wounds. For a long time, I adhered atavistically to this role and even assumed a position of leadership. The atrocities we heard and read about each day spurred us on to greater efforts. But after a time I began to see things from a different perspective. Day and night I was tormented by the horror of what was going on. Fortunately, the Dutch government was a peaceable one, but had that not been the case, its resolve to join in the war would have been inevitably strengthened by the fact that it could count on its women's support. I myself was involved with philanthropic work that, rather than hastening a cease-fire, was actually helping to prolong hostilities because all we did was to ease the burden of war.

I became increasingly convinced that we women had a higher mission to fulfill. It was our duty to protest against the mindless destruction of art treasures, the breaking up of families, the barbaric sacrificing of young lives. It was up to us to oppose the insanity of war. Once I came to this decision, I did whatever I could to ensure that women's protests were heard. The conference that was held in The Hague in April 1915 was the direct expression of this spirit. Chapter 8 describes this conference in greater detail as well as my subsequent trip with Miss Jane Addams from Chicago to contact various governments, and my journey to North America, which culminated in an interview with President Wilson.

Meanwhile I still maintained the task I had adopted at the beginning of the war, which at that time did not seem to conflict with my pacifist beliefs. As I mentioned at the end of chapter 8, my work consisted of helping foreign women and girls who found themselves stranded in the Netherlands. I am returning to this subject because it involved some particularly extraordinary cases. For instance, one day a young woman who was black as pitch turned up on my doorstep clutching a letter. She spoke a little French but with such a heavy accent that it was impossible to understand her. The letter was from a London woman who had heard of me through the woman's movement and also knew many of my London acquaintances. This Negro woman had come from London and was traveling to Cologne where she had friends and family. She originally came from Madagascar and the letter asked me to help her reach Germany. This proved to be extremely tricky, but after a couple of weeks I managed to get her across the border where she was to be met by someone she knew. Despite her promises, she never wrote to inform me of her safe arrival. But four years later I was amazed to receive a letter from Cologne from the very same young woman, who went by the delightful name of Razanamanga of Madagascar. In awkward but adequate German, she reminded me of how I had helped her to reach Germany. In a few weeks' time she would be arriving in Holland and was again requesting my help in order to reach either England or France and return to her native country. I was also approached by female members of the English and German aristocracy who found themselves stranded with neither money nor passports and who needed a helping hand.

Nineteen hundred and fifteen was almost entirely devoted to the pacifist cause, yet somehow we still found time to continue our suffrage campaign. The constitutional reform bill had been prepared and would soon be debated in parliament. In early 1916, our association's plans included holding large-scale demonstrations in Amsterdam and The Hague to involve voters in our cause. A major problem was that, during the war, the authorities usually did not permit such events to take place on the street. But when women set their sights on a particular goal, they usually succeed in achieving it. Amsterdam presented no problems as the chief of police immediately decided to override all objections so that the first demonstration could be held there on June 16. Those involved included not only our own members but many individuals from other associations that represented a wide range of interests. For two and a half hours, we marched through the most densely populated districts and were greeted with great enthusiasm. The event was a tremendous success.

But The Hague was another story entirely. The mayor was determined not to allow any wartime demonstrations, including our own peaceful march. As soon as I heard this, I traveled from Amsterdam to The Hague where Mrs. Kehrer-Stuart, president of the local branch, and I went to speak with the police commissioner. He neatly evaded the issue by referring us to the mayor in his capacity as chief of police. So, thirty minutes later, we found ourselves sitting in the mayor's office. He attempted to explain why he had decided not to allow any demonstrations in the city for the duration of the war. Despite the fact that we disproved all his arguments, he refused to change his mind. I then pointed out that this event was vital to our campaign because a decision was about to be made in Parliament that would profoundly affect the interests of Dutch women. Our plan was simply to organize a meeting at the Zoological Gardens where a motion would be proposed, passed, and collectively presented to the leader of the Dutch parliament. If the mayor as chief of police was willing to ensure that we would able to march freely, I would be prepared to assume personal responsibility for the consequences of our actions.

The police commissioner was summoned at this point. We agreed that I was to guarantee that the event would be orderly at all times and that, for their part, the police would ensure that nothing untoward would be allowed to occur. This second demonstration took place on October 18, 1916, without incident. We had asked the leader of the Dutch parliament to meet with us on that day so we could present him with our proposal. We appeared at the parliament building at the appointed time, when Parliament normally would have been in full swing, and were astonished to find just one member there. All the others had escaped through a back door! Courage is certainly a masculine quality.

From that day on, until the end of the suffrage debate, women maintained a constant vigil outside the parliament building so members would always be reminded of the fact that women were demanding the right to vote. Even so, we were not at first granted direct suffrage, although we were allowed to run for office, a solution that proved to be unique among constitutional governments. The 1918 elections were held on the basis of the revised constitution, which included universal suffrage for men and also women's eligibility to hold office. Many political parties included female candidates, and I was put forward by the Liberal Democrats. Yet somehow all parties carefully managed to avoid electing a woman. But women now had the opportunity to address vast audiences of voters and to draw attention to the new constitution's idiotic provisions. Only the Social Democrats succeeded in getting a woman candidate elected, a phenomenon that occurred in all countries where woman suffrage or eligibility for office had been instituted for the first time.[2]

We were far from discouraged by all this. In fact we were convinced that most people now supported our cause and that victory was in sight. By November 1918, almost every country was dominated by the spirit of revolution, and Holland was no exception. In a state of panic, the government asked for the revolutionaries' demands, of which only two were clearly articulated: an eight-hour working day and woman suffrage. The reactionary government, composed of Christian parties, promised to grant both demands. The leader of the Liberal Democrats, Mr. Marchant, had introduced a bill at the beginning of the parliamentary session in September that would ensure that women become men's political equals. This bill was passed by a large majority and received royal assent on September 18, 1919.

I was immediately inundated with flowers and congratulatory messages from all parts of the country, and the large party organized in Amsterdam's Concertgebouw was held primarily in my honor. Among the many presents I received was a copy of the woman suffrage emblem crafted in gold by an artist, which I still treasure and wear almost every day. I also received many letters and telegrams from abroad. But I must promptly add that none of this would have been possible without the help of our many sterling supporters. I will not mention names, for fear of making too many omissions, but I would like to make just one exception. Mrs. Clara Mulder van de Graaf-de Bruijn is both a strict Catholic and one of our most diligent campaign leaders.[3] She has often visited the southern provinces to defend woman suffrage from the Catholic viewpoint, despite the opposition of local priests and bigots.

How did I feel now that my fervent desire for suffrage had finally been fulfilled? I will answer by remembering the days I spent in Manila with Mrs. Chapman Catt. Our hotel rooms looked out over a small house that served as some sort of office. It was located in a garden where there was a tree with a large monkey whose sole purpose in life seemed to be to amuse the local officials. The animal would periodically climb down to the ground where it was forced to remain near the tree because of a chain that tied him firmly to the trunk. This upset me each time I looked out the window, for I would have loved to have helped the poor creature to escape. One day I pointed the animal out to Mrs. Catt. She looked at me mischievously with her beautiful blue eyes and said, "That monkey is just like us. Aren't we tied fast to the suffrage tree? When will we be freed?" I can best describe my initial happiness at the granting of woman suffrage as a sense of delicious relief. At last I had broken free of the suffrage tree to which I had been chained for so many years!

But I soon began to wonder about what I would do next. My first act was to move from Amsterdam to The Hague, where, I hoped, I would no longer be caught up with the association and would be able devote myself to many kinds of work I had always wanted to do but had never had the time for. I also wanted to leave Amsterdam because many of my dearest friends had either died or moved away. I knew that I was bound to make many new friends in The Hague. Everything went according to plan except that the quiet and retiring life was to elude me for some time to come. Before I had even unpacked my things, I found myself cajoled into going to Zurich to help organize a peace conference. I have already covered this event and our five-day trip from The Hague to Zurich in chapter 8, as well as my journey to Germany immediately afterward and all the other pacifist work that kept me just as busy as the earlier suffrage work.

Although life in The Hague may be less than relaxing, I also know full well that this is really the way I wanted it to be. I have found many dear and sincere friends among the Broese van Groenou family. I feel more attached to them, including numerous children and grandchildren, than I do to many of my own relatives. One of these grandchildren is also my own godchild, so now I feel as if I am a real grandmother. In addition, since Clara Mulder van de Graaf also moved to this neighborhood shortly after my arrival in The Hague I can relax in the knowledge that I will never be a lonely old woman.

Since 1919, I have devoted myself to work for peace and, time permitting, to certain areas of the now very extensive woman's movement. On both a national and an international level, I am particularly involved with the issue of married women's nationality, which has once again assumed prominence. Another concern, although this is as yet beyond the scope of the woman's movement, is planned motherhood. Over the last few years, family planning has become an important topic in America, England, and Scandinavia. It is frequently discussed by economists and doctors and has also aroused much public interest. Indeed, answering all the letters I receive on this subject has become a major undertaking. I am also frequently visited by experts from the above-mentioned countries, who regularly ask my advice. Right now—in the spring of 1924—I am preparing to leave for the United States and have been bombarded with requests for appointments or for my American address to facilitate future contact.[4]

In 1921, as I have already mentioned, I participated in the peace conference in Vienna. That year was a particularly significant one for me, for it marked the fiftieth anniversary of my entering the university. My friends in The Hague decided to organize a day of celebrations. For this I will be eternally grateful to them. It was a day filled with flowers and affection. The high point for me was a procession of young girls, representing the six universities of Holland, who arrived to convey their gratitude and to commemorate the moment when Dutch universities first reluctantly opened their doors to women. This innovation was due to one young girl, and now, years later, these modern students had come to thank her in person. I particularly treasure their present of a bracelet-cum-watch. In fact I am never parted from it. This watch not only keeps perfect time but is also tangible proof that young girls are now better educated, able to live more freely, and achieving far more than we ever dreamed possible in my youth.

The last few years seem to have been one long celebration. And I have to admit that all the warmth, friendship, and tributes have more than made up for the abuse I once suffered from many of my compatriots.

In 1922, I again found myself the center of attention, during the first general election in which women could exercise their right to vote. Since I was just recovering from a serious illness, it seemed unlikely that I would be well enough to go to the polls in person. I was still confined to bed until shortly before the great day itself. But my friends in The Hague did everything possible to enable me to cast that precious first vote. Laden with flowers presented by grateful women voters, I carefully placed my ballot in the box and the polling official came over to shake my hand and convey his best wishes. That day I was inundated with congratulatory letters and telegrams from throughout the country, sent by women who had just voted for the very first time. More than anything else, I was particularly touched by a letter from a group of Christian women who admitted that they had always opposed woman suffrage. But they realized that, now that they had the vote, they were in a far better position to fulfill their Christian duty toward society.

In 1923, I attended the International Woman Suffrage Alliance conference in Rome.[5] From there I journeyed to Paris and had scarcely returned home before I set out once again for several international meetings in Dresden and Berlin. There I was deeply affected by the dreadful conditions in which most of the German people were forced to live. Probably that was the reason I took on more than I could cope with. Whatever the cause, when I went to stay with the Manus family shortly after I returned to Amsterdam, I suddenly fell sick. I had been aware of the symptoms of this illness for quite some time, but now I was forced to stay in bed for weeks on end. At first I thought I would never recover, although my long-suffering physician, Dr. O. J. Wijnhausen, assured me otherwise. Due to to his patience, his obstinate charge did indeed recover and was able to celebrate her seventieth birthday.

During my illness and subsequent convalescence, Miss Rosa Manus and my other friends began elaborate preparations to celebrate my seventieth birthday.[6] This tribute was organized by a large committee with an executive subcommittee that consisted of Rosa Manus, Mrs. F. W. van Wulfften Palthe-Broese van Groenou, Mrs. H. van Biema-Hijmans, Mrs. C. Mulder van de Graaf-de Bruijn, Mrs. B. van den Bergh-Willing, and C. S. Groot. They made sure that everyone, both at home and abroad, was made aware of the fact that I would be celebrating my seventieth birthday on February 9, 1924. That day made me realize how many friends from throughout the world actively appreciated me, even some who had once been my opponents!

The great day began with stacks of letters and presents brought to my home. And there were so many flowers—magnificent, sweet-smelling flowers. The committee arrived at 11 a.m. to present me with a gift of immense value. I was informed of the day's program, which had been thoughtfully planned to include sufficient rest, since I was still recovering from my illness.

To describe the events of that wonderful, glorious afternoon, I can do no better than to quote the words of that excellent reporter, Miss Emmy J. Belinfante, as they appeared in two successive issues of *de Nieuwe Courant*.

Dr. Jacobs's 70th Birthday
The Reception

There were glowing tributes at the 70th birthday celebration of Dr. Aletta Jacobs, the pioneering equal rights campaigner. Among the many bouquets, which had virtually turned the hall into a sea of flowers, was a thoughtful token of appreciation from Dr. and Mrs. Siemens: a photograph decorated with sprigs of beautiful orchids showing the house in Sappemeer where Dr. Jacobs was born. The Association of Noncommissioned Officers had also marked the occasion with a flower arrangement. There was piano music as Dr. Jacobs made her entrance and little girls strewed her path with flowers.

It would be impossible to report on all the speeches in any detail, but the general tone was one of gratitude for Dr. Jacobs's achievements: for women as a feminist pioneer; for science through her medical work; for the peace movement as a pacifist; for morality through her campaign against the double standard [for men and women]; for women students by being the first woman student; for housewives through her own experience as a housewife. A number of men spoke on behalf of the Liberal Democrats and drew attention to Dr. Jacobs's role in founding their party. Mr. Merens of The Hague branch of the Freedom Union declared that her crusade to improve women's legal status was greatly appreciated by the men of the Union whose manifesto also included full civil and economic rights for women.

Not only did those who shared her views concerning politics, the woman's movement, and pacifism pay tribute to her. Women with opposing political or feminist beliefs were also quick to acknowledge the importance of her contribution.

MISS ROSA MANUS, in her capacity as president of the executive subcommittee, conveyed messages of congratulations from women abroad (including the president of the International Woman Suffrage Alliance) and also from those who were unable to attend such as Mrs. Rutgers-Hoitsema, whose absence was due to illness. Miss Manus remarked that Dr. Jacobs had had an extraordinary life: she had managed to achieve many of her ideals through a combination of daring, determination, and sheer energy. She reminded the audience that our guest of honor is also a well-known figure abroad, a fact that was immediately greeted with enthusiastic applause. Miss Manus also mentioned that the committee had already presented Dr. Jacobs with a token of their esteem and felt that there could be no better tribute than to publish her book on her birthday (to the extent that it was ready to go to press). Finally she gave Dr. Jacobs a large laurel wreath.

MRS. V. D. HOEVE-BAKKER (Dutch Association of Women Citizens) said that the secret of her influence lay in her personality, "You are like a diamond that leaves its trace on every other stone."

MRS. DOORMAN-KIELSTRA (The Netherlands' National Women's Council) praised Dr. Jacobs as one of the mainstays of her organization and hoped that she would continue to work at her present level so as to help the council achieve its goal.

DR. DEKNATEL (on behalf of The Hague branch of the Dutch Society for the Advancement of Medicine) assured Dr. Jacobs that she had practised her profession in an exemplary fashion. Her work had been a godsend to countless women.

ANNA POLAK (National Association for Working Women) declared that Dr. Jacobs had opened the way to one of highest and most noble forms of work. Both the scientific world and the women of Holland would be eternally indebted to her.

MRS. RAMONDT-HIRSCHMANN (Dutch Committee of Women for Permanent Peace) paid tribute to Dr. Jacobs the pacifist and added that the foreign women in London had specifically asked her to convey their greetings.

MR. WERKER (chairman of the Liberal Democratic Union) chose not to praise her in terms of any one area but as "representing a higher unity."

MR. MARCHANT (chairman of the parliamentary faction of the Liberal Democratic Union) emphasized her qualities of leadership in an organization that had always bowed to her wishes in terms of women's rights.

MISS WESTERMAN (member of parliament, the Freedom Union women's group) commented that we especially needed to honor Dr. Jacobs at a time when so much that she had fought for could easily still be lost. She hoped that other women would emulate Dr. Jacobs and help to reverse this trend.

MRS. ROS-VRIJMAN (the executive committee of the Liberal Democratic women's club) stated that we could all be proud of Dr. Jacobs and wished her many happy returns. She thanked her on behalf of the women and mothers of Holland for what she had done for their children and hailed her as a builder in the temple of humankind. She concluded her speech with the builders' benediction: "I wish you safety, blessings and prosperity, wisdom to make plans, strength to realize them, beauty to give them a form that is both pleasing and harmonious."

JONKVROUW DE JONG VAN BEEK EN DONK (the University Women Students' Association) assured Dr. Jacobs that young women today would make themselves worthy of what she had achieved.

MRS. JACOBS-ZOETHOUT (the Dutch Association of Housewives) described Dr. Jacobs's hospitality in Amsterdam.

MRS. MARIE VAN DIJK (the Women's Club Building) spoke of the indirect contribution Dr. Jacobs had made to the founding of the building and hoped that she would soon honor the club's members with a personal visit.

This was followed by speeches by Sister VERWEY MEJAN of Nosokómos, Mr. WINKEL of The Hague branch of the Liberal Democratic Union and, as already mentioned, by Mr. MERENS of The Hague branch of the Freedom Union.

Other speakers included: MRS. CARNO-BARLEN of the Association of Free Women, MRS. VAN HEEMSKERCK VAN BEEST and BARONESS VAN REEDE TOT TER AA of the Dutch Women's Association for Moral Advancement and MRS. VAN SCHAIK-DOBBELMAN of the Association for Women's Mutual Protection. Messages were also read out by representatives of the Dutch Association for Women Citizens from Alkmaar, Amersfoort, Amsterdam, The Hague, Groningen, Haarlem, Rotterdam, and Voorburg. MRS. BAKKER-NORT spoke as a member of parliament, and MRS. NINCK BLOK-GRUYS conveyed the good wishes of The Hague branch of the Liberal Democratic Women's Club, as did MRS. COHEN TERVAERT-ISRAELS for The Hague Women's Council, MRS. ALBARDA-KNOCK for the Social Democratic Women's Clubs, MRS. TH. HOVEN for "Work Ennobles," and MRS. ROMEIJN-TUCKERMAN for the Cooperative Women's Union and for the Dutch Committee of Women for Permanent Peace in The Hague.

Each speech was greeted by loud applause.

DR. JACOBS was clearly moved and said that she had been surrounded with so much love, friendship, and admiration that she now found it difficult to express her feelings. But first and foremost she felt a deep sense of happiness that she had been able to live to see this day. She had been able to discover just how much Dutch women today differed from their mothers and grandmothers. Had she been born fifty years later, she would have been considered quite ordinary: "I was just doing what you all do now. (Shouts of 'No, no!') I was a woman just like you; I felt the way you do. And if even one woman in this country was unfairly treated because of her gender, I felt personally insulted. And that's how you all feel nowadays." She then demonstrated just how much had changed by quoting examples of women's dependence in those dreadful "good old days."

Dr. Jacobs said that the committee's decision to turn her birthday into a party had been brilliantly successful. She had realized that, however different women today may be, they were determined to work just as hard as their predecessors who could bask in the knowledge that the younger generation would maintain the woman's movement a hundred times more efficiently because they were better prepared and did not have to waste time on campaigning for the right to vote. Suffrage gave them the necessary weapon to achieve additional rights for women in the near future.

She then added the following for the younger members of the audience: "With regard to our failures, do not forget that the problems we encountered were not the same as yours, that we had to fight our way through a barrage of prejudice." She concluded by saying, "We have fought to ensure that in the future women will be able to enjoy happier and more carefree lives!"

This was immediately followed by thunderous applause and a rendition of "Lang zal zij leven" [May she live long].

The reception ended as all those present filed past Dr. Jacobs to convey their congratulations in person. Tea was served in the salons of the Club Building and guests prepared for an intimate dinner in Witte Brug.

The Dinner

Dr. Jacobs's arrival was greeted by a welcoming song. Then, when everyone was seated and before dinner was served, a "Minister Thorbecke" appeared on stage to recite an ode to the guest of honor, an act that was particularly successful, for it alluded to the current political situation. MRS. VAN WULFFTEN PALTHE then read a welcoming speech written in rhyme that was also greeted with great enthusiasm.

The mistress of ceremonies, MISS ROSA MANUS, read out a congratulatory telegram from the Sappemeer Council and mentioned that there had been a veritable mountain of telegraphic messages including those from: Lady Aberdeen, the president of the International Council of Women, countless associations both Dutch and foreign, Suze Groeneweg, Mrs. Marie van Eysden-Vink, Rosa de Guchtenaere and many other individuals and organizations connected with the national and international women's world.

There is little that I can add to this report. I received so many telegrams that it was impossible to read more than the most prominent ones aloud. A number of these have already been mentioned, but I would like to add that I was particularly moved by the congratulatory messages from the senate of the University of Groningen, from Sappemeer Council, and from the doctors who wrote to me both in groups and individually. I particularly appreciated the speech given by Dr. Deknatel, the chairman of The Hague branch of the Society for the Advancement of Medicine, who also presented me with a magnificent bouquet of flowers. Although they were already well represented at the reception, many female students from the various universities sent me telegrams as well. In addition, I was congratulated by a number of well-known personalities who deserve to be mentioned here. They included: Mr. J. Limburg, a reformer with whom I particularly sympathize and who is also the leader of the Social Democratic Workers' Party; Mr. and Mrs. P. J. Troelstra; and Mr. D. Hans, the chairman of the Dutch Union of Journalists. The chairman of The Hague branch of this union, Mr. J. J. van Bolhuis, also conveyed his best wishes. Among the many telegrams I received from the women of Holland, Dr. Mia Boissevain's message stated that she knew she was but one of the many now celebrating my life and that she hoped that whatever pain I may have experienced would be transformed into joy by all these tributes. Apart from those organizations that were present at my birthday celebrations, others who did not attend wrote to convey their respect and admiration. Among these I particularly remember the groups whose political or religious beliefs I do not share, including the Women's Group of the Freedom Union, the Christian Nursery School Teachers, and the Jewish Women's Council.

Of the many foreign telegrams, I would especially like to mention the messages I received from Mrs. Chapman Catt, who served for twenty years as the president of the International Woman Suffrage Alliance, and from her successor, Mrs. Corbett Ashby; from Lady Ishbel Aberdeen, the president of the International Council of Women, and from the entire council board; from Miss Jane Addams, the president of the Women's International League for Peace and Freedom, and also from the league's board. I was also congratulated by countless associations from Finland, Denmark, Norway, Flemish-speaking Ghent, Hungary, Czechoslovakia, Germany, France, Spain, and Italy. The stream of letters from both home and abroad thanked me for my work in general and specifically for the ways in which I had been able to help particular organizations.

When I surveyed the plethora of tributes the next day, I found myself wondering: had I really done all this? Then I looked at the picture I had been given that depicted my parents' house. My gaze was drawn first to the room where I had studied as a young girl and had sat pondering an uncertain future. Had I really lived through all this? A mass of experiences far too complex to be squeezed into this one book . . . ? So I simply sat there quite alone, dizzy from the emotions of the previous day, staring at my picture. Then I was suddenly struck by the somber thought that neither my parents nor my many brothers and sisters, who had so often worried about my future, had lived to witness my wonderful day.[7] And, looking at that room, where my father had taught me so much, I spoke to him silently, "Father, it's all right. You often worried that I'd end up landing myself in real trouble. But the little I still have to do is really no cause for concern. My work has been successfully completed, thanks to your help and advice. Women can now look forward to a brighter future!"

ALETTA JACOBS IN
HISTORICAL PERSPECTIVE

A pioneering physician and feminist, Aletta Jacobs had twentieth-century vision, even though she lived most of her life during the Victorian era. As the first woman to attend university and receive a medical degree in the Netherlands, who then managed to combine a career with a companionate marriage and political activism, she can serve as a role model for modern professional women, although her example was difficult for other women of her own generation to emulate. Jacobs established what is often considered the first birth control clinic in the world. She also spearheaded campaigns for the deregulation of prostitution, the improvement of working conditions for women, and the introduction of woman suffrage in Holland. She was a prominent leader in both Dutch and international suffrage organizations and in the women's peace movement during World War I. Aletta Jacobs's *Memories* documents what one courageous woman can accomplish through a lifetime of dedicated work on behalf of other women.

Much of what we know about Aletta Jacobs, her life and her work, is based on what she chooses to tell us in her memoir. *Memories* presents her experiences in her own words and helps us understand strengths and weaknesses of the nineteenth-century women's movement and some of the foundations upon which late twentieth-century feminism has been built. Although Jacobs has received wide recognition in the Netherlands as a very important figure in first-wave feminism, she is relatively unknown to an English-speaking audience, since until now most of what has been written by and about her has appeared only in Dutch. General works dealing with European women's history frequently make brief mention of Aletta Jacobs's contributions to birth control and the 1915 Women's Peace Conference in The Hague, but to date only one source available in English, Mineke Bosch and Annemarie Kloosterman's *Politics and Friendship,* provides the U.S. reader with insights into Jacobs's role within the International Woman Suffrage Alliance and her personal life through her correspondence with other suffragists.[1]

Jacobs was an extraordinary individual, but she was not alone in her endeavors. She was fortunate to have lived at a time when new choices and opportunities were becoming available for women. She was part of the first generation of European women physicians and feminists who helped push open educational and professional doors for themselves and for others and fought on behalf of women's rights and woman suffrage.

Jacobs defied many of the conventions of her day and refused to live the life of a typical Victorian woman. Middle-class girls in the mid-nineteenth century were expected to remain within the domestic sphere as wives and mothers, but Jacobs rebelled against following in her mother's footsteps as a homemaker. Education for girls was segregated, except at the elementary level; Jacobs strongly advocated coeducation. Girls' high schools, often known as "finishing schools," taught modern languages, music, art, and handicrafts to prepare "young ladies" for marriage, but did not offer mathematics, physics, Greek, or Latin, which were prerequisites for admission to the all-male universities. Jacobs, however, hated attending a private school for girls and was not at all interested in learning etiquette and housekeeping skills; she decided to study medicine instead. The only acceptable career for a middle-class, single woman was teaching, whether as a governess or in a girls' school. Married women teachers had to relinquish their employment. Jacobs helped pave the way for women to become doctors, and she continued to practice medicine after her marriage, despite the fact that it was not regarded as proper for a middle-class married woman to work outside the home except as an unpaid volunteer.

Aletta Jacobs was by no means a revolutionary by temperament, and she certainly did not wish to scandalize her neighbors, but her views and personal behavior were clearly ahead of her times. In late nineteenth-century Amsterdam, respectable women were not supposed to skate on the canals in winter or walk down certain major thoroughfares in the afternoon, let alone appear in public unescorted or walk alone after dark. A "streetwalker" was assumed to be a prostitute, since a proper young woman would surely have a chaperon. Jacobs, however, enjoyed skating and insisted upon visiting her patients and her family, day or night, on foot. She also attended the theater by herself and participated in political meetings, often as the only woman. Before the turn of the century, when sex and sexuality were absolutely taboo subjects for discussion in middle-class circles, and birth control and prostitution were not mentionable in polite company, especially by a woman, Jacobs provided contraceptive information and devices and delivered speeches on prostitution and women's rights.

Married Dutch and other European women lost their legal status as individuals and their right to own property, becoming the property of their husbands instead. Jacobs strongly objected to marriage as an institution that demeaned women. She desperately wanted to bear a child, but feared the stigma of illegitimacy.[2] At the age of thirty-eight, after more than a decade of an intimate relationship, Jacobs decided to marry Carel Victor Gerritsen, but she retained her name, her bank account, and her own living quarters within their shared home, a highly unusual arrangement in the 1890s. As her reminiscences show, their friendship and marriage represented a genuine intellectual partnership based on equality and mutual respect. They particularly enjoyed traveling together and writing collaboratively.

A widow after 1905, Jacobs continued to travel extensively in Europe and around the world, by herself and with female companions. By the early twentieth century, such independent behavior had become more acceptable for women, especially older women, and aroused little comment. European and American upper- or upper-middle-class women in Jacobs's day, including many of her colleagues in the woman's movement, often traveled extensively, whether for pleasure or to attend international conferences. Although traveling by ship, train, or horse-drawn carriage was extremely slow, it could generally be done in leisurely comfort, with the help of servants and porters, except during wartime. By the time of her death in 1929, at age seventy-five, Jacobs's advanced views and lifestyle would have raised many fewer eyebrows than during her younger years.

BECOMING A MEDICAL DOCTOR

Aletta Jacobs was a medical pioneer; she did not have female role models to emulate. As a girl, she wanted to become a physician not because she had ever seen or even heard of a woman doctor but because her beloved father and oldest brother were both physicians. It was not unusual for members of the first generation of women doctors to choose to study medicine because of the example of a close male relative. Franziska Tiburtius (1843–1927), an unmarried teacher who was one of the first German women to obtain a medical degree in Switzerland in 1876, opted to study medicine rather than establish a school for girls because of the urging of her physician brother.[3] Jacobs, Tiburtius, and other medical pathbreakers provided the missing female role models for later generations to follow.

Growing up in a Jewish household that valued learning greatly increased the odds that Aletta and her sisters would receive a higher education to prepare them for careers that would allow them to become self-supporting. Advanced

studying for girls required, in addition to a middle-class upbringing, exceptional personal motivation and considerable parental support, both financial
and moral. As was quite common among early university women, the strongest
influence on Jacobs's early life was unquestionably her father.[4] A committed
democrat, antimilitarist, and liberal, Abraham Jacobs was "the prototype of the
Jew in those days when the Netherlands was governed by [Johan] Thorbecke,"
the Liberal prime minister until 1872.[5] He provided his five daughters, as well
as his six sons, with the best education available. Unlike many fathers, Abraham
Jacobs supported his favorite daughter's unconventional aspirations and, together with several of his Jewish medical colleagues, provided her with mentor-
ing and tutoring both before and during medical school. Although she briefly
attended a boys' gymnasium (high school), she did not complete standard
matriculation requirements, but qualified for university on the basis of passing
an assistant pharmacist's examination instead. Thanks to her own determination and her father's personal intervention, Aletta Jacobs received special
permission from Prime Minister Thorbecke to be admitted provisionally to the
University of Groningen at the age of seventeen.[6] An exceptional first case
whose example proved difficult to follow, she was considerably younger than
most other European women who sought entry into the medical profession in
that era.

In the late nineteenth century, medical education in the United States,
Britain, and Russia tended to be segregated by sex; elsewhere in Europe,
however, separate training programs for women doctors never developed.
Many of the early Russian, German, British, and American women physicians,
such as Nadezhda Suslova, Franziska Tiburtius, Elizabeth Garrett (Anderson),
and Mary Putnam (Jacobi), received their doctorates from Zurich, Bern, or Paris
because they were unable to gain access to medical schools at home or because
they considered the training provided by women's medical courses to be
inferior. It was only in the early twentieth century that coeducation such as
Jacobs received became the norm and nearly all European medical schools,
including those in Germany and Austria, became accessible to women.[7]

Jewish women made up a disproportionately large percentage of the female
students attending European universities in the late nineteenth and early
twentieth centuries. Like Aletta Jacobs, many of them seemed particularly
attracted to the study of medicine.[8] Among the early European female physicians were Varvara Kashevarova-Rudneva (1842–1899) of Russia, Rosa Welt of
Czernowitz, Austria, and Irma Klausner (1874–1959) of Berlin. Like Jacobs,
Kashevarova, a midwife, had to receive special permission to attend the Medical
Surgical Academy in St. Petersburg in 1863. Ten years after qualifying as a
physician, having overcome many obstacles, she became the first woman to
receive her medical doctorate in Russia in 1878.[9] Varvara Kashevarova-Rudneva
did not pave the wave for medical coeducation in Russia; instead, separate
medical courses were established to train women as doctors. Due to restrictions

and quotas in their homeland, many Russian women, especially Jews, went to Switzerland and, later, Germany and Austria for their medical training.

In 1878 also, a year before Aletta Jacobs obtained her doctorate, Rosa Welt became the first Austrian woman to receive a medical degree from a Swiss university. Just as two of Jacobs's sisters also helped blaze trails for women, one as a pharmacist and another as a high school teacher, two Welt sisters followed in Rosa's medical footsteps within the next decade, while another sister became a chemist. Like Jacobs, Rosa Welt (Strauss) continued her medical practice after her marriage and became an active feminist involved in suffrage campaigns in both the United States and Palestine.[10]

The experiences of Irma Klausner in Germany almost twenty years later also paralleled those of Aletta Jacobs. Although women were not allowed to enroll in German universities before the turn of the century, except as auditors with special permission from their instructors, Klausner's father strongly supported her desire to study medicine and used his political connections to help push a law through the Prussian Landtag (state assembly) that enabled his daughter to take her preclinical state board examination at the University of Halle in 1899; this law allowing women to take German medical examinations became known as "Lex Irma." As a married woman, and then as a widow, Irma Klausner-Cronheim continued to practice medicine for over half a century. In contrast to Jacobs, Klausner-Cronheim never became involved in politics or feminism, but one of her sisters became a high school teacher and feminist politician, while another eventually became a judge.[11] The Klausner sisters, like the Jacobs and the Welt sisters, illustrate the strong support for higher education for women among middle-class European Jewish families in the late nineteenth century.

Aletta Jacobs was fortunate that, unlike so many of her contemporaries, she did not have to leave her homeland in order to obtain her medical degree and she received exactly the same training as her male counterparts. As in the cases of Elizabeth Blackwell at Geneva Medical College in New York in 1847, Varvara Kashevarova in St. Petersburg, and Nadezhda Suslova in Zurich in the 1860s, and Irma Klausner in Halle or Rahel Goitein Straus in Heidelberg at the turn of the century, Jacobs was the only woman studying medicine in Groningen, and then in Amsterdam, but she neither requested nor received any form of special treatment. By and large, her professors and her fellow students accepted and even helped her; like most of these early women who studied medicine in Europe, she did not complain about overt discrimination or harassment, although such incidents undoubtedly occurred.[12]

After Jacobs received authorization to continue her medical studies in 1872, Dutch women encountered no legal obstacles preventing their access to institutions of higher learning in the Netherlands, as long as they could pass the same matriculation examinations as men, but few possessed the necessary secondary education to take advantage of this opportunity. The second woman to qualify as a medical doctor in Holland was Catherine von Tussenbroek (1852–1925), who, after pursuing a teaching career, entered the University of Utrecht in 1880 and received her degree in 1887.[13] By 1900, there were only ten women medical doctors in Holland; by 1923, around the time that Jacobs began writing her memoir, there were 175 female physicians and many more women studying in the medical faculties of Dutch universities, following in Jacobs's and Tussenbroek's footsteps.[14]

PRACTICING WOMEN'S MEDICINE

It was often assumed by both men and women that women doctors were best suited to treat other women who were too modest to seek gynecological help from a male physician. Women frequently justified their entry into the medical profession on that basis. Indeed, both Russia and Austria tolerated the training and hiring of their first women doctors precisely for the purpose of treating Muslim women in such outlying provinces of their empires as Orenburg and Bosnia.[15] When Jacobs first began her medical studies, she did not intend to specialize in treating women or children. Near the end of her training, when she substituted temporarily for her brother and considered taking over her father's rural practice, she handled male patients as well as female. Nevertheless, after she established her own practice in Amsterdam in 1879, she, like Catherine van Tussenbroek a few years later, followed the same pattern as virtually all nineteenth-century and most early twentieth-century women physicians by focusing her attention almost entirely on the health of women. Like Franziska Tiburtius and Emilie Lehmus in Berlin in 1876, and other women medical practitioners, Jacobs set up a private practice, where she charged standard rates to patients who could afford them, and also a clinic for poorer women, whom she treated gratis when necessary.[16]

In limiting her practice largely to women, Aletta Jacobs made a choice that was perhaps not entirely voluntary, but she quickly found her own niche. By openly dispensing birth control devices in both her clinic and her private practice after 1881, Jacobs differentiated herself from virtually all of her medical colleagues, including van Tussenbroek and Tiburtius. She is frequently referred to as the founder of the first birth control clinic; her small-scale twice-weekly dispensary for women preceded the better known, more publicized clinics of Margaret Sanger in the United States and Marie Stopes in England by at least thirty-five years.[17]

Jacobs wanted to enable women to space their children and avoid having large families they could not afford. Around 1882, once she had learned of, and tested, the Mensinga pessary, which had been developed in Germany, she began fitting her patients with this new variety of diaphragm, which became commonly known as "Dutch caps." She had adopted what was probably the most effective form of birth control then available to women, the same type of diaphragm that Sanger was later to distribute. Jacobs did not publicize her clinic widely, but she continued to provide free birth control services for roughly twelve years, until after the birth and death of her own infant in 1893. The Dutch Neo-Malthusian Union continued to operate birth control dispensaries in the Netherlands after Jacobs's retirement, providing a model for other clinics established in the twentieth century.[18] After her death, the Aletta Jacobs House, the most highly respected center for birth control and sexology in Holland, was named to honor her.[19]

In the 1880s, however, Jacobs's open advocacy of birth control scandalized Dutch society. Within medical circles, providing contraception was as controversial an issue in the late nineteenth and early twentieth centuries as abortion was to become later on. Although the practice of birth control was becoming more widespread, distribution of contraceptive information was not legal in most countries, as evident from the famous trials of Annie Besant and Charles Bradlaugh in England in 1878 and Margaret Sanger in New York in 1917.

Although many patients requested contraceptive advice from their female physicians, most early women doctors, unlike Jacobs, were unwilling to provide such help in the nineteenth century because they feared jeopardizing their professional reputations. Jacobs's insistence that medical doctors should be in charge of the dissemination of birth control brought her into conflict with her colleague Catherine van Tussenbroek, who objected to such a policy on the basis of medical ethics and reluctance to give husbands and doctors the right to control women's bodies.[20] This situation began to change by the interwar years, when many women doctors, especially young socialists, supported the sex reform movement and helped establish family counselling clinics in Germany, England, and the United States.[21] Abortion, however, remained illegal and beyond respectability in the medical world. The French physician Madeleine Pelletier (1874–1939), a woman who dressed in mannish clothing, had short hair, and associated with anarchists, was a rare example of a medical doctor who publicly supported and performed abortions in the early twentieth century.[22] Aletta Jacobs was by no means as radical as Pelletier either politically or personally, but she too demonstrated considerable courage and the strength of her convictions by openly advocating and supplying birth control at the outset of her career.

Once she had relinquished her medical practice, Jacobs played down her association with contraception and became more actively involved with other feminist causes instead, but long after she retired in 1904, she was still consulted as a respected authority in this field. She never became prominent in birth control organizations, however. Although she had learned about contraception from the Neo-Malthusians whom she had met in England, she did not continue to support the Dutch Neo-Malthusian Union because she strongly believed that only medical doctors should provide contraceptive aids. When Margaret Sanger tried to arrange a meeting with her in 1915, Jacobs refused to see her, evidently because Sanger was a trained nurse, not a physician. In 1925, however, she made peace with Sanger at an international birth control conference in New York.[23] By that time, Jacobs had undoubtedly become the "grand old lady" of birth control, but it had not been one of her priorities for many years.

FIGHTING FOR WOMEN WORKERS' RIGHTS

Through her medical practice, Jacobs became aware not only of the need for planned motherhood but also of the plight of prostitutes and sales clerks. Her concern for working-class women was as a progressive reformer, not a socialist. She did not try to organize either the salesgirls or the prostitutes to fight for their own rights; nor did she personally intervene to help them individually through philanthropic means, although she did provide them with medical care. Her preferred solutions to social problems were education and legislation.

Perhaps because Holland was not yet heavily industrialized and relatively few women worked in factories, Jacobs became concerned about improving the working condition of saleswomen in shops and department stores. She launched a publicity campaign for seats behind counters, more frequent breaks, and a shorter working day. Her efforts, which began as a rather idiosyncratic private crusade and expanded into a threatened consumer boycott, eventually achieved at least limited success.

It took far more personal courage to combat prostitution and venereal disease, topics that were even more taboo in the Victorian age than birth control. Somewhat on the model of Britain's Josephine Butler (1828–1906), Jacobs sought to deregulate prostitution by closing down state-run brothels and eliminating humiliating medical examinations for registered prostitutes.[24] When Jacobs attacked prostitution, she was fighting against a double standard of morality, but she seems to have emphasized the medical aspects of the problem even more than the moral issues. She never became involved in the campaign against "white slavery" or other efforts aimed at preventing young girls from falling into the clutches of traffickers in women or rescuing prostitutes from a life of ill repute. In this, she differed not only from Britain's Josephine Butler but also from Bertha Pappenheim (1859–1936), the German-Jewish feminist who established the *Jüdischer Frauenbund* (League of Jewish Women) in 1904.[25]

Most medical doctors in Holland, as well as elsewhere in Europe, supported state regulation of prostitution as a means of curtailing the spread of sexually transmitted diseases.[26] Jacobs, however, viewed the existing regulations, which were directed against prostitutes but not their patrons, as completely ineffective, since they stigmatized women but did not solve the rampant medical problems that resulted from prostitution. Seeking to get rid of prostitution as a legal institution through a process of education, Jacobs spoke publicly and published articles on this subject both at home and abroad. As was the case elsewhere in Europe, although prostitution was never abolished in the Netherlands, official brothels eventually disappeared and mandatory medical examinations of prostitutes ceased at least temporarily. In part due to the efforts of Aletta Jacobs and other Dutch feminists, Holland served as a European model for the declining incidence of venereal diseases in the early twentieth century.[27]

LIBERALS AND DUTCH POLITICS

Aletta Jacobs was both a liberal and a feminist. Her political outlook was shaped largely by the influence of liberal men, such as John Stuart Mill. She shared the progressive, democratic views of her father, Abraham Jacobs, and her husband, Carel Gerritsen. Gerritsen was an active social reformer who held strong feminist convictions even before he met his future wife and amassed an extensive collection of literature and documents on women and women's rights. Like Aletta Jacobs, both of these men were liberal freethinkers who had broken away from their religious roots, Jacobs from Judaism and Gerritsen from Dutch Calvinism. Intermarriages between Jews and Protestants in Holland were relatively rare in the late nineteenth century. Although civil marriage was uncommon, Aletta and Carel opted for a civil ceremony because neither identified with any religious community.[28]

By the early twentieth century, Dutch society had become segmented into four political camps, the Protestants, the Catholics, the liberals or "neutrals," and the socialists. The right wing within Dutch politics included three explicitly Christian parties, the Christian Historical Union and the Anti-Revolutionary Party, among the Protestants, and the Catholic Party. The left was splintered into various liberal factions, the Liberal Union, the Radical Union, and, later, the Liberal Democratic Union as well as the Social Democratic Workers' Party.[29] Aletta Jacobs and Carel Gerritsen belonged to the left-liberal wing within this political spectrum.

In Holland, as in Germany and Austria, most Jews of Aletta Jacobs's generation could be categorized as liberals. Dutch Jews had acquired civil rights in 1796, in the aftermath of the French Revolution, which had brought about the emancipation of French Jewry several years earlier. Although a majority of Dutch Jewry were poor and lived in Amsterdam, during the course of the nineteenth century many middle-class Jews, especially those in the provinces, had become increasingly "Netherlandized," or assimilated. In the second half of the nineteenth century, virtually all Dutch Jews supported the liberals; by the twentieth century, many of the Jewish diamond workers in Amsterdam and some Jewish intellectuals had gravitated farther left toward the socialists.[30] Jewish women activists from Eastern Europe, like many of the younger generation of Jewish university women in Germany and Austria in the early twentieth century, tended to become radicals and socialists rather than liberals or feminists; Jacobs, however, remained in the liberal camp, as did nearly all nineteenth-century Western European feminists of Jewish origin.[31]

Together with Gerritsen, Aletta Jacobs was actively involved in the left-liberal Radical Union, which was the first Dutch political party to admit women and to advocate universal suffrage; it also supported social reform and separation of church and state within the public schools. Gerritsen served as a Radical alderman on the Amsterdam City Council and a member of the Dutch parliament (or Tweede Kamer). Both Jacobs and Gerritsen were among the founding members of the Liberal Democratic Union, the successor to the Radical Union, in 1901. In 1918, a year before Dutch women were granted the right to vote, Jacobs ran for parliament on the Liberal Democratic ticket, but, much to her disappointment, failed to win election.

VOTES FOR WOMEN

Although Jacobs was involved in many different feminist activities at various stages of her life, the cause to which she devoted herself for the longest period of time was woman suffrage. For Jacobs, unlike most continental European feminists, obtaining the vote, and hence direct access to political power, was the key to improving women's lives. Aletta Jacobs described herself primarily as an equal rights feminist who fought for the political and legal emancipation of women, although she sometimes utilized relational feminist arguments emphasizing female superiority and motherhood. In her outlook and her activities, she had much more in common with Anglo-American individualist feminist activists, such as Millicent Garrett Fawcett (1847–1929) and Carrie Chapman Catt (1859–1947), than with prominent European defenders of motherhood, such as Swedish Ellen Key (1849–1926) or French Nelly Roussel (1878–1922).[32] Nevertheless, she supported many of the same causes as did leading German radical feminists such as Anita Augspurg (1857–1943), Lida Gustava Heymann (1868–1943), and Helene Stöcker (1869–1941), founder of the German *Bund für Mutterschutz* (League for the Protection of Motherhood), as well as Hungarian feminists Rosika Schwimmer (1877–1948) and Wilma Glücklich (1872–1927).[33] She firmly believed that if women gained political power, they would help bring about a better and more harmonious world.

In the late nineteenth and early twentieth century, Europe witnessed a proliferation of organizations devoted to improving the status of women; some were concerned with promoting educational and professional opportunities for middle-class women, others aimed at protecting the rights of working-class women, while still others, both moderate and militant, focused on voting rights for women. From the time she attempted to register to vote in 1883 to the day she was allowed to cast her first ballot almost forty years later, Aletta Jacobs engaged in a suffrage campaign based on moderation and legality. She was a suffragist, not a suffragette, and was firmly opposed to the militant tactics of the British Women's Social and Political Union, which included property damage and often resulted in arrests and forced feedings as well as a great deal of publicity. While Jacobs acknowledged that such militancy drew attention to the common cause, she preferred lobbying and involvement in the political process, as well as speaking tours and peaceful demonstrations. The Dutch

Woman Suffrage Association, founded in 1894 and headed by Jacobs, was very much in the mainstream of the International Woman Suffrage Alliance, to which it belonged as an affiliate. Jacobs never held office in the IWSA, which was established in 1904 and presided over by her close friend, Carrie Chapman Catt, but she regularly participated in its congresses as the head of the Dutch delegation and often traveled on its behalf.[34]

By the time Aletta Jacobs wrote her memoir, women had obtained the right to vote in Holland and many other European states, but not France, Italy, or Spain. Once suffrage was achieved in various countries, the international women's movement, especially the International Woman Suffrage Alliance, but also its more conservative and broadly based antecedent, the International Council of Women, began to disintegrate. In the interwar years, women won election to European national and provincial parliaments, as well as municipal councils. Most were elected as socialists or communists, but a few as liberals as well. In the Dutch elections of 1918, although Jacobs's candidacy met with defeat, a Social Democrat, Suze Groeneweg, became the first woman member of parliament in Holland;[35] Betsy Bakker-Nort, a Jewish lawyer closely associated with Jacobs in the suffrage movement, was elected as a Liberal Democrat in 1922. Although European women legislators from all parties generally promoted and supported measures to improve the status of women, they were unable to effect major changes within the political system. Female socialists or communists tended to consider themselves as socialists or communists first and feminists second, if at all.[36] Although Jacobs remained optimistic at the end of her life that suffrage would soon result in true equality for women, her hopes were not to be realized.

ACTIVIST FOR PEACE

Before the outbreak of World War I, Jacobs had not been actively engaged in pacifist activities; unlike Bertha von Suttner (1843–1914), the Austrian woman who had been the prime mover in the international peace movement until her death, Jacobs's top priority was woman suffrage.[37] The war created a serious schism within the various national suffrage organizations, as it did within most European socialist parties. A majority of suffragists, especially moderate leaders such as Anna Shabanova in Russia, Millicent Garrett Fawcett in England, and Carrie Chapman Catt in the United States, but also more militant suffragettes, including Emmeline and Christabel Pankhurst, opted for patriotism and backing their national war efforts rather than supporting the peace movement, which some felt might jeopardize women's chances of gaining suffrage. By contrast, a relatively small minority of radical feminists, including the Hungarian Rozika Schwimmer, the Germans Anita Augspurg and Lida Gustava Heymann, and the British Chrystal Macmillan and Emmeline Pethick-Lawrence, along with some Americans such as Anna Garland Spencer, Fannie Fern Andrews, and Crystal Eastman, became convinced that women's primary obligation was to stop the carnage of war as soon as possible.[38] Once the IWSA conference scheduled to be held in Berlin in 1915 was canceled because of the war, Aletta Jacobs decided to take it upon herself to issue invitations to women from both neutral and belligerent countries to attend a special congress to discuss strategies for peace. The resulting April 1915 International Congress of Women in The Hague represents the most significant women's gathering to promote peace and bring an end to World War I.[39]

Like its much smaller socialist counterpart held in Bern in March,[40] the Hague Congress, attended by almost twelve hundred women, most of whom were Dutch, is remarkable not so much for its actual accomplishments but for the fact that it took place at all. Under extremely difficult wartime conditions and against much opposition, women who were citizens of countries on both sides of the battle lines were able to meet together in neutral Holland and agree upon proposals to try to resolve the conflict and prevent future wars. As the chief organizer, Aletta Jacobs delivered the opening address in The Hague and helped draw up the congress's resolutions, while Jane Addams, the much respected American social reformer, chaired the proceedings.[41]

In the aftermath of this congress, as Jacobs relates, two delegations traveled to various European capitals to present their proposals to leading government officials, with Jacobs and Addams heading one delegation and Rozika Schwimmer and Chrystal Macmillan the other. Although Jacobs uses this material with dramatic effect in her reminiscences, these efforts at personal diplomacy, whether in Europe or subsequently in the United States, like the congress itself, had little or no impact on the war situation.[42] The most concrete result of the International Congress of Women at The Hague was the establishment of what was eventually called the Women's International League for Peace and Freedom (WILPF), which is considered the most important women's peace organization in the twentieth century. Aletta Jacobs was instrumental in founding this group and served as one of its vice presidents in its early years; Jane Addams, its first president, received a Nobel Peace Prize in 1931.[43]

Once woman suffrage had been achieved in Holland in 1919, Jacobs continued her efforts on behalf of lasting world peace. She was very concerned about the dire economic situation in postwar Germany and the long-term negative effects of the Treaty of Versailles. By this time, however, Jacobs was approaching seventy years of age and in poor health; her financial situation had also deteriorated. Although she still attended international conferences as often as possible, she lacked the strength to embark on yet another personal crusade.

A COMPARATIVE PERSPECTIVE

Although she is generally recognized for her important role in both birth control and the women's peace movement during World War I, what most clearly distinguishes Aletta Jacobs from other pioneering women physicians and first-wave feminists is the number of different women's causes she personally espoused and actively championed. She cannot be easily compared to any other single individual, although she shares many characteristics with a variety of other pathbreaking women doctors and suffragists.

Most nineteenth century women physicians devoted their lives to the practice of medicine. Although medical pioneers like Elizabeth Blackwell, Elizabeth Garrett Anderson, and Franziska Tiburtius promoted women's medical education and often sympathized with and supported various feminist causes, they generally did not assume leadership positions in women's organizations. Similarly, the better known early feminist leaders, such as Susan B. Anthony and Elizabeth Cady Stanton in the United States and Josephine Butler and Emily Davies in England, tend to be associated with one, or perhaps two, aspects of the woman's movement. Jacobs's traveling companion, Carrie Chapman Catt, for example, was primarily involved in suffrage work for most of her life, although she later engaged in women's peace activities as well.[44] By contrast, Jacobs was prominent in multiple spheres, both as a physician and as a feminist, often internationally as well as in Holland.

At least one other early continental European feminist doctor, the Russian gentrywoman Anna Shabanova (1848–1932), managed to combine a medical career with leadership in a national woman's movement. In choosing to become a liberal feminist prominent in the suffrage movement, rather than a radical or socialist, Shabanova resembled Jacobs but differed from many other Russian women physicians of her day. A member of the first graduating class of the Women's Medical Academy in St. Petersburg in 1877, she was a practicing pediatrician, researcher, teacher, and writer as well as a social activist and pacifist before World War I. Although she was personally and politically more conservative than Jacobs and never active in such causes as birth control and prostitution deregulation, Shabanova's career and goals paralleled Jacobs's quite closely, at least until 1914; both women avoided militancy and preferred to work through legal channels and personal connections to bring women political and economic equality with men.[45]

Another European feminist leader with whom Aletta Jacobs had much in common was her younger protégée, Rozika Schwimmer. Schwimmer came from an assimilated Hungarian Jewish family, but she received no higher education. A prolific journalist and fiery public speaker, Schwimmer was involved in organizing working women and founded the Hungarian woman suffrage association. Like Jacobs, she campaigned on behalf of birth control and marriage reform and was deeply committed to pacifism as well as woman suffrage. Schwimmer played a vital role in shaping the development of the feminist movement in Hungary before World War I and was active within the IWSA. Jacobs and Schwimmer met in 1903 and developed a close friendship, corresponding regularly and participating in many conferences together until 1915. Their personal styles were different. Much more militant than Jacobs in her behavior and political views, Schwimmer's personality was more domineering and abrasive. Schwimmer spent the last years of her life as an emigrée and an outcast in American society, whereas Jacobs in her old age found honor in her own homeland.[46]

JEWISH IDENTITY

One of the ties binding Jacobs and Schwimmer was their shared awareness of their Jewishness. Aletta Jacobs kept her identity as a Jew very private. Others clearly perceived her as being Jewish and she did not deny her Jewish origins, yet she preferred not to discuss this subject publicly. She referred to herself as a "wandering Jewess" in her personal correspondence and identified others as Jews in her letters to Schwimmer, but she seems to have completely lacked a public Jewish persona and considered herself a "citizen of the world."[47] Like most Jewish women of her time, she received no formal Jewish education; she makes no mention of her grandparents or of any Jewish observances in her childhood home. As a freethinker, she belonged to no organized religious community and disliked religion of any kind. She was certainly never a Zionist or a Jewish nationalist; when she traveled in Palestine, she exhibited no special interest in Jewish sites or the development of a Jewish homeland.[48] During a visit to Sarajevo, she was intrigued by the customs of Sephardic women there, but she refers to them as Spaniards rather than as Jews, just as she prefers to call Bosnian Muslims Turks, despite the fact that virtually no ethnic Turks or Spaniards lived in Sarajevo on the eve of World War I.

Like Jacobs and Schwimmer, many Jewish feminists, as well as socialists, of the late nineteenth and early twentieth century tended to minimize their identification with Judaism and the Jewish community, even though they often associated with other like-minded Jews. Some Eastern European Jewish revolutionaries and Western European social reformers rejected their Jewish family backgrounds completely. Rosa Luxemburg (1879–1919), the brilliant Polish-born Social Democratic theoretician with a doctorate in political science from Zurich, was interested in neither Jewish nor feminist matters. As she once wrote to a Jewish friend, "Why do you come to me with your special Jewish sorrow? . . . I cannot find a special corner in my heart for the ghetto. I feel at home in the entire world. . . ."[49] Anna Kuliscioff (1855–1925), the Italian socialist feminist physician who began life as Anna Rozenstein in Russia and studied medicine in Zurich and Pavia, also broke off ties with the community of her birth, but she occasionally expressed sympathy with persecuted Jewry.[50]

Like modern Jewish women in general, the early generation of Jewish women physicians and feminists demonstrated a broad range of Jewish identities, but most had largely abandoned traditional religious practices. At the opposite end of the spectrum from Jacobs, Rahel Goitein Straus (1880–1963), the first woman medical student at Heidelberg at the turn of the century, maintained a kosher Jewish household for her husband and five children and was actively involved in both the Zionist movement and the German Jewish feminist organization, the Jüdischer Frauenbund (League of Jewish Women), while continuing her private medical practice and giving lectures on sexuality and reform of antiabortion legislation. Rahel Straus's strong commitment to the Jewish community was more exceptional among Jewish women with higher education than Aletta Jacobs's noninvolvement.

Breaking away from one's Jewish roots did not shield one from antisemitism, however. Among the assimilated Jewish social reformers who were active within the German woman's movement, the most prominent was Alice Salomon (1872–1948). The creator of the modern social work profession in Germany, with a doctorate in sociology from the University of Berlin, Salomon became alienated from Judaism at a young age and was baptized as a Protestant in 1914. Nevertheless, although she had served as secretary and vice president of the Bund Deutscher Frauenvereine (Federation of German Women's Associations) and also as corresponding secretary of the International Council of Women for many years, she was prevented from assuming the presidency of the Bund Deutscher Frauenvereine after World War I because of antisemitism.[51] Jacobs does not mention antisemitism, but even if she did not experience it personally, she was undoubtedly aware of this problem, which adversely affected the lives of other Jewish feminists, including not only Salomon, but also Rozika Schwimmer and Rosa Manus.[52]

CONCLUSION

In *Memories*, Aletta Jacobs comes across as a very self-confident, energetic, and forceful leader, who is determined to achieve her goals and much prefers to give orders rather than to follow them. Although she occasionally acknowledges the contributions of other women who worked with her, particularly within the suffrage and peace movements, she often presents herself as a one-person crusader. She tries to look at the bright side of things, emphasizing the positives and playing down the negatives that she encountered; she does not wish to expose her weaknesses or her personal misfortunes. In her extensive correspondence, some of which has been published in English, we can catch glimpses of a somewhat less formal and more vulnerable Aletta Jacobs.[53] Nevertheless, she remains a very private person whose inner thoughts and fears remain undisclosed.

Jacobs spoke English, German, and French, in addition to her native Dutch, and gave lectures in German and English during her many travels. Nearly all of her published works, however, except for some of her travelogues, are in Dutch. Although she went on frequent speaking tours in Holland and elsewhere while campaigning for woman suffrage, she never felt very comfortable as a public speaker and much preferred to transmit her ideas in written form. She published many popular articles advocating women's rights in various Dutch newspapers and magazines, and wrote the text that accompanied anatomical illustrations in a book dealing with the female body so that Dutch women could learn about the position and function of their genital organs. In her efforts to raise awareness concerning the economic plight of women, she translated Charlotte Perkins Gilman's *Women and Economics* and Olive Schreiner's *Women and Labor* into Dutch. She also wrote a book of biographical sketches of six of the leading women in the international woman's movement, all of whom were either American or British. She kept detailed diaries of her journeys with Gerritsen and with Carrie Chapman Catt, parts of which appeared in serial form in newspapers and later on as books. Most of her writings, including *Memories,* her last significant opus, focus on women and their status in society.

How did others view Aletta Jacobs in her lifetime? Carrie Chapman Catt, one of her closest friends, with whom she traveled in Africa and Asia for fifteen months, describes Jacobs with considerable affection and respect: "We were both strong-willed, stubborn, opinionated, yet we came through firm friends, and I at least with a warm and sincere admiration for her. Her devotion to the cause of her sex, her fund of general information on side lines, her strong memory, her calm judgment, her unceasing energy, combine to make her a truly wonderful and great woman."[54] Alice Hamilton, an American physician who accompanied Jane Addams and Jacobs on their diplomatic mission in 1915 and again in 1919, was less generous when she depicted Jacobs as "an elderly woman, very decided, fairly irritable and quite able to see that her own comfort is attended to."[55] Other evaluators of Jacobs also occasionally temper their praise. While one biographer of Margaret Sanger refers to Jacobs as "heroic," another calls her "imperious" because she did not "deign" to meet with Sanger.[56] Although her contemporaries generally respected and admired Jacobs, they were not always fond of her as a person and sometimes found her to be difficult, especially in her later years.

In a letter she wrote to Carrie Chapman Catt in 1928, a year before her death, Aletta Jacobs summed up the changes she had helped bring about during her lifetime:

> I feel happy that I have seen the three great objects of my life come to fulfillment during my life . . . They were: the opening for women of all opportunities to study and to bring it into practice; to make Motherhood a question of desire, no more a duty; and the political equality for women.
>
> With these three newly obtained rights the women are able to get their full legal, social, and economic equality easily if they really wish it. And I feel it, every day more, it will not take a long time before the women of the world have reached that goal. No, my dear Carrie, I feel sure we have not lived for nothing. We have done our task and we can leave the world with the conviction that we have left it in a better condition than we have found it.[57]

Jacobs and her colleagues had indeed made important contributions toward improving women's lives, but her assessment of the achievements of the first wave of feminism that she represented was overly optimistic. Women had gained access to higher education, but not acceptance in the male professional world. By the time of Jacobs's death, birth control clinics had become more widespread in both Europe and America and the birthrate had declined considerably, but effective contraception was not yet readily available and abortion was illegal. Working conditions for women had improved somewhat, but women were still exploited and underpaid. Prostitution had been deregulated but not eradicated, and sexually transmitted diseases continued to be prevalent. Women had won the right to vote, but woman suffrage had made little impact on the political process. The women's peace movement that emerged during World War I would be helpless to combat the rise of Nazism and the onslaughts of World War II. Thanks to the hard work of Jacobs and other nineteenth-century feminists, women had come far, but they still had a very long way to go to accomplish their goals.

HARRIET PASS FREIDENREICH
Temple University

PATTERNS OF REMEMBRANCE: A LITERARY AFTERWORD

W omen's memoirs are comparatively rare in this country," Jacobs writes in her preface. She had few models for portraying the sweep of her life with its exceptional richness of activities, causes, and relationships. In *Memories* she sought a form suited to that diversity and created an autobiographical text she deemed appropriate to place before the public.

Its structure is partly chronological and partly thematic. The first four chapters chronicle her childhood, her student years, and the first years of her medical practice. Each of the five middle chapters, which I like to call the "struggle chapters," is devoted to a major cause to which Jacobs committed herself. The last four chapters, like the first four, form a chronological sequence: from the beginnings of her relationship with her husband, Carel Victor Gerritsen, to her seventieth birthday celebration.

Jacobs's professional, political, and personal commitments were thoroughly intertwined and overlapping. Her commitments were worked on over time, sometimes with the same allies or adversaries and through related organizations. As a result, in a number of instances Jacobs tells about the same event in two different chapters. Sometimes one telling is simply much more elaborate than the other; sometimes different aspects of the same experience are highlighted. Far from being an occasional quirk, these doublings offer glimpses of

Jacobs's process of sorting, of integrating and separating, of crafting episodes and narratives.

For example, the 1899 London conference of the International Council for Women, a thrilling experience for Jacobs and an important juncture in her suffrage and women's advocacy work, has its elaborated telling in chapter 10, "My Union with Carel Victor Gerritsen." There is a shorter account in chapter 6, "The Campaign for Woman Suffrage," where the conference might more plausibly seem to "belong." There she emphasizes her memorable first meeting with Susan B. Anthony and other international suffrage leaders. In chapter 10, Jacobs stresses that she and her husband went to the conference together. She reports with pride that he was one of the few male speakers, and that the experience of being repeatedly introduced as "the husband of Dr. Jacobs" made him realize what it is like to be seen only as an appendage of one's spouse. Each version is "at home" in its chapter; Jacobs's embedding the more elaborate version of this important suffrage experience in the Gerritsen narrative suggests the blending she so cherished of her love-partnership and her work.

Jacobs's identity as a physician, so much desired and so dilligently pursued in her student years, nowhere appears as one "chunk" of her adult life. It is in a sense subdivided or dispersed among a range of causes and activities, beginning in chapter 4, "The Early Years of My Practice." Far from being limited to her practice of medicine in any narrow sense, this highly episodic chapter also contains spirited vignettes about women's particular difficulties at the time, such as being restricted to seats in the balcony at the theater and looked at askance for walking alone at night. Yet despite her choice not to make the twenty-five years of her medical practice one focused narrative, Jacobs repeatedly makes clear that it was attending to her patients that led her to champion causes such as family planning, better working conditions for sales-girls, and the elimination of sexually transmitted diseases; this dispersed physician identity is seen as crucial in many of her political struggles. She also recounts humorous or dismaying incidents from her travels in which her identity as a physician remains significant even though she had long since given up active medical practice.

I have discussed more fully elsewhere how the rich material she has to work with seems to resist becoming either one continuous story or a series of separable stories.[1] Yet the overall impression is one of conviction and direction. A sense of purposefulness unites the disparate elements; the cross-referencing and episodic quality are balanced by a very consistent and controlled self-presentation.

Interestingly, this self-presentation is evoked not only by her own words but by a very large proportion of quotations and references. Perhaps affected by having composed the autobiography in a study filled with print memorabilia, Jacobs includes in *Memories* entire newspaper articles, excerpts from articles, short quotations, paraphrases of published material, and numerous references to published and unpublished work, including Jacobs's own and Gerritsen's. She draws on her private correspondence as well as on professional journals and feminist publications. At times her story seems almost a collage of sources, through both direct quotation and such phrases as "I was constantly in the papers" and "Piles of letters and telegrams arrived and were dispatched each day."

Through frequent reference to her international correspondence, Jacobs includes the words of many activists with whom she was in frequent touch; more private mementoes let us hear voices of her dear ones. Her account of her relationship with Gerritsen is particularly laden with references to their writing: constant correspondence whenever they were apart, drafts of articles they always shared with one another before sending them off for publication, jointly written travel diaries. Taken together, this profusion of other voices, yet voices that she chooses, allows Jacobs to include evidence of an adulation that would sound pretentious in the first person. It also situates her as a very public figure and places her in the history of her day.

Memories has its characteristic presences and absences. Three related motifs that occupy much of the narrative space are international conferences, travel, and female friendships. There are characteristic omissions, and there are silences about certain difficult relationships and about being Jewish.

The book is replete with many sorts of international conferences; clearly Jacobs reveled at all periods in her adult life in these gatherings of like-minded people. Here she was in her element; she loved the professional recognition, the conviviality, the festivities and excursions, the opening up of vistas of thought, the encounters with luminaries of all sorts, the reunions with friends, the occasional chance to speak out in a compelling or striking way, and sometimes to be fussed over.

The pulse and emotional meaning of the conferences changed as she matured and aged, but not her wish to go. She writes of being dazzled by the 1879 international medical conference in Amsterdam, the very first she attended, as a young woman of twenty-five. There she experienced the thrill of professional recognition and a chance to mingle with some famous physicians. Her account of the 1908 conference of the International Woman Suffrage Alliance (IWSA) in Amsterdam, almost three decades later, emphasizes her energy and her pride at being in charge, organizing Dutch suffragists to host the whole event: she dwells on the mundanities of committee structure, hospitality, and publicity. Conferences Jacobs attended in her later years, especially those of the IWSA and WILPF, became energizing reunions, one more chance to see cherished, aging friends who lived thousands of miles away.[2]

Accompanying her husband, for years a Dutch legislator, she attended many of the yearly conferences of the Interparliamentary Union; Jacobs writes that she herself was not a peace activist at that time and used the occasions mainly to make international suffrage contacts.[3] Nonetheless, these yearly experiences of seeing delegates from many nations trying to build institutions and practices that would support peace no doubt also contributed to what she was later able to envision and accomplish amid the overwhelming catastrophe of European war.

For during those prewar years, and especially through managing the 1908 IWSA conference, Jacobs was first observing, then herself developing the administrative, organizing, and networking skills that she would use most potently in what was perhaps her finest hour—organizing the April 1915 International Congress of Women at The Hague in which twelve hundred women from belligerent and neutral nations came together to protest the war.

Besides her accounts of suffrage and peace conferences, Jacobs also writes about attending numerous international medical and medicine-related conferences, not only during her years of practice but for the rest of her life. By including so many of these international events, she balances the many pages devoted to internal Dutch politics and the situation of Dutch women and presents an international yet very Dutch identity.

As surely as she thrived on attending and organizing international conferences, Jacobs adored traveling. As early as her girlhood fantasy of running away to America disguised as a boy, distant vistas beckoned. All freedom of movement was important to her, whether across borders or, in the early years of her practice, simply around the streets of Amsterdam, at times and in places where "respectable" women had not felt free to walk. Wry, nostalgic, a bit pedantic, lyrical, hilarious, and incisively observant by turns, Jacobs dwells on her travel memories at every opportunity.

In a book full of meetings with the great and near great, from presidents to popes, she lingers nostalgically over trip mishaps that go on for pages. Indeed, her important and close friendship with Carrie Chapman Catt is portrayed with particular verve through one such tale: the time she and Catt, on a suffrage tour in 1906, took the wrong train out of Prague, slept in a loft, and had a horrendous day thereafter. Similarly, Jacobs situates much that is important in her relationship with Gerritsen as occurring during their many travels. On a walking tour in Switzerland, they decide to commit to one another, but not to marry. Some years later, they take a long vacation trip to the isles of Jersey and Guernsey in order to make choices about their future, and on the trip decide to marry yet maintain economic independence.

Describing her travels, Jacobs often portrays herself as doing what we might call amateur ethnography/sociology—observing, learning, comparing other cultures with her own, and writing. She illustrates the depth of her bond with Gerritsen by explaining how they jointly wrote up their observations after each day of bicycle touring. They often carried their previous travel notes with them on their bikes, the better to make comparisons and learn. She comments on the diverse contents of the articles they each wrote for Dutch newspapers while on their 1904 U.S. trip. And she refers readers who want more than what is in chapter 12, "A World Tour," to her *Reisbrieven* (Travel Letters), a collected reissue of the twice-weekly articles she faithfully wrote during that trip for *De Telegraaf*, a Dutch newspaper.[4]

A third central motif is friendship with women. Paradoxically, Jacobs's relationships with women are partly submerged in the narrative despite her topical emphasis on women's issues. She often stresses the importance of her female friendships; yet because much of her memoir is organized around "struggles," the development and continuity of these relationships is most often only glimpsed—or unseen. She writes with feeling about long-lasting friendships, but the accounts aren't fleshed out. Extended narratives are reserved for causes, journeys, and Gerritsen.

Her treatment of her friendship with Carrie Chapman Catt, which extended from 1904 to Jacobs's death, seems to be an exception; a whole chapter is devoted to their 1911–1912 trip through Africa and Asia, with Jacobs offering a warm tribute to Catt at the chapter's end. She affirms that this was the first year she had been been happy since her husband's death and praises Catt's almost saintly nature. And almost half of "The Campaign for Woman Suffrage" is devoted to their 1906 travel and suffrage adventures in Austria-Hungary. However, the travels *are* the friendship; the growth of intimacy, caring, and a very special playfulness, all of which made such long stretches of time together very significant for both women, does not itself become a subject.[5]

A more typical example of friendships mentioned but undeveloped begins in "The First Years of My Practice." Jacobs writes that her new fame brought her into contact with four women—Hélène Mercier, Elise Haighton, Catherina Alberdingk Thym, and Cornélie Huygens—whom she had known only from their published works, "but the friendships we forged were to last a lifetime." Yet except for one later mention of these "dear friends," and two brief anecdotes about Hélène Mercier, she does not write again about these obviously important friendships.

Her friendships with Miel Coops and Mien van Wullften-Palthe, the members of the Broese van Groenou family with whom she was most intimate, are similarly not exposed to view. She does say in the final chapter that when living in The Hague, she was blessed with the family's friendship and felt more attached to them than to many of her own family. However the relation with Mien and Miel, which goes back to 1908, does not have its lineaments drawn.[6] In fact Miel is never even mentioned by name, and Mien only as Jacobs's travel companion for the visits to heads of state after The Hague conference, again as a travel companion to the 1919 Zurich conference, and as a planner for the seventieth birthday celebration.

Certain other women are similarly mentioned once or twice in the context of their international work and praised, but the long-standing private friendship that so often went along with the public international work—a theme thoughtfully developed in Bosch—is left out.[7] For instance, German feminist leaders Anita Augspurg and Lida Gustava Heymann are mentioned as founders of the International Woman Suffrage Alliance, again in connection with the 1915 Hague conference, and not thereafter. But in a 1926 letter to Miel Coops, Jacobs writes about them as "Anita and Lyda" who have just sent her a book for Christmas.[8]

Jacobs herself was well aware of the difference that could exist between a public and a private persona. In this regard she writes to Miel Coops, in a long chatty letter with a whole section on what she is reading, "If you are interested later in the letters that Rosa Luxemburg wrote to Louise Kautsky and those to Sonja Liebknecht, letters that she wrote from prison, I can lend you those too. They're very much worth reading. They let us see this woman quite differently than the picture we have formed of her from newspaper stories. The woman hid a treasure of tenderness and a loftiness of character behind her quick-tempered spirit."[9] Interestingly, this letter was written during the period when Jacobs was at work writing her life story. Jacobs's own correspondence indeed offers, as Inge de Wilde has pointed out, a different and often softer side than she has chosen to share in her public memoir.[10]

Jacobs's accounts of international conferences, travel, and important friendships with women come together in a distinctive way in the sweeping Hague conference narrative that occupies the physical center of the text and is a major emotional center as well. Without attributing to the actual conference more significance than it may have had in Jacobs's long and busy life, one can observe that in *Memories* the prominence of the conference narrative is subtly heightened by the way the three recurrent narrative elements are transformed: going to international conferences becomes creating a conference; travel becomes a diplomatic mission; and friendship networks among women become bold alliances.

This Hague narrative, so central thematically and structurally to the memoir, is a useful place to notice what Jacobs characteristically omits from her narration of public events. This is very much a memoir about *her* involvements; while often giving credit to coworkers and volunteers with whom she worked directly, she feels no need to refer to the accomplishments of other groups— those further to the left, or with a different rationale, or operating elsewhere— in the name of historical balance or completeness. She does not put The Hague conference in the context of other contemporaneous peace efforts such as the activities of her more radical Dutch contemporary Bart de Ligt at home, the formation of the Women's Peace Party in the United States, and initiatives by various European women.[11] Awareness of such other initiatives, however, can frame Jacobs's narrative differently for the reader.

Her engrossing narrative of crossing the Atlantic in wartime to see Woodrow Wilson could give the impression that hers was a unique effort, whereas he had in fact already been beseiged by a whole series of peace activists trying to get him to intervene and mediate. These included Jane Addams and Emily

Balch, the very people who were helping and encouraging Jacobs as she rushed back and forth to see his assistants Colonel House and Robert Lansing and, finally, disappointingly, the president himself.[12]

One other such unmentioned initiative forms a fascinating parallel: a women's international peace conference that preceded her own. A month before Jacobs's great moment, a much smaller group of twenty-eight women gathered in Bern, Switzerland. Like The Hague conference, the Bern conference arose from a network of women that predated the war, but from a different, left-socialist network. Among those present were prominent Dutch socialists Heleen Ankersmit and Carry Pothuis-Smit. Jacobs surely knew about this event, for the group sent "greetings" to The Hague gathering in the form of a fiery letter stressing the need for the international proletariat to rebel against the capitalist warmakers.[13]

Both networks of women, suffragists and socialists, had been at work in the spring of 1914 preparing international women's conferences that had to be canceled because of the war. In both networks a tiny subgroup of women from warring nations was willing to come together, even against the wishes of their own parties or organizations. Though Jacobs did not choose to mention the Bern conference, historical awareness of it as a small left "cousin" adds a particular resonance to our reading of her account.

Silence about a difficult relationship with her one-time close friend and coworker, Hungarian suffragist and pacifist Rosika Schwimmer, also affects the version of history given in *Memories*.[14] Schwimmer was a key figure at The Hague conference and in fact was the one who proposed the postconference missions; she, U.S. pacifist Emily Balch, and several others constituted the delegation to the neutral nations. But Jacobs became intensely angry at Schwimmer and British Hague conference participant Chrystal Macmillan because they left for the United States on their own just after Jacobs left to see Wilson; she feared that the publicity they would create could damage her chances of success.[15] After returning from her trip, Jacobs abruptly and permanently broke off the friendship.[16]

In the memoir, the flamboyant and caustic Rosika, powerful speaker, recipient of many of Jacobs's confidences, is reduced to one bland mention. Neither the intense affection nor the later anger is there. Omission of Schwimmer's crucial role obscures the fact that there were two equally significant missions that traveled to heads of state after the conference, for the delegation to neutral countries, which included Schwimmer, is almost left out.

Another once close but ultimately painful relationship in Jacobs's life is also missing. Charles Jacobs, son of her adored older brother Julius, came from the Indies to the Netherlands as a boy in 1894; after Julius's death in 1895, Jacobs and Gerritsen raised Charles as their foster son. Away at school after 1900, he returned to live with Jacobs soon after she was widowed in 1905 and remained until 1909, when he left for law school.[17]

Ample evidence of their intimate tie and Jacobs's delight in his youthful spirit is in Jacobs's correspondence; Catt calls him "your splendid son." But, in July 1909, Jacobs writes to Rosika Schwimmer that "Charles was more than rude to me," that he had been alienated from her by his fiancée and her family, and that she has spent "sleepless nights, dark days." He moved out. Subsequently he asked and was given forgiveness, but Jacobs writes to Schwimmer that "he is not the same boy to me as he was before. There is something broken."[18]

Not only is Charles never mentioned, but, for example, her decision to vacation in the Tatra mountains in the summer of 1909, which a consoling letter from Catt relates to seeking comfort after the initial rupture in their relationship, is ascribed to other causes.[19]

Also deeply upsetting was Charles's subsequent role in her financial reverses. Probably he gave her unwise investment advice. After still other financial problems in 1922 resulted in a declaration of bankruptcy, she was supported for the rest of her life by members of the Broese van Groenou family and another well-to-do friend.[20] Yet, about the year 1922, which brought her so much despair, she records only recovering from illness in time to have the thrill of casting her first ballot.

Memories is not a book in which difficulties and conflicts are omitted. Jacobs does not hesitate to convey her anguish when the child born to her and Gerritsen lived only one day, or the depth of her despair after Gerritsen's death. But close relationships gone sour and feelings of shame do not fit into the life story she crafted for her public.

One other intriguing silence deserves comment. In her account of the 1879 international medical conference in Amsterdam, at which she received much acclaim, Jacobs quotes a Dr. Petithan's subsequent ebullient article about her in the Belgian medical journal *Le Scalpel*. "It is impossible to imagine science in a more charming form than that of this pretty twenty-five-year-old Jewess, listening to even the most delicate discussions with utmost tact and serenity."[21] This is, strangely, the only reference in the autobiography to her Jewish background. It is quoted in French, translated into Dutch, and passed over without comment.

If Jacobs actively wanted to conceal her Jewishness she could have left "Jewess" out altogether. To leave it in and then say no more about her background elsewhere in the memoir strikes me as even more dismissive than concealment; with this gesture, she almost outdoes herself in making her Jewishness nonsignificant. But was it?

Available evidence suggests that many of her associates did see Jacobs's Jewishness as a component of her identity. Fellow freethinker Carrie Chapman Catt recorded in her diary that upon their arrival in Djakarta in the Dutch East Indies they were met by Jacobs's pharmacist sister Charlotte, "a handsome, well-preserved Jewess."[22] And pacifist Emily Balch, a long-time associate of Jacobs in the Women's International League for Peace and Freedom (WILPF), described her in a talk some years after her death as a "Dutch Jewish physician."[23]

Yet in her autobiography, Jacobs at one point dissociates herself from any personal connection with Jewish communal life. Commenting on the piles of telegrams and good wishes she received on her seventieth birthday, she writes, "And here I am particularly thinking of the groups whose political and religious beliefs I do not share such as the . . . Christian Nursery School Teachers and the Jewish Women's Council," as if her psychological distance from the two groups felt the same. Perhaps it did.

Jacobs was a freethinker who disdained missionaries and any display of religious dogmatism; in her last extant letter to Miel Coops she writes, "Damned religion gives so many people kinks in the brain. If we could just rid the world of the whole mess, how much calmer and more peaceful it would be."[24]

But this outburst does not explain her silence about her heritage as she recounts her life story. For she writes with empathy about her husband Carel Gerritsen's early rejection of the fervent Protestantism of his parents and with approval and admiration about her friend Clara Mulder van de Graaf's courageous proselytizing for suffrage in her mostly disapproving Catholic milieu.

Surprisingly, in view of this silence in her memoir, Jacobs in fact had, from childhood on, associations with Jewish physician-mentors who managed to combine professional assimilation and advancement with maintaining ties to their ancestral heritage. Levi Ali Cohen, a close family friend in whose presence Jacobs threw a memorable tantrum of frustration about having no future because she was a girl, was a Hebraist who started a lecture series on Jewish subjects. Renowned professor Samuel Rosenstein, another family friend who facilitated her entry to the University of Groningen, was the son of a Berlin rabbi and "an observant Jew who used to pass his clinic on his way home from the synagogue on the Sabbath clad in his frock coat and black hat, which were in fashion in those days."[25]

She also knew the Israëls family. Physician and medical historian Abraham Israëls, a close friend of Ali Cohen, was sufficiently learned in traditional Jewish texts to write his medical doctoral thesis on references to obstetrics in the Babylonian Talmud; his younger brother, the noted painter Jozef Israëls, often painted Jewish subjects.[26] And internationally acclaimed Professor Barend Stokvis, who treated her when during her medical studies she fell seriously ill with typhoid fever, manifested his Jewish attachment in a different way as president of the board of several Jewish charitable institutions.[27]

Jacobs did not follow these models of people involved with Jewish learning and Jewish institutions and also successful and assimilated in their professional worlds. Many other prominent Jewish women of her era, reformers and revolutionaries, similarly did not practice their faith in the traditional way. Besides Rosa Luxemburg and Emma Goldman,[28] two towering figures Jacobs knew about but does not mention in her memoir, there were scores of others in Europe and the Americas whose attitudes toward their Jewishness were varied and complex—including downright rejection, disinterest, on-and-off recognition, on-and-off pride, nostalgia, and surreptitious embracing.

One letter written in 1906 to Rosika Schwimmer, who was also Jewish, does reveal Jacobs tacitly and indeed proudly acknowledging their shared Jewish identity. In a passage especially noted by Bosch she writes, "We have . . . recruited some good young [suffrage] workers. It is remarkable that they are always Jewish girls. With us and everywhere else. Courage and spirit are found most in these girls."[29] And to Lucy Anthony she writes with a mixture of humor and sadness in 1928, just a year before her death, "I am going to sell my house and my belongings and than [then] I will become the wandering Jewess, perhaps a tramp. But it is possible that I shall die before it is so far. One does not know."[30] These two comments, twenty-two years apart and so different in mood, indicate that Jacobs's relation to her Jewish roots was complex. But about that complexity her memoir is silent.

After Jacobs completed her autobiography, with its "sunset" feeling that her active life is almost over, she continued, despite recurrent health problems, traveling and attending international conferences. She embarked for the United States twice in two years, arriving in May 1924 for the WILPF meeting in Washington, and then returning in March 1925 for a birth control conference in New York and thereafter for the May meeting of the International Council of Women in Washington. Jacobs planned visits to old friends at their homes before and after the various conferences.[31]

Even two months before her death, slowed down by illness, Jacobs was still in motion; in June 1929 she was off to two meetings in Berlin, one on behalf of women workers and the other the twenty-fifth anniversary celebration of the IWSA. She died on August 10, and was mourned and remembered at the late August WILPF conference in Prague, which she had planned to attend.

ABBREVIATIONS

BOOKS

BWN   *Biografisch Woordenboek van Nederland*
BWSAN   *Biografisch Woordenboek van het Socialisme en de Arbei-
            dersbeweging in Nederland*
DSAB   *Dictionary of South African Biography*
NAW   *Notable American Women*
NAWM   *Notable American Women: The Modern Period*
NNBW   *Nieuw Nederlandsch Biografisch Woordenboek*
WPV   *Winkler Prins Encyclopedie "Voor de Vrouw"*

ORGANIZATIONS

ICW   International Council of Women
IWSA   International Woman Suffrage Alliance
NUWSS   National Union of Women's Suffrage Societies
VVVK   Vereeniging voor Vrouwenkiesrecht (Dutch branch of
            IWSA)
WILPF   Women's International League for Peace and Freedom

NOTES

Editor's Foreword

1. This family consisted of Wolter and Jeannetta (Wieseman) Broese van Groenou, their seven children, and the children's families. Jacobs was especially close to the two oldest daughters, "Mien" (Wilhelmina) van Wulfften Palthe (1875–1960) and "Miel" (Emilia) Coops (1876–1966), both of whom she first met in 1908 when the girls volunteered to help with preparations for the conference of the International Woman Suffrage Alliance in Amsterdam (see chapter 11). Inge de Wilde's *Brieven van Aletta H. Jacobs aan de familie Broese van Groenou* (1992) provides a rich overview of the evolving relationship, including the five years between the completion of the autobiography and Jacobs's death.

2. (De Wilde, *Brieven* 50–51) Translations in the editor's foreword and "Patterns of Remembrance" are mine, with the assistance of Charlotte Loeb.

3. Addams papers, Swarthmore College Peace Collection. Numbers in parentheses in the text refer to reel and frame numbers of the microfilmed papers.

    The passage about Jacobs's memoirs is embedded in a letter covering many topics: Jacobs's relief that Addams left Tokyo before a major earthquake and her concern about their acquaintances there, current Dutch citizen efforts to oppose construction of a large navy, her recovery from a stomach ulcer, the divorce of a fellow activist, and her dissatisfaction that an article she wrote for the *Woman Citizen* arguing for U.S. membership in the League of Nations was published in shortened form and she was not consulted. Such wide-ranging letters were typical of this network of women whose friendships and political activities were inextricably linked.

    The Jacobs-Addams material in the Addams papers goes back to 1915 and the International Congress of Women at The Hague; however, the two women knew each other before that through the international suffrage network. They were both prominent at the 1913 International Woman Suffrage Alliance conference in Budapest. Addams writes, in *Peace and Bread in Time of War,* that, among the women who had signed the invitation to the Hague Conference, "I had long warmly admired Dr. Aletta Jacobs of Amsterdam, whose name led the list." (12)

4. On Cor Ramondt, see chapter 8, note 20. On Emily Balch, see chapter 8, esp. note 34.

5. Sophonisba Breckenridge attended The Hague conference as a representative of the University of Chicago branch of the Women's Peace Party. On Rosa Manus's relationships with Jacobs and Catt, see Bosch.

6. Davis 226–68.

Foreword (1924)

1. There is no equivalent in current medical training for *de verkrijging van den doctoralen graad* (receiving her medical doctorate). After completing the study and training required to practice medicine, Dutch students of Jacobs's day had a choice as to whether to write and defend a thesis; this scholarly attainment entitled the student to a doctoral degree in medicine.

   After she successfully took over her ailing father's practice, Jacobs considered not doing a thesis, but was urged on by friends and mentors; see below, chapter 2.
2. Jacques Oppenheim (1849–1924) was Jacobs's cousin on her mother's side. He studied law at the University of Groningen and eventually became a professor there; later he held important public office in The Hague. (De Wilde, *Aletta Jacobs in Groningen* 33)

Chapter One: The Childhood Years

1. Aletta Jacobs's older sister Charlotte (1847–1916) started her study of pharmacy in 1877 at the University of Groningen, where she, Aletta, and Frederika were at times referred to as "de Sappemeertjes" (the girls from Sappemeer). After finishing her studies in 1881 in Amsterdam and working as a pharmacist in a Utrecht hospital for two years, she sailed for Batavia [Djakarta] in the Dutch East Indies. There, after six years assisting another pharmacist, she was able to set up her own practice. She hired only female assistants, was a leader in the suffrage movement in the Indies, and worked for better education for native girls. In 1913, she returned to the Netherlands and participated with her sister in peace activities, including the 1915 Hague conference. (De Wilde, "Minder opvallend")

   Inge de Wilde's article about Charlotte Jacobs—to date the only article about another Jacobs sibling—also contains much information about the lives, travels, and careers of the rest of the family.
2. Johan Rudolf Thorbecke (1798–1872), a major figure in modern Dutch history, was the chief author of the 1848 constitution that gradually transformed the Netherlands into a constitutional monarchy in which Parliament controlled executive and legislative powers; becoming prime minister in 1849 as head of the liberals' party, he strengthened and consolidated the new system. During his several ministries, Thorbecke sponsored measures to extend the franchise, supported nondenominational schools over sectarian schools, and was involved in a number of other reforms. (NNBW)
3. See note 1 to the foreword.
4. Though there were at this time in the Tweede Kamer (Second Chamber, comparable to the U.S. House of Representatives or the British House of Commons) groupings of like-minded political figures, nationwide political parties with specific programs and mass support emerged only gradually in the 1880s and 1890s. (Gladdish 15–25)
5. Levi Ali Cohen (1817–1889) was a state health inspector in Groningen. He was also a medical historian and author of the highly regarded *Handbook of Public Administration and State Medicine*. (Hes 8–9; Lindeboom 358; De Wilde, *Brieven* 24) See also "Patterns of Remembrance."
6. Samuel Siegmund Rosenstein (1832–1906) studied and practiced medicine in Berlin, then went to the University of Groningen in 1865 to take the chair of internal medicine. As rector magnificus in 1870 and 1871, he was in a key position to assist Jacobs. He left Groningen in 1873 to become professor of medicine and pathology at the University of Leiden. Rosenstein was renowned as an extraordinary teacher who

modernized internal medicine in the Netherlands. (Hes 142, Lindeboom 1675–1676; De Wilde, *Aletta Jacobs in Groningen* 282–289) See also "Patterns of Remembrance."
7. For a discussion of changes in the laws regulating the training of pharmacists and their assistants, and of attitudes toward women in pharmacy, see De Wilde "Minder opvallend" 60–66.
8. A close examination of the correspondence between Jacobs and her father and Minister Thorbecke, noting some discrepancies between what Jacobs recalls and what is in the official files, is in De Wilde, *Aletta Jacobs in Groningen* 18–22, 29–32, 43–45; photographs of several of the letters are included.
9. A Dutch women's movement developed in phases familiar to students of U.S. women's history—first philanthropic, church-based groups where women took on progressively more responsibility, then gradually a range of organizations often separate from the church and from men with specific educational, health, and political goals—but for a variety of reasons these developments came later in the Netherlands than in the U.S.

   By 1865 women were just beginning to lecture in public; in 1870, Betsy Perk, one of the first Dutch women to struggle for women's right to work, started a women's paper, *Ons Streven* (Our Struggle); two important early women's organizations, *Arbeid Adelt* (Work Ennobles) and *Tesselschade* (named for Maria Tesselschade Visscher [1594–1649], a poet and scholar) were founded in 1870 and 1871 respectively to address the problem of finding meaningful activity for upper-class women. (Posthumus-van der Goot and de Waal, *Van Moeder* 63–109; Naber/Jansz)

Chapter Two: Student Years

1. De Wilde (*Aletta Jacobs in Groningen* 35–37) discusses the impact of J. S. Mill's *The Subjection of Women*, which appeared in Dutch in 1870, on liberal circles in Groningen. A lively discussion about women's education was already taking place in newspapers, pamphlets, and public discussions. Mill's work, too radical even for most Groningen liberals, stimulated and deepened this discussion. The ongoing debate offers a context for the welcome Matthijs Salverda (1840–1886) and others offered Jacobs at this time. Salverda subsequently served as inspector of secondary education in several provinces of the Netherlands until his death. (NNBW)
2. Jacobs's defender Heike Kamerlingh Onnes (1853–1926) was awarded the Nobel Prize in Physics in 1913 for his research on the properties of matter at low temperatures.
3. On Jozef Israëls, see "Patterns of Remembrance," note 26.
4. Multatuli was the pen name of Eduard Douwes Dekker (1820–1887), a major figure in Dutch literature. His novel *Max Havelaar* (1860) was a devastating critique of Dutch colonial administration. His atheism and his iconoclastic views on many subjects, together with the irregularities of his personal life, were disturbing to many with traditional views; his often aphoristic style, wonderful sense of irony, and desire to unsettle the thinking of his readers brought him a multitude of admirers, especially among the young. (NNBW)
5. In her later efforts to combat state regulation of prostitution, Jacobs was part of an international movement spearheaded by British reformer Josephine Butler, who, like Jacobs, was totally repelled by the medical "examinations" forced upon women and rejected the double standard. Butler led the successful campaign in England to repeal the Contagious Diseases Acts. (Banks) See also chapter 9.
6. Barend Joseph Stokvis (1834–1902) was a major and multifaceted figure in Dutch medicine, distinguishing himself in chemical physiology, pharmaceutics, and tropical

medicine as well as in the brilliance of his teaching. (Hes 157–58; Lindeboom 1890–1891)

7. As a physician Jacobs was very much concerned with raising the level of nursing care both by recruiting able candidates and by professionalizing their training. She was involved in founding a Dutch organization, Nosokómos (Greek for "hospital"), devoted to these purposes, and wrote articles for their journal of the same name about nursing in Switzerland, Madeira, Egypt, South Africa, and the Philippines. (De Wilde, *Brieven* 79–80; BWSAN)

   The low status of nursing in the Netherlands partly accounts for Jacobs's refusal to see U.S. birth control advocate and nurse Margaret Sanger when Sanger came to the Netherlands in 1915 seeking information; Jacobs felt strongly that physicians, not nurses or lay people, should be in charge of dispensing contraceptives. (Sanger, *An Autobiography* 142, 148)

8. A stanza of the Dutch text gives a sense of the poem's language: "Niet tot het dag'lijksch, huislijk leven / Voeldet g'U geroepen of verplicht, / Uw geest was op een hooger streven, / Uw oog op edeler doel gericht."

9. Hendrik Albert Kooyker (1832–1904), who supervised Jacobs's doctoral dissertation, was professor of pathology and forensic medicine at the University of Groningen from 1873 to 1900; he succeeded her mentor Rosenstein when the latter accepted a professorship in Leiden. (De Wilde, *Brieven* 67; Lindeboom 1075)

10. Most probably Jacobs had read *The Englishwomen's Review,* which often reported on women's struggle with the medical profession. (Personal communication from David Doughan, Fawcett Library) A number of excerpts from such articles are in Blake. Most Russian women who studied medicine abroad in fact went to Switzerland, not Vienna or Paris as Jacobs indicates. Women were not admitted to the medical faculty of the University of Vienna before 1900. On women students in Switzerland and Paris, see Bonner.

Chapter Three: My Stay in London

1. Sir Lawrence (Dutch: Laurens) Alma-Tadema (1836–1912) was a Dutch painter who settled permanently in England. He was extremely popular, especially for his paintings of Greek and Roman antiquity and Egyptian archaeology; in 1879, the year of Jacobs's visit, he was elected a member of the Royal Academy. His English second wife, Lady Laura Theresa (Epps), was also a successful painter.

2. This was the London School of Medicine for Women, which had opened in 1874 under the leadership of Sophia Jex-Blake. (Blake 167–168)

3. This four months in London was clearly a period of extraordinary growth and horizon-widening for Jacobs; not only had she never before left her native land, but her formative years had been spent in intense study and in convalescence from several bouts of serious illness.

   From her own account—for there is as yet no scholarly study specifically of this period in her life—she indeed met major and highly controversial reformers: Annie Besant, later widely known for her allegiance to Theosophist Madame Blavatsky; George Drysdale, a physician who perhaps served as an affirming role model in that he espoused family plannning, denounced state regulation of prostitution and was a freethinker; and Charles Bradlaugh, a hero to many secularists for refusing to take a religious oath in order to assume his seat in Parliament. This was surely a heady dose of reform activism. Jacobs arrived not long after the notorious Besant-Bradlaugh trial (1877), which occurred because the two had deliberately sold a pamphlet containing explicit information on human sexuality and the prevention of conception. Besant was among the founders of the Fabian Society, which was not founded until 1883, so Jacobs may be referring to meetings of people who later were Fabians.

4. Jacobs refers to the New Hospital for Women, which Elizabeth Garrett Anderson had opened above the St. Mary's Dispensary for Women and Children in Marylebone Road in 1872; the hospital moved to the larger quarters Jacobs visited in 1874. (Blake 150, 170)

5. Though she is not mentioned in either book, a sense of Jacobs's 1879 experiences in the circles of Elizabeth Garrett Anderson (1836–1917) and her sister Millicent Garrett Fawcett (1847–1929) can be gained from the appropriate sections of Jo Manton's biography of Anderson and David Rubinstein's of Fawcett.

6. *Gedenkboek* 41–42

7. The British medical journal the *Lancet* has a brief report of this meeting of the International Medical Congress in its September 20, 1879 issue. The article describes the welcome by the internationally esteemed Dutch physician Donders, and summarizes Sir Joseph Lister's much applauded talk on antisepsis as well as a presentation by Jacobs's mentor Rosenstein on Bright's disease.

8. British surgeon Sir Joseph Lister (1827–1912), the founder of antiseptic medicine, had by 1879 attained international fame for his introduction of carbolic acid to prevent infection during surgery. Ambroise Paré (1510–1590) was in his own time a famous and innovative surgeon who served four French kings.

9. The article appeared in the December 7, 1879 issue of *Le Scalpel*, a Belgian medical journal written in French. Charles Petithan was a Belgian physician who also wrote for the *Journal Belge des Sciences Medicales*. (De Wilde, personal communication) In the Dutch text, Jacobs quotes the French; her translation into Dutch is at the foot of the page. The present English translation is of her Dutch version, which is not always precise; in particular, his final phrase, which she renders as "a copy of her erudite thesis" would be more accurately translated as "a learned treatise on localizations in the cerebrum."

Chapter Four: The Early Years of My Practice

1. A *leesmuseum,* of which there were several in the Netherlands in Jacobs's day, combined elements of a public library and a private club. Materials did not circulate, as they do in a modern lending library, but they were freely available in the reading rooms to all who became members. Comfortable surroundings encouraged quiet perusal and some social interchange. There is still a *damesleesmuseum* (women's leesmuseum) in The Hague. (De Wilde, personal communication)

2. Hélène Mercier (1839–1910) was one of the first Dutch women to speak out in favor of education and employment for women from the upper classes. Spurred into action by the deplorable conditions in Amsterdam's slums, she not only wrote movingly about these conditions but set up a public soup kitchen, founded the sociocultural center Ons Huis (Our House) in 1892, and was deeply involved in establishing the first School for Social Work in the Netherlands in 1899. (De Wilde, *Hélène Mercier* 1985) See also chapter 9.

   Catharina Alberdingk Thijm (1849–1908), the daughter and sister of noted literary men, was founder and for some years editor of two periodicals for girls and young women, and wrote historical novels. Becoming interested in her later life in social questions, she was involved in the opening of a home for homeless women and girls in Amsterdam. (NNBW)

   Like Alberdingk Thijm, Cornélie Huygens (1848–1902) wrote a series of historical novels, most of which dealt with the plight of young women from the wealthy bourgeoisie. She later became an ardent socialist active in the Social-Democratic Workers' Party and successfully turned her literary talents to writing political pamplets and articles. In 1897 she published the socialist novel *Barthold Mervan*, which became a bestseller. She drowned herself just a few weeks after her marriage to a fellow socialist. (BWN)

Elise Haighton (1841–1911), who wrote under the pseudonyms Brunhilde and Hroswitha, was a devoted student of Doorenbos (see below) and edited a four-volume collection of his acclaimed lectures on history. An outspoken freethinker and prolific writer of articles on women's issues, she moved gradually into international work and participated in a number of conferences of the ICW and IWSA. Her article about Aletta Jacobs, "A Dutch Lady-Doctor"—probably the first in an English-language publication—appeared in the *Phrenological Journal* in 1883. (199–205, 259–261)

3. Born into poverty, Bernardus Hermanus Heldt (1841–1914) rose to become leader of the Algemeen Nederlandsch Werklieden-Verbond (ANWV; General Dutch Workers' Association) at its founding in 1871, and in 1885 became the first working-class member of the Tweede Kamer. He was a fervent supporter of universal suffrage. (BWN)

Willem Doorenbos (1820–1906), scholar of classical and Eastern languages, was an important literary critic and journal editor. A secondary school teacher of history and literature in Amsterdam, he gave in 1872–1875 an exceptional series of public lectures on history to which women were invited. Doorenbos served as mentor to a whole circle of writers, including feminists like Haighton and Mercier. (NNBW)

Chapter Five: Planned Motherhood

1 George Drysdale, whom Jacobs does not name here, was the author of *The Elements of Social Science, of Physical, Sexual, and Natural Religion: An Exposition of the True Cause and Only Cure for the Three Primary Social Evils: Poverty, Prostitution, and Celibacy.* A Dutch translation was published in Rotterdam in 1873 by Nijgh and van Ditmar.

2. A biographical sketch by Armin Geus of German physician and birth control pioneer Wilhelm Peter Johann Mensinga (1836–1910) is in Mensinga ix–xxi. I have not located the 1882 journal article Jacobs mentions; perhaps she is referring to his 1882 pamphet "Das Pessarium Occlusivum und dessen Applikation", described as a supplement to "Über Facultative Sterilität" (Neuwied und Leipzig). He published that pamphlet as well as some other works of the 1880s under the pseudonym "Carl Hasse."

3. Jacobs is here adapting German philosopher Friedrich Wilhelm Nietzsche (1844–1900) to her own goals. Nietzsche was quite unconcerned with social welfare issues such as allieviating the suffering of working-class mothers, and was indeed antisocialist and antiliberal; his concern was with cultural issues.

4. In fact, Jacobs and Gerritsen were among the founders of the NMB. Her negative comments here reflect the complicated way the birth control debate evolved in the Netherlands. She and the other physicians who favored some form of birth control nonetheless objected to the NMB's clinics because they were staffed by trained lay people; physicians, Jacobs and her colleagues asserted, should be the ones dispensing contraceptive information and devices. (Bosch, personal communication)

5. Eleanor Kinsella McDonnell, "Keeping the stork in his place." The article appeared in the December 1919 (not 1920, as Jacobs states) issue of the *Pictorial Review*. McDonnell produces an engaging but romanticized and in some respects inaccurate story about Jacobs.

Close to one hundred letters to Jacobs elicited by this essay are preserved in her archive in Amsterdam.

6. Jacobs refers to the Fifth International Neo-Malthusian and Birth Control Conference, held July 11–14, 1922, in London. In her biography of Margaret Sanger, Chesler comments that this conference had much broader participation than previous meetings of European Neo-Malthusians, attracting "the attention of mainstream economists, demographers, social theorists and physicians." (236)

Chapter Six: The Campaign for Woman Suffrage

1. Here Jacobs errs. Mill's tract was published in 1869; a Dutch translation first appeared in 1870 (not 1868), with a foreword by A. J. Vitringa, which placed Mill's text in the context of the discussion of girls' and women's education that had been going on in the Netherlands since the mid-1860s. The work had a very powerful effect on liberals throughout the Netherlands. (De Wilde, *Brieven* 33–42; see also chapter 2, note 1)

2. It is interesting to compare Jacobs's account here with her assertions at the end of chapter 1 about her ignorance, at the time she entered the University of Groningen, of feminist struggles.

3. B. D. H. Tellegen (1823–1885) taught constitutional law and international law at the University of Groningen from 1860 to 1885. His pamphlet "De toekomst der vrouw," influenced by Mill (see above, note 1), was published in 1870. (De Wilde, *Brieven* 33–35) For brief biographies of these and many of the other Dutch male politicians Jacobs mentions, see BWN and BWSAN.

4. Samuel van Houten (1837–1930) was an outstanding liberal thinker and politician who championed electoral reform, anticlericalism, and Neo-Malthusianism as well as feminism. A founding editor of the important journal *Vragen des Tijds* and a member of the Tweede Kamer for many years, he sought a unifying, scientifically based liberalism that would integrate changes in gender and class relations. (Stuurman; BWN)

5. Active suffrage is the right to vote; passive suffrage the right to run for office, i.e., to be voted for. As Jacobs points out in chapter 13, the Netherlands was unique among Western democracies in awarding women passive suffrage the year before they were granted active suffrage.

6. From a prominent Swedish family in Finland, writer and activist Baroness Alexandra von Gripenberg (1857–1911) attended the founding meeting of the International Council of Women (ICW) in Washington, D.C., in 1898 and thereafter established an ICW branch in Finland. When woman suffrage was instituted in Finland in 1906, she became a member of the Diet, where she continued to work for women's rights. (Schmidt 167)

   Gina Krog (1847–1916) coordinated the Norwegian feminist movement in its first phase; she was involved in founding the major national organizations and edited the feminist periodical *Nyloende* from its beginnings in 1887 until her death. She brought Norway into the ICW in 1904 and encouraged Norwegian connections with U.S. feminists. (Rasmussen 652–653)

7. Statesman Herbert Samuel (1870–1963), one of the first Jewish members of the British cabinet, served from 1920 to 1925 as high commissioner of Palestine, which had come under British control after World War I. At the time the Samuels hosted Jacobs and Gerritsen, he was a social worker in the slums of East London; three years later he was elected to the House of Commons as a Liberal and rose to prominence in a long and versatile career.

8. The Vrije Vrouwenvereeniging (Free Women's Movement), an organization deliberately unaffilated with any party or dogma, was founded in 1889 by Wilhelmina
Drucker (see chapter 10, note 12). On its early years, see Posthumus-van der Goot
and de Waal, *Van Moeder* 92–96.

9. See chapter 10 for Jacobs's meeting with feminist philosopher Gilman at the 1899
conference of the International Council of Women in London. Notwithstanding her
difficult experience lecturing on Gilman, in 1905 Jacobs successfully arranged for
Gilman to speak in Amsterdam despite the unwillingness of local organizations to
sponsor her, and put Gilman up for several days at her home. (Bosch 57) On
Gilman, see NAW.

10. On the founding of the International Woman Suffrage Alliance (IWSA), see Bosch
6–9, 285. The Washington meeting Jacobs refers to above was organized by Carrie
Chapman Catt in 1902 to coincide with the annual meeting of NAWSA (North
American Woman Suffrage Association). Before the meeting, Catt sent out question-
naires to get information about the status of the woman suffrage question in other
countries. Susan B. Anthony chaired the meeting, in which women from ten
countries participated.

    Bosch and Kloosterman argue persuasively that the dominance of American
suffragists in the IWSA's own chronicles has obscured the role of Heymann and
Augspurg in 1899 while magnifying that of Catt in 1902. Jacobs's account, here as
often elsewhere, provides balance by giving a European perspective.

    On Augspurg and Heymann, and on Catt, see "Patterns of Remembrance."

11. On the Interparliamentary Union, see "Patterns of Remembrance," note 3.

12. See chapter 9, note 2, on the Vrouwenbond tot Verhooging van het Zedelijk
Bewustzijn (Women's Association for Moral Advancement).

13. Austrian women were not granted the right to organize for political purposes until
1908. The women Jacobs met circumvented the prohibition by giving their group a
name that made it appear apolitical and unaffiliated with any party.

14. On Rosika Schwimmer, see "Patterns of Remembrance," esp. note 14, and "Aletta
Jacobs in Historical Perspective."

15. At this time the surging vitality of the Czech nationalist movement made it very
difficult for the Czech and German women Jacobs and Catt met to see one another
as allies in a common international struggle for women's rights. On issues of
nationalism and feminism in the situation of Czech women, see David 1991.

16. In Richard Wagner's opera *Die Meistersinger,* Beckmesser is a pedantic clerk who
is given the task of writing down all the "errors" of the competitors in a singing
contest.

    This comment is Jacobs's only mention of a musical work in her autobiography;
however, here again her letters reveal a different sensitivity; just a few months before
her death she writes from Nice to Miel Coops: "I was . . . the other night at the opera
Butterfly. It was an especially dazzling production. I lived once again in the pure
Japanese atmosphere and suffered with Butterfly the long hours of waiting and the
disillusionment as if I had to go through all that myself." (De Wilde, *Brieven* 97)

17. As this episode illustrates, the many translations of Swedish feminist Ellen Key's
Barnhets århundrade (*The Century of the Child*), first published in 1900, made her
internationally famous. A prolific writer and lecturer who stressed the sanctity of
motherhood while attacking conventional expectations of marriage and sex roles,
Key (1849–1926) was an enormously inspiring, controversial, and at times ambig-
uous figure.

    Though she was often hailed as champion of a new and freer sexual morality,
Key's ideas could be appropriated by antifeminist as well as reform circles. In the

Netherlands, for example, the 1898 Dutch translation of her *Missbrukad kvinnokraft* (Misused Womanpower) was, because of its emphasis on motherhood, most often cited by opponents of feminism. A pacifist who hoped women's growing influence would bring an end to war, Key became progessively more distressed during World War I by the nationalism and war support of most women in the warring nations. (Josephson; Bosch, personal communication)

18. Austrian Social Democrat Victor Adler (1852–1918) was a major figure in the Austrian Social Democratic Party, a multinational party that advocated federalism and autonomy for the diverse peoples of Austria-Hungary. He was a leader in the struggle for universal suffrage.

19. This was not quite correct, since Austrian women were allowed to belong to political organizations after 1908. See also note 14, above.

20. Jacobs gives an extended discussion of the 1908 IWSA congress in Amsterdam in chapter 11.

Chapter Eight: My Involvement with Pacifism and Antimilitarism

1. Beginning in 1873, the Dutch fought a long and bloody war to subdue the peoples of Atjeh, a province in northern Sumatra (now part of Indonesia).

2. In his study of Dutch colonial policy, Kuitenbrouwer places Julius Jacobs's writings on Atjeh in the context of the ongoing military activity that was engendering fierce debate; Jacobs "noted considerably more religious influence and less moral decadence in Atjeh than the leading government adviser had recorded" and ascribed "unfavorable" Atjeh traits such as secretiveness and mistrust to their twenty-year struggle to resist the Dutch. (267–268)

3. The Dutch peace movement was indeed small and quiescent until 1898, when it was galvanized by the aristocratic Johanna Waszklewicz-van Schilfgaarde (1850–1937); she was inspired in part by Tsar Nicholas II's call that year for an international initiative for disarmament. At the First Hague Conference in 1899 (Jacobs writes 1898) she entertained lavishly, turning her spacious home into a place where peace activists could mingle with diplomats and Dutch citizens. (Cooper, *Patriotic Pacifism* 72, 98; Josephson)

4. Bertha von Suttner (1843–1914) was part of the lobby of pacifist leaders at the 1899 First Hague Conference. One of the most famous women of her time, she wrote prolifically, lectured on behalf of peace throughout Europe and the United States, and had a leading role in establishing and convening peace societies internationally. Her novel *Die Waffen Nieder* (1889; *Lay Down Your Arms*), often referred to as the *Uncle Tom's Cabin* of the peace movement, had, by her death on the eve of World War I, been translated into sixteen languages and read by millions. Over time, she developed a more positive relation to feminism and the suffrage struggle than would be apparent from Jacobs's anecdotes. (Josephson)

5. Marie Quam (1843–1935) helped found the Norwegian suffrage movement in 1898. She served as vice president of the Norwegian Council of Women from 1904 to 1913.

6. This is probably the same conference Jacobs refers to in chapter 13 (see note 1), which coincided with the August 1913 opening of the Peace Palace in The Hague. Both the Interparliamentary Union and the Congrès Universel de la Paix scheduled their 1913 conferences to coincide with this gala event.

7. Crusading English editor William T. Stead (1849–1912), former editor of the popular *Pall Mall Gazette* and founder of the influential *Review of Reviews,* had just attended the May 1899 Hague peace conference (see above). There, he and two other journalists published a daily report that became indispensable to other journalists and to

diplomats. Before the conference he undertook a controversial and much publicized journey to European capitals to ensure that the meeting would occur and to to promote an emphasis on arms reduction. His odyssey can be seen as an interesting precursor in "citizen diplomacy" to the journeys Jacobs and other women took after their 1915 Hague conference. (Cooper, *Patriotic Pacifism* 98–99; DSAB)

8. Norwegian journalist and orator Bjørnstjerne Martinius Bjørnson (1832–1910) moved during decades of activism from Scandinavian nationalism to international-ism and peace work. His many social and political activities included circulating a worldwide peace petition after the 1892 World Peace Congress in Berne. A prolific writer of novels with a social message, he was awarded the Nobel Prize for Literature in 1903. Bjørnson was greatly admired by peace prize initiator Alfred Nobel (Josephson)

9. War was not declared until October 1, 1899; however, in the months before that declaration Great Britain engaged in a number of hostile diplomatic and military moves against the two Boer republics: the Transvaal and the Orange Free State. It is to these actions that Jacobs refers. In response, the Boers armed and mobilized troops. In the ensuing conflict, known as the Boer War, the Anglo-Boer War, or the South African War, the British defeated the Boers. The war ended on May 31, 1902.

10. At this point Dreyfus was having a second trial. First tried for treason in 1895, found guilty by a military court and imprisoned on Devil's Island, he was brought back to France in 1898 on the basis of new evidence and a huge public outcry in which novelist Émile Zola was a principal actor.

11. Jacobs was far from a lone voice in condemning England's role in the Boer War. Many Dutch identified with the Boers because of cultural and linguistic ties. Continental peace leaders also spoke out, as did a number of brave British activists, including Jacobs's friend William Stead. After the elation in the peace community brought about by the First Hague Conference, the outbreak of the Boer War almost imme-diately thereafter was a source of anguish. (Cooper, *Patriotic Pacifism* 104, 175–77)

12. Vrede door Recht (Peace Through Justice) was an existing organization, founded in the wake of the Franco-Prussian War, which Johanna Waszklewicz-van Schilfgaarde had galvanized and merged with her own women's peace network. See above, note 3.

13. Preacher, temperance leader, and suffragist Anna Howard Shaw (1847–1919), men-tioned several times in the autobiography, had a rich and intense relationship with Jacobs lasting until Shaw's death. Susan B. Anthony's niece Lucy Anthony was Shaw's intimate friend from 1890 on. In Bosch, Shaw is one of five women in the IWSA—the others being Jacobs, Catt, Rosa Manus, and Rosika Schwimmer—whose interrelationships are explored; her letters to Jacobs in that collection flesh out the glimpses in this memoir. (See NAW)

14. Jacobs's references to British/South African feminist, philosopher and peace advocate Olive Schreiner (1855–1920) are in three different chapters. For Jacobs's comments on Schreiner's *Woman and Labor,* which she translated into Dutch, see chapter 11. For her long overland detour to visit Schreiner in South Africa in 1911, see chapter 12. The South African visit is more extensively described in *Reisbrieven* 102–108.

15. Chrystal Macmillan (1872–1937) was for decades a key organizer and activist in a range of suffrage, peace, and labor organzations in Great Britain and interna-tionally. An outstanding graduate in mathematics and natural philosophy from Edinburgh University, she served on the executive committee of the National Union of Woman Suffrage Societies (NUWSS) but resigned, together with Kate Courtney (see below, note 19) and others in disagreement with Millicent Garrett Fawcett's pro-war stand. She was secretary of the IWSA from 1913 to 1920. After the war she studied law and in 1923 became one of the first women called to the bar. She was

especially concerned with equal employment opportunities for women and the nationality of married women. See Banks, vol. 2; Wiltsher.

16. *Jus Suffragii* continued publication under enormous difficulties all during the war, under the dedicated editorship of Mary Sheepshanks. It was one of the very few means by which women were able to maintain their international contacts. (Oldfield 176–198)

17. From a wealthy Amsterdam family long in the forefront of social and cultural life, Mia Boissevain became the first Dutch woman to earn a Ph.D in biology. She began her studies in Amsterdam and completed them in Zurich. Drawn to feminism through the determined community of women from all over the world pursuing higher education in Zurich, upon her return to the Netherlands she sought out Aletta Jacobs and eventually set up, with Rosa Manus, the Dutch suffrage association's highly successful publicity committee. (WPV; Bosch, personal communication)

On Rosa Manus, see the editor's foreword. Boissevain and Manus were intimate friends and coworkers for many years; after Manus was killed by the Nazis, Boissevain wrote a memoir (unpublished) that includes anecdotes revealing Manus's pain about her Jewishness. (Bosch 219–220)

The exhibition "Woman 1813–1913" was an important event in Dutch women's history. Like the earlier National Exhibition of Women's Work in 1898, it gave many talented women a chance to develop organizational and leadership skills and a sense of community, and served as an awakening for countless attendees. (Posthumus-van der Goot and de Waal 146–153)

18. Those who attended this planning meeting are listed in International Congress, p. xxxix. The proceedings and Anita Augspurg's account (Heymann and Augspurg 127–128) each list four Belgians, with a discrepancy as to the fourth. Wiltsher's list (63,294) differs in several particulars.

19. Suffrage leader Kathleen Courtney (1878–1974) played a key role in the 1912 rapprochement between the NUWSS and the British Labour Party, but then in 1914 resigned from the NUWSS executive because of her antiwar views. She was a founding member of the Women's International League for Peace and Freedom (WILPF) and served for many years as chairman of the English section. In the post-World War I years she held significant positions in the League of Nations Union and the Women's Peace Crusade, and lived on to become chairman of the United Nations Association. See Banks, vol. 2; Wiltsher.

20. All three of these women were long active in women's organizations and in peace work. The most prominent and the closest to Jacobs, Cornelia (Cor) Ramondt-Hirschman (1871–1957), participated in the Hague Congress delegation to neutral nations; after the war she was, for many years, president of the Dutch branch of WILPF and from 1917 to 1937 a member of the WILPF board (WPV). Jeanne van Lanschot Hubrecht (1864–1918) was active in suffrage work and in the nurses' advocacy group Nosokómos. Hanna van Biema-Hijmans (1874–1937) pioneered in social work among working-class girls and in innovative approaches to helping unwed mothers. (WPV)

21. The conference met from April 28 to May 1.

22. A list of the American women who attended, with their professional credentials and the organizations they were representing, is in the official conference report. (266–270) Forty-two came on the Noordam and five more arrived by other means. Among the more eminent participants not mentioned by Jacobs (Balch, Hamilton) or in the editor's foreword (Breckenridge) were author Fanny Fern Andrews, lawyer Madeline Doty, trade unionist Leonora O'Reilly, and author Mary Heaton Vorse.

23. No French women attended the Hague conference, but Jacobs's remark here seems to suggest that, as with the British, a significant group might have come had they been able to get there. This was not so. Partly because of the particular history of women's activism in France and its relation to nationalism and to specific parties, and partly because of the individual situations of the minuscule number of French women publicly questioning the war, no potential French delegation materialized.

   Antiwar socialist Louise Saumoneau, who attended the March 1915 socialist women's peace conference in Bern (see "Patterns of Remembrance") was not considered an appropriate choice by Jacobs and other key organizers, and peace activist Jeanne Mélin, whom Jacobs and Macmillan repeatedly telegrammed urging her to come to The Hague, was a refugee and may not have received the telegrams. Indeed, a leading group of French suffragists sent a message "deploring the holding of such a gathering while their country was under invasion." (Sowerwine, "Women," *Sisters*; Cooper, *Patriotic Pacifism* 200) On Jeanne Mélin see chapter 13, note 1.

24. Emmeline Pethick-Lawrence (1867–1954) was deeply involved beginning in 1906 with the militant Women's Social and Political Union (WSPU); she and her husband Frederick Pethick-Lawrence edited *Votes for Women* and were close to WSPU leaders Emmeline and Christabel Pankhurst. A break with them occurred in 1912. After World War I erupted, she and Hungarian pacifist Rosika Schwimmer (see "Patterns of Remembrance") traveled through the U.S., speaking sometimes together and sometimes separately to oppose the war. She was a founding and long-time member of WILPF. Her autobiography, *My Part in a Changing World* (London, Gollancz, 1938), contains colorful anecdotes of the Hague and Zurich conferences.

25. On the delegation to neutral nations, barely mentioned here, see "Patterns of Remembrance."

26. On Mien Palthe, see the editor's foreword and "Patterns of Remembrance."

27. Pioneer industrial toxicologist and social reformer Alice Hamilton (1869–1970) played a greater role in the events unfolding in this chapter and in chronicling them than Jacobs's brief references would indicate. Initially skeptical about the whole venture, but then deeply affected, she joined with Jane Addams and with Emily Balch, who had participated in the delegation to the neutral contries, to write *Women at The Hague* (1915). Hamilton attended the 1919 Zurich conference and went to Germany, as Jacobs relates later in this chapter, to assess the famine in relation to the postwar Allied food blockade. Her letters about the Noordam voyage, The Hague conference, and the Zurich conference (Sicherman 221–232, 233) are extraordinary documents. See NAWM.

28. Eduard Bernstein, a leading member of the German Social Democratic Party (SPD), was a staunch advocate of internationalism in the prewar years; after initially supporting Germany's war effort, he became an outspoken critic. He was an early advocate of an international organization of peoples. See Josephson.

29. Gertrude Woker, professor of chemistry at the University of Bern, attended the 1919 Zurich conference, subsequently became a member of the WILPF Committee on Chemical Warfare, and spearheaded efforts to get scientists to condemn the use of scientific research for war and destruction. More than three decades later, in 1955, she was still active in WILPF, drawing attention to the horrors of nuclear weapons. (Bussey and Tims 65–66, 212–13)

30. Jean Longuet, a son of Marx's daughter Jenny Marx Longuet, was a close associate of French socialist leader Jean Jaurès and a significant figure in French socialism.

31. The key participants in this French imbroglio all had long involvements in a range of peace and/or suffrage ventures.

    Madame de Witt Schlumberger (1856–1924) was from 1914 on the chairperson of the French branch of the IWSA. She participated in the Inter-Allied Suffrage Conference held in Paris during the peace conference at the initiative of Lady Aberdeen. (Bosch 173)

Ghenia Avril de Sainte-Croix (1855–1939) was for years chairperson of the ICW committee on White Slave Traffic; after the war she was active in the League of Nations. (De Wilde, *Brieven* 64)

Though she did not attend the Hague conference, Gabrielle Duchêne (1878–1954) organized a national committee of the International Committee of Women for Permanent Peace (ICWPP) during the war and subsequently became active in WILPF. She was for decades a champion of women's and workers' rights in France. Confronted with the rise of Fascism in the 1930's, like some other European WILPF leaders she moved away from pacifism and toward resisting force with force. (Josephson; Bussey 27)

Belgian pacifist Paul Otlet (1868–1944) with his collaborator Henri LaFontaine, undertook numerous international projects ranging from an international bibliographers' association (1895) to "The Mundanum," a center in Brussels intended for documentation of all global projects (1923) and part of his dream of a "world city." (Josephson, Cooper, *Patriotic Pacifism* 71)

32. From a family that had distinguished itself in public service, Emily Hobhouse (1860–1926) devoted enormous effort to alleviating the suffering of civilians, especially women and children, in the Boer War. Deeply shocked by her visits in 1900 to internment camps for Boers, she prodded the British government for changes and was consequently labeled a traitor and agitator by many Britons.

During World War I she once again created a furor by visiting German-occupied Belgium, POW camps inside Germany, and even Berlin, and urging the Britsh government to put out peace feelers. Hobhouse had the dubious distinction of being closely watched by both British and German intelligence. Her efforts form an interesting counterpoint to those of Jacobs's circle. (DSAB)

33. Having lost her position in the economics department at Wellesley College in 1919 because of her prominent antiwar activities, Emily Balch (1867–1961) then became the first international secretary-treasurer of WILPF. In that role she sought to influence the then young League of Nations to take a range of humanitarian and democracy-fostering steps. Balch was awarded the Nobel Peace Prize in 1946. Mercedes Randall's biography of Balch provides a stirring and important account of The Hague conference and its aftermath. See NAWM.

34. English economist Norman Angell (1873–1967) tried in his most famous work, *The Great Illusion* (1910), to show the fallacy of the notion that war and conquest brought great economic advantage. The book was translated into over twenty languages. Angell was awarded the Nobel Peace Prize in 1933.

35. In a memory slip, Jacobs wrote "Bar Harbor," a nearby town on the island, but from the context clearly meant Mt. Desert Island.

36. From a prominent Chicago family, Mary Hawes Wilmarth (1837–1919) was a member of the first board of trustees of Hull House and a continuing supporter. She was the founder and first president of the influential Women's City Club, led the Illinois branch of the Consumer's League, and was an active suffragist. Jane Addams eulogized her in *The Excellent Becomes the Permanent* (97–109). See the article about her daughter Anna Wilmarth Thompson Ickes in NAW.

37. It is striking that Jacobs says nothing about the Zurich conference itself, yet from the recollections written by Addams, Balch, and Hamilton (see above, note 28; Randall 261–272) it is clear that the conference was a heart-wrenching, enormously powerful experience for those who attended.

38. Norwegian explorer and oceanographer Fridtjof Nansen (1861–1930) led several expeditions to the Arctic. He headed the first Norwegian delegation to the League of Nations. Assigned the immense repatriation problem Jacobs describes, he was able to report in 1922 that almost half a million prisoners had returned home. Beginnning in 1921 he also was high commissioner of a huge effort to mitigate the effects of widespread famine in Russia. He was awarded the Nobel Peace Prize in 1922.

39. At this Conference for a New Peace, according to WILPF historians Bussey and Tims, "In addition to many leading WILPF members, delegates were present from 111 national and international organizations from 20 countries, estimated to represent a total membership of over 20 million men and women.

    "The conference demanded the convening of a World Congress to draw up new international agreements on which a new, and genuine peace might be based.... Jane Addams, Catherine Marshall and Jeanne Mélin were deputed to seek personal interviews with statesmen in Britain, France, Holland and Scandinavia, and were received by high officials in all those countries." (31–32) Note the interesting echo of the 1915 Hague conference in the sending of a postconference delegation to meet with statesmen. In the difficult postwar climate, this WILPF effort at outreach was of very limited effect.

Chapter Nine: Prostitution

1. Theologian and pedagogue Hendrik Pierson (1834–1923) was inspired by the mid-nineteenth–century Dutch Protestant movement known as the Réveil and also by the international movement launched by British reformer Josephine Butler to combat state regulation of prostitution. (*Winkler Prins Encyclopedie*)

    In the 1870s, several of Butler's brochures were translated into Dutch and created a great stir in the Netherlands; Pierson organized the first public meeting on the subject of prostitution in 1878, just one year before Jacobs set up her practice. Butler herself came to the Netherlands for an international conference in 1883 and encouraged further organization and public outcry against state regulation. (Posthumus-van der Goot and de Waal 84–85)

2. The Vrouwenbond tot Verhooging van het Zedelijk Bewustzijn (Women's Association for Moral Advancement) was founded in 1884 by Marianne de Klerck-van Hogendorp (1831–1909) and her two sisters. The Van Hogendorp women—Marianne's mother, Marianne, and her sisters Anna and Wilhelmina—were an important force in women's charitable and social work. (Posthumus-van der Goot and de Waal 85–91) However, their fervently Christian approach to aiding prostitutes and unwed mothers was apparently considered too restrictive by the freethinking Jacobs.

3. The Vereeniging ter Behartiging van de Belangen der Vrouw (Society for the Advancement of Women's Interests), which she founded in 1895, was only one of numerous spheres of activity for M. W. H. Rutgers-Hoitsema (1847–1934). She was among the founders of the Woman Suffrage Association (VVVK), organized help for unwed mothers, served for thirteen years as president of the NMB (Neo-Malthusiaansche Bond), and fought against protective legislation for women workers. (BWSAN)

4. In contrast to today's emphasis on identifying fathers of out-of-wedlock children and insisting that they pay child support, the legal situation Jacobs describes was one in which it was actually against the law even to seek to determine paternity.

5. This is the sixteenth meeting of the International Congress of Medicine.

6. This was Baroness Lipthay, whom Jacobs names when she reminisces about this conference again in chapter 11.
7. Here and in the *Reisbrieven,* Jacobs uses *Turkish* to refer to Muslims living within the Ottoman empire, as well as in Egypt.
8. In addition to her antiprostitution work, Julia Frances Solly (1862–1953) was active in a number of movements. She was a temperance worker, pacifist, and ardent conservationist. She was the moving spirit in founding the Women's Enfranchisement League in Cape Town in 1907, the first suffrage organization in South Africa. Solly was a close friend of Olive Schreiner. (DSAB)
9. In fact only one of the formal sessions at the Budapest conference, entitled "The White Slave Traffic," was devoted to prostitution. The discussion was introduced by Catt and directed toward the question, "What have women voters accomplished toward the solution of this problem?" (International Woman Suffrage Alliance 11). Jacobs perhaps means that the topic dominated informal conversation among the delegates. "White slavery" had been discussed at ICW meetings for years, but was an unusual topic for the suffrage-focused IWSA. See also Schreiber and Mathieson 23.

Chapter Ten: My Union with Carel Victor Gerritsen

1. There is to date no biography, or even a full-length article, about Gerritsen. See the brief biography in BWSAN, also De Wilde, "De bibliotheek," on his extraordinary library, and Nabrink 66–77 on his activities in the NMB (Nieuw-Malthusiaansche Bond).
2. At this time anyone elected to the British parliament had to take a Christian oath of office. Bradlaugh, a freethinker, could not in all conscience take the oath; he sought to be seated without taking an oath and was ejected. As Jacobs writes below, Gerritsen was instrumental in changing a similar Christian oath in the Netherlands to a simple pledge.
3. *Antirevolutionary* here means a specific political group rooted in Calvinist belief, the Anti-Revolutionary Party (ARP), which had existed in nucleus in opposition to the Liberals since the advent of parliamentary government in 1849 and took shape as a national mass-based party in the 1870's. (Gladdish 15–25)
4. The Geuzen were a sixteenth-century group of Dutch patriots who opposed Philip II and the Roman Catholic Church.
5. At this time, Gerritsen was well on his way to amassing an exceptional collection of books and periodicals in women's history and feminism, economics, and sociology, which by 1892 included thirty thousand titles. It is clear from Jacobs's international correspondence that she also actively solicited materials for the collection. Sold in 1903 to the John Crerar Library in Chicago and resold in 1951 to the University of Kansas, it is known as "The Gerritsen Collection of Women's History" and is available on microfilm. (De Wilde, "De bibliotheek")
6. Pieter Jelles Troelstra (1860–1930) was in 1893 and 1894 one of the founders of the Social Democratic Workers' Party (SDAP). His rich oratorical gifts, charisma, and deep identification with the working masses gave him a very special leadership role in the Netherlands; he was also important in the Second International. A legislator in the Tweede Kamer until 1925, he fought for universal suffrage and unsuccessfully sought a proletarian revolution after World War I. He was also an accomplished poet in Frisian, the language spoken in his native province of Friesland. (BWN)
7. It is puzzling that no record of these "Travel Letters" exists in any extant list of Jacobs's or Gerritsen's publications, nor have Dutch scholars researching Jacobs and

related topics encountered them. Perhaps some were published in newspapers or privately printed.

8. Gavin Brown Clark (1846–1930), a Liberal member of Parliament from 1885 to 1900, wrote and spoke tirelessly on behalf of the Boers. A Scot, he favored home rule in Scotland and Wales and frequently was an advocate for smaller groups without their own nation-state and for the poor. (DSAB)

9. Leading Russian feminist Anna Pavlovna Filosofova (1837–1912) began her activism in the 1860s and went on to cofound the Mutual Philanthropic Society, an important and broadly active group, in 1895. Her later years were devoted to trying to unite all the women's clubs in Russia into a National Women's Council that would be an affiliate of the International Council of Women, but because of political problems she was unsuccessful. (Stites 67–71, 193–197)

   The proceedings of the 1899 ICW conference mention Dr. Kazekévitch Stefanovska (note difference in spelling) as a Russian from St. Petersburg.

10. The committee included several women who played important roles in the Dutch women's movement. Wilhelmina E. Drucker (1847–1925), born out of wedlock and raised in difficult circumstances, took the initiative to organize the Vrije Vrouwenvereeniging (Free Women's Association) in 1889 and to cofound (with Theodora Haver) the journal *Evolutie* in 1893; her work was crucial in laying the foundation for an independent women's movement. Because of her often radical views and her disapproval of cooperation with male political organizations, she distanced herself both from more cautious contemporaries and from many socialist feminists yet served as an inspiration to Dutch feminists of the 1970s; the activist Dolle Mina's (Rebellious Minas) were named after her. (Dieteren; Bosch 55)

    Drucker's close friend and coeditor Theodora P. B. Haver (1857–1912) was one of the founders of the VVVK (Woman Suffrage Association) and chair of the Amsterdam section. (Bosch 69; WPV)

    A prominent member of the IWSA and the VVVK, Martina G. Kramers (1863–1934) was active internationally, editing the IWSA's *Jus Suffragii* from 1904 to 1913 and leaving only under difficult circumstances. As corresponding secretary for the Dutch National Council of Women, she delivered a report at the 1899 ICW conference in which she summarized the achievements and struggles of Dutch women for the previous fifty years. (International Congress of Women, vol. 1 121–125; Bosch 31–32, 125–129, 287–288)

11. After Gerritsen's death in 1905, Jacobs arranged to have the articles he and she wrote published together in one volume, *Brieven uit en over Amerika*. See chapter 11.

12. Unitarian clergyman and reformer Samuel June Barrows (1845–1909) served one term in Congress (1896–98), but was not a congressman at the time of Jacobs's visit. Appointed prison commissioner for the United States in 1895 after spearheading prison reform in New York State, he was a major force for change, visiting prisons in many countries and carrying on a worldwide correspondence. He was an official U.S. representative to the Interparliamentary Union.

Chapter Eleven: From 1905 to 1911

1. Anna Polak (1849–1939) was director of the Bureau voor Vrouwenarbeid (Bureau of Women's Work) from 1908 to 1937, and was instrumental in greatly expanding employment possibilities for women. (WPV)

2. Cornelia Sara ("Kee") Groot (1868–1934) was active in social work and in the VVVK. On her VVVK propaganda tours throughout the Netherlands she was

extremely effective making speeches in dialect, wearing a traditional costume, and calling herself "Marijtje," a name common in rural areas. (WPV)

3. Betsy Bakker-Nort (1874–1946) was active in the VVVK from its inception in 1898 till Dutch women gained suffrage in 1919. A prolific translator of Danish, Swedish, and Norwegian literature, she studied law while in her thirties and already married—very unusual at that time—and obtained her degree in 1914. In 1922 she became the first woman elected to Parliament on the slate of the Vrijzinnig Democratische Bond (Liberal Democratic Union). In Parliament she was especially concerned with the legal position of married women. A Jew, she survived imprisonment in Theresienstadt during World War II. (De Wilde, "Betsy Bakker-Nort" 29–32)

4. The Christian-Historical Union was a political party that began as the conservative wing of the already conservative Anti-Revolutionary Party (ARP) (see chapter 10, note 3) and between 1898 and 1909 gradually emerged as a separate entity under the leadership of A. F. de Savornin Lohman. (Gladdish 22)

5. In the Netherlands, it is customary to celebrate a twelve-and-a-half-year anniversary (half of twenty-five) of a significant event.

6. Jacobs is obliquely referring to a split in the Dutch suffrage movement; in 1907, a group headed by journalist and editor Esther W. W. Francken-Dyserinck (1876–1956) and several others broke away to form the Nederlandsche Bond voor Vrouwenkiesrecht (NBV). A combination of personal incompatabilities and dis-agreements about suffrage tactics and philosophy caused the split. (Bosch 44, 71; De Wilde, *Brieven* 34, 65; WPV)

7. Feminist historian Johanna W. A. Naber (1859–1941) was for decades a major figure in a broad range of Dutch women's activities. Already the author of a prize-winning manual on needlework, she was awakened to feminism by the 1898 Exhibition of Women's Work. Many of her over 250 publications are biographical studies of well-to-do, deeply religious women from the sixteenth to the early twentieth centuries who struggled for autonomy and socially oriented achievement. Naber was the first Dutch woman on the board of the IWSA and served for some years as secretary and successful publicist of the VVVK. Always concerned with continuity and the trans-mission of women's history across generations, she joined Rosa Manus and Will-emijn Posthumus-van der Goot in setting up the International Archives of the Women's Movement (IAV) in which Jacobs's papers now reside. (Bosch 287; Grever)

8. The "Spaniards" Jacobs refers to are Sephardic Jews, descendents of the Jews who were expelled from Spain in 1492 and resettled in many Mediterranean and North Atlantic cities and towns. They spoke Ladino, a language melding elements of Spanish and Hebrew. The "Turks" are Bosnian Muslims who had converted to Islam while under Ottoman rule.

9. This quote is in English in the original text, as are all other direct quotes from English-speaking friends.

10. Adela Stanton Coit was on the board of the IWSA from 1907 to 1920, serving as treasurer. German-born, she married U.S. settlement house pioneer and author Stanton Coit and settled with him in England.

11. Maximilian Bircher-Benner (1867–1939) established his private clinic on the Zurichberg in 1897 and was chief physician there for forty-two years. Ahead of his time in promoting raw vegetables for health, he can be remembered through the ubiquitous boxes of Bircher-muesli for sale in many healthfood stores in the United States.

12. *Uit het leven van merkwaardige vrouwen.* The six sketches originally appeared in the *Maandblad voor Vrouwenkiesrecht* and their subjects were Elizabeth Cady Stanton,

Frances Power Cobbe, Anna Howard Shaw, Carrie Chapman Catt, Helen Loring Grenfell, and Lady Henry Somerset. Of the six, only Catt was still alive.

13. *De vrouw, haar bouw en haar inwendige organen* (Deventer: Kluwer, 1898).

Chapter Twelve: A World Tour

1. Except for the opening section about how she and Catt planned the trip, this chapter contains material more fully explored in Jacobs's *Reisbrieven,* a series of articles she wrote for the Dutch paper *De Telegraaf* and collected in two volumes running to over seven hundred pages. That collection of articles is not systematically summarized here; rather, Jacobs chooses to dwell on certain experiences from the trip and skip over others. She writes expansively about South Africa, for example, but she leaves out their time in India almost completely and gives very little space to their sojourn in the Dutch Indies. For an analysis of the *Reisbrieven,* see Feinberg, "Jacobs's *Reisbrieven.*"

2. Noted Swedish novelist Selma Lagerlöf (1858–1940) was the first woman to win the Nobel Prize for Literature (1909). Early in the *Reisbrieven,* Jacobs tells of hearing her give a powerful speech at the 1911 IWSA conference in Stockholm; in a later letter, describing her stay at the communal Swedish-American colony in Jerusalem, Jacobs praises Lagerlöf's description of it in her book *Jerusalem.* (9–10, 209)

3. Readers wanting to explore the careers and beliefs of Steyn, Herzog, and Smuts, all very important in South African history, can start by perusing the detailed articles about them in the *Dictionary of South African Biography* (DSAB).

4. This was probably feminist leader Huda Shaarawi, whose removal of her veil at the Cairo train station upon her return from the Rome conference was a dramatic and important moment for Egyptian feminism. The photographs in Margot Badran's edition of Shaarawi's memoirs include one from Carrie Chapman Catt with the handwritten note "Success to the new women of Egypt! . . . Rome, May 19, 1923." (Feinberg, "Pioneering" 76; Shaarawi 7, 128–129)

5. For Carrie Chapman Catt's recollections of their travels together, see Van Voris 85–105.

Chapter Thirteen: From 1913 to 1924

1. Jacobs knew all four speakers through her years of involvement in international organizations. On Bertha von Suttner, see chapter 8, note 4. Christian socialist and pacifist Sandor Giesswein (1856–1923) was active in the Interparliamentary Union. He spoke out for peace during World War I, and afterward especially championed peace education and Esperanto. (Josephson) Carl Lindhagen (1860–1946) was mayor of Stockholm from 1903 to 1930. He is best known for encouraging development in the rural north of Sweden, for his efforts to get all the Scandinavian countries to pass a uniform code of laws enhancing women's rights, and for advocating a Swedish republic, without royalty. A long-time advocate of woman suffrage, he espoused the cause of peace later in his career. A favorite slogan urged "conscience politics, not just interest politics." (Personal communication from Brita Stendahl) Prominent U.S. suffragist May Wright Sewall (1844–1920) was president of the ICW from 1899 to 1904 and chaired the ICW's Committee on Peace and Arbitration from 1904 to 1914. A leader of the Women's Peace Party, she vigorously opposed U.S. involvement in World War I. (Josephson; NAW) French feminist and peace activist Jeanne Mélin did not attend the 1915 Hague conference; her late arrival at the 1919 Zurich conference precipitated, according to several

accounts, a moment of riveting drama. Traveling from a devastated region of the Ardennes, she managed to get to Zurich only on the last day of the conference. German delegate Lida Gustava Heymann, who was seated on the platform, sponta-neously rose to embrace her, crying, "A German woman gives her hand to a French woman," and pleading for bridge-building between the nations. Mélin responded eloquently in kind, whereupon U.S. delegate Emily Balch, followed by all the women present, solemnly rose and raised their hands in a pledge to dedicate themselves to ending war. (Randall 275–276; Bussey and Tims 30) On Heymann, see "Patterns of Remembrance." Mélin was active in WILPF for some years after the war, participat-ing with Jane Addams in one of the delegations sent out by the 1922 Conference for a New Peace. See chapter 8, note 40.

2. The Social Democratic woman who was elected in 1918 was Suze Groeneweg. (Bosch 170, note 1) See "Aletta Jacobs in Historical Perspective."
3. The first Catholic member of the VVVK, Clara A. M. Mulder van de Graaf-de Bruijn (1865–1945) was on the VVVK's board from 1911 to 1919. She also served for sixteen years on the board of the Dutch section of WILPF. (De Wilde, *Brieven* 24)
4. For a letter Jacobs wrote during this trip, which included visits to Jane Addams in Chicago and to Carrie Chapman Catt in New York state, see De Wilde, *Brieven* 53–36.
5. At the time of the Rome conference, Mussolini had already come to power. See Jacobs's letter from the conference in Bosch, 194–195. The Dutch original is in De Wilde, "Inleiding" 37–38.
6. Space does not permit comment on the dozens of people named as participants in this festivity except to say that they represented a broad but not comprehensive cross section of Dutch organizations and causes.

    Ironically, one organization conspicuously not represented was the Dutch orga-nization of university-educated women, the Vereeniging van Vrouwen met Aca-demische Opleiding (VVAO), which at that time still found Jacobs's espousal of birth control displeasing to its conservative-leaning members. Within two years and under new leadership, the organization moved to include and indeed honor Jacobs. (De Wilde, "Aaneensluiting")
7. Jacobs's last surviving sibling, her brother Eduardo, who had been a witness at her wedding, died in 1921 at sixty-six. Two of her siblings, Frederika and Herman, died in their thirties, and four of the others in their fifties; Charlotte, the longest-lived, died at sixty-nine in 1916. So it is not surprising that at seventy Jacobs, just after a serious illness, writes here as if her life is drawing to a close. (De Wilde, "Minder opvallend")

Aletta Jacobs in Historical Perspective

1. Bosch.
2. In a similar case, Helene Rosenbach Deutsch (1884–1982), who trained as a physician in Vienna and later became a prominent Freudian psychoanalyst, decided to have an abortion in 1911 rather than have a child out of wedlock, even though, like Jacobs, her personal life was rather unconventional and she very much wanted a child. Shortly thereafter, she married and had a son. (Roazen 184) By contrast, Anna Kuliscioff (1855–1925), a Russian-born revolutionary and physician, had two long-term liaisons, the first of which resulted in the birth of a much loved daughter, but she never married. (Shepherd 84–100)
3. Unlike Jacobs, Tiburtius had a sister-in-law who had already received a degree in dentistry in the United States. (Tiburtius 108–111; Brinkschulte 26–28)
4. Other examples of Jewish women physicians who received strong paternal support can be found in Deutsch; Mahler; Wolff; Morantz.

5. Hes 71.
6. This loophole for special admission to medical school was only temporary and hence did not benefit others. In England, Elizabeth Garrett (Anderson) used the stratagem of a pharmacist's license to allow her to begin practicing medicine in 1865; she had difficulties completing her medical training in England, however, and eventually studied in Paris. See Bonner; Blake.
7. For further details, see Bonner; Blake; Morantz-Sanchez.
8. Jewish women, most of whom were in the medical school, made up a majority of the Russian women studying at Swiss universities in the late nineteenth century. On the eve of World War I, Jewish women comprised 30 percent of the first generation of female medical students attending Prussian universities and 60 percent of the women medical students at the University of Vienna. The number and proportion of Jewish women at Dutch universities was considerably lower, however. See Neumann; Heindl 139–149.
9. Tuve 46–56.
10. Albisetti 11–12; Rohner 42, 81–82; Bernstein 276.
11. Widowed at a young age, with two children, Irma Klausner-Cronheim maintained a very busy private practice in Berlin, caring for men and women of all classes. Personal correspondence with Georg Cronheim, Woodland Hills, California, 1994.
12. See Bonner; Straus.
13. De Lange 99–100.
14. Lipinska 465, 546–547; Potter 5–6. At least fifteen of these women were of Jewish origin. Although Jewish men never made up more than 5 percent of the Dutch medical profession, Jewish women accounted for roughly 8 percent of the women physicians in interwar Holland. These figures far exceed Jews' proportional representation within the Dutch population, although they are less than half the proportion of Jewish men and women in the German and Austrian medical profession. See Hes; Daalder 188.
15. Stites 56; Tuve 46–56; Forkl and Koffmahn 24.
16. Tiburtius; Brinkschulte.
17. Anderson and Zinsser 176; Riemer and Fout 204, 214–217; Leathard 6; Usborne 121–122; Hall 176–177; Rose. See also McLaren.
18. Sanger, *My Fight* 107–116; Douglas 81–84; Chesler 145–146, 183; Evans, 124–127.
19. Douglas 211; Hes 82.
20. Bosch, personal communication, May 1995.
21. Grossmann 183–217; Woycke 51–55 and 119–123; Usborne 118–123, 128–133; Leathard 11–20; Evans; Chesler.
22. Gordon; Smith 347; Offen, "Defining Feminism" 144–145.
23. Sanger, *My Fight* 113; Douglas 184; Chesler 145)
24. See Walkowitz; Anderson and Zinsser; Smith.
25. Pappenheim campaigned widely against the international traffic in women, particularly Jewish women, and also ran a home for unwed Jewish mothers and their children. The *Jüdischer Frauenbund*, like its American counterpart, the National Council of Jewish Women, adopted a case work approach to solving the problems of women, including prostitution. See Kaplan, *The Jewish Feminist Movement* and *The Making of the Jewish Middle Class*; Shepherd; Rogow.
26. See Blake 110–113.
27. Sanger, *My Fight* 108; Douglas 83. The most important Dutch organization combatting prostitution was the Protestant Dutch Women's Association for Moral Advancement. (Bosch, personal communication, May 1995)

28. Around the turn of the century, the rate of mixed marriages between Jews and Christians was roughly 6 percent of marriages involving Jews. (Michman, "Jewish Essence" 4–5)
29. For information on the Dutch political system, see Gladdish; Verkade.
30. See Daalder 175–194; Michman, "Jewish Essence," 1–22; Leydesdorff; Michman, *Pinkas*.
31. See Shepherd; Fassmann.
32. For a discussion of the distinctions between individualist and relational feminists, see Offen, "Defining Feminism" and also "Liberty, Equality and Justice for Women."
33. Gelblum 207–225; Josephson; Woycke 55–56; Bosch.
34. See Bosch, which includes letters between Aletta Jacobs and other members of the IWSA.
35. Bosch 170n1.
36. See Usborne; Wickert, *Unsere Erwählten* and "Frauen im Parlament" 210–240.
37. Von Suttner, who died just before the outbreak of World War I, was never actively involved in feminist activities; her chief concern was peace, not women's rights. (Carroll 6–7) See chapter 8, note 4, and also Josephson 921–924; Cooper, *Patriotic Pacifism* and "Women's Participation" 51–75.
38. Carroll 8–9; Wiltscher.
39. Cook 237–241; Foster 10–11; Bussey and Tims 18–19.
40. See "Patterns of Remembrance" for more details.
41. For details and evaluations on the 1915 Hague Conference, see Addams, Balch, and Hamilton; Wiltscher; Bussey and Tims; Foster; Cooper, "Women's Participation."
42. See Addams, Balch, and Hamilton; Wiltscher; Foster.
43. A second American woman and WILPF leader, Emily Greene Balch, won the Nobel Peace Prize in 1946. See Bussey and Tims; Foster.
44. See Van Voris.
45. See Stites 191–232; Tuve 65–73.
46. See "Patterns of Remembrance"; Bosch; Wiltscher; Wenger 66–99.
47. Bosch 33, 66, 202.
48. Feinberg, "Pioneering" 71.
49. Shepherd 69–88.
50. Straus; Schmelzkopf 471–480. See also Freidenreich; Kaplan, *The Making of the Jewish Middle Class.*
51. Salomon; Peyser; DÜrkop 140–150.
52. See Bosch; Wenger.
53. See Bosch.
54. As quoted in Voris 104–105.
55. Sicherman 192.
56. Douglas 81; Chesler 145.
57. Bosch 204.

Patterns of Remembrance: A Literary Afterword

1. Feinberg, "Pioneering." There has been much discussion of the meaning of what appear to be discontinuities and episodic writing in many autobiographical works by women. Even an overview of recent scholarly activity on women's autobiography is beyond the scope of this afterword, though I would like to mention as especially useful sources the volumes by Brodzki and Schenck; Benstock; Heilbrun; and the chapter "Writing a Life" in Wexler.

2. The Women's International League for Peace and Freedom (WILPF) was founded in 1919 in Zurich by a core of women who had participated in The Hague conference. Jacobs knew many of the WILPF women from her suffrage work. See chapters 6 and 8.

3. A forum for elected officials from many nations who wanted to promote arbitration and other nonviolent approaches to international problems, the Interparliamentary Union held eighteen international congresses in European and U.S. cities between 1889 and the outbreak of World War I. Theodore Roosevelt welcomed participants in the 1904 St. Louis meeting, the last one Jacobs and Gerritsen attended before his death, at the White House. Twice interrupted by worldwide conflict and then reorganized, the IU still exists; its offices are currently in Geneva. See Cooper, *Patriotic Pacifism*, esp. 85–87.

4. "A World Tour" is a selective distillation of those articles with some added commentary. See chapter 12, note 1.

5. See epecially Bosch 120–121 for a display of the playful aspect.

6. Both women were active in a range of causes. Mien, for over twenty years secretary of the Dutch section of WILPF, shared especially Jacobs's pacifist commitment. Miel propagated the educational ideals of Maria Montessori; the first Montessori class in the Netherlands was in her home. Fortuitously, through this friendship Jacobs was thus brought into some contact with another noted woman physician-pacifist.

Van den Dungen and Lewer compare Jacobs, Montessori, and three other antiwar woman physicians (Alice Hamilton, Anne-Marie Pelletier, and Anna Kuliscioff) in their article "Frauendiplomatie—ärztinnen gegen den Krieg."

7. See especially 21–42.

8. Jacobs further writes, "Lyda and Anita were together twenty-five years on December 18 and as a gift Lyda invited her friend on a trip of about two months to Constantinople, Greece, Egypt, and Jerusalem." (De Wilde, *Brieven* 89) This is interesting evidence that Jacobs and Miel at some level accepted Augspurg and Heymann's lifelong female partnership. On Augspurg and Heymann, including examinations of their relationship within a lesbian history context, see the bibliography in Bosch.

9. De Wilde, *Brieven* 49. Polish-born German revolutionary Rosa Luxemburg (1871–1919) was imprisoned during World War I because of her agitation against the war and for a proletarian revolution. She and Karl Liebknecht, leaders of the underground Spartacus League, were murdered by counterrevolutionaries. Sonja Liebknecht was Karl's wife and Luise Kautsky the wife of Marxist theorist Karl Kautsky.

10. De Wilde, "Inleiding" 19. Readers of Dutch have access to De Wilde's beautifully edited collection of the often intense letters Jacobs wrote to her intimate friends Mien and Miel and other members of the Broese van Groenou family (De Wilde, *Brieven* 1992). Readers of English are now fortunate to have Bosch and Kloosterman's *Politics and Friendship*, a revision and translation of their *Lieve Dr. Jacobs*, which presents a rich correspondence among Jacobs and four close associates in the suffrage struggle: Carrie Chapman Catt and Anna Howard Shaw from the U.S., Rosika Schwimmer from Hungary, and Jacobs's faithful Dutch assistant, Rosa Manus. This book provides a historical/organizational context for Jacobs's autobiography and a wealth of biographical data on the women in her networks. Bosch and Kloosterman drew on the wealth of letters and other materials in the Aletta Jacobs archive at the International Archive of Women's History (IIAV) in Amsterdam.

11. On Dutch anarchist Bart de Ligt (1883–1938), who was dismissed from his pulpit and eventually imprisoned because of his antiwar speeches and tracts, see Peter van

den Dungen's introduction to De Ligt, *The Conquest of Violence,* and BWN. On the Women's Peace Party, which sponsored the American delegation to The Hague conference, see Degen. See also Bosch 136.

12. Randall 193–196.
13. International Congress of Women 118–119 (in German). Ankersmit and Pothuis-Smit had attended the Second Conference of Socialist Women in Copenhagen in 1910; Ankersmit developed a friendship with Clara Zetkin, a leading German left-wing socialist and head of the International Women's Secretariat, and subsequently wrote articles for Zetkin's periodical *Die Gleichheit* (Equality). When Zetkin and Inessa Armand, a close associate of Lenin, subsequently planned the Bern conference, Ankersmit and Pothuis-Smit were among the delegates.

    The Hague conference was much larger, was planned entirely by women, and did produce a set of published resolutions; the Bern conference, however, was stymied by efforts of Armand and the Bolshevik minority to put forward their own agenda; according to Armand biographer R. C. Elwood, "Lenin spent most of the conference sitting in the cafe of the Volkshaus waiting for reports from his female subordinates" and fuming over the proceedings. (157–158)

    Although both conferences served as meeting places for a mix of belligerents and neutrals, the Bern conference had a different "mix"; it did have French and Russian participation, but no Americans.

    On the Bern conference see Elwood 153–158 on ideology and planning, especially differences between Zetkin and Armand; Sowerwine, "Women" and *Sisters* 144–150 on French participation and on the Bern meeting in relation to the later and much better-known Zimmerwald conference of male socialists against the war; and Outshoorn on the Dutch socialists. See BWSAN on Ankersmit, BWSAN and BWN on Potuis-Smit.

14. Before the war, Rosika Schwimmer (1877–1948) played a leading role in organizing Hungarian women and in the IWSA. During the war, she met twice with Wilson to urge mediation and was a key figure in Henry Ford's much-maligned "Peace Ship" venture. Schwimmer spent her later years in the United States, but was denied citizenship because of her pacifist views.

    Brief biographies are in NAW and in the *Dictionary of American Biography,* supplement 4, 1946–1950, 724–738. For an insightful recent treatment, see Wenger. A number of Jacobs's letters to Schwimmer are in the Schwimmer-Lloyd Papers. On Macmillan, a key Hague conference organizer, see chapter 8, note 15.

15. Bosch 141, 157–160.
16. Scholars differ as to the deeper causes of the rupture. (Bosch 295–296; Wiltsher 163) Jacobs even sought to remove all mention of Schwimmer from her personal papers.
17. De Wilde, *Brieven* 19, 24n.
18. Bosch 86, 105.
19. Ibid. 87–89.
20. Bosch 170; De Wilde, *Brieven* 19–20.

    The Broese van Groenous could readily support Jacobs; paterfamilias Wolter had become a very wealthy sugar planter in the Dutch East Indies before returning to the Netherlands. This unusual and generous man espoused pacifism and woman suffrage, even lending his automobile and chauffeur to a 1910 traveling suffrage campaign. He encouraged his children to learn Esperanto in hopes of fostering worldwide understanding, giving the home his architect son Dolf built for him an Esperanto name, Hejmo Nia (Our House). Support for their aging activist friend was in this case a natural expression of family ideals. (De Wilde, *Brieven* 8–12)

21. Jacobs quotes in French: "Il n'est pas possible de se figurer la science sous une forme plus charmante que celle de cette jolie juive de 25 ans, suivant les discussions les plus délicates avec un aplomb et un tact parfait . . ." See chapter 3, note 9.
22. The comment reads: "The leader [of the group of women who met them] was the Doctor's sister who has been an apothecary here for thirty years. She is sixty-five years old, a handsome, well-preserved Jewess, and she was clad in a beautiful white gown which far outclassed anything we had." (Catt papers, Library of Congress, box 2, Java diary 1912, p. 1) Thanks to Jacqueline van Voris for making her notes of Catt's diary available to me. On Charlotte Jacobs, see chapter 1, note 1.
23. "In 1936, at the height of the Hitler madness, Emily Balch, in a speech describing the small group of women who called together the Hague conference, said that 'Dr. Aletta Jacobs, a Dutch Jewish physician, was the most outstanding figure. I refer to the fact that she was a Jew because I recognize that in her life-long work for peace and internationalism, for humanitarianism and justice, she was engaged in a service markedly characteristic of her people. In what strange ways is that service repaid.'" (Randall 309) No reference is given for the talk.
24. De Wilde, *Brieven* 99. Jacobs was expressing irritation to Miel at a woman she met who in hopes of bringing about world peace was giving all her money to missionaries.
25. Hes 8–9, 142.
26. Ibid. 80–81; *The Jewish Encyclopedia*; BWN. Jozef was especially known in his time for genre scenes and landscapes. One of his most noted paintings is *A Jewish Wedding*. Jozef's more assimilated painter son Isaac Israëls painted three portraits of Jacobs in 1919–1920; they are reproduced in De Wilde, *Brieven*.
27. Hes 57–58.
28. Goldman (1869–1940) began her own thousand-page autobiography, *Living My Life*, the year before Jacobs's death, while in exile in France. Miel Coops was a great admirer of Goldman and put her up at her home in 1933. (Wexler 134; De Wilde, *Brieven* 17)
29. Bosch 33, 66.
30. Ibid., 202.
31. De Wilde, "Aletta" 54; De Wilde, *Brieven* 53–66.

BIBLIOGRAPHY

ARCHIVES

Archives and Special Collections on Women in Medicine, Medical College of Pennsylvania, Philadelphia.

Jane Addams Papers. Swarthmore College Peace Collection, Swarthmore College, Pennsylvania.

Schwimmer-Lloyd Papers. Rare Books and Manuscripts Division, New York Public Library, New York.

BOOKS AND ARTICLES

Aberdeen, Countess of, ed. *The International Congress of Women of 1899.* 7 vols. London: Unwin, 1900.

Addams, Jane. *Peace and Bread in Time of War.* New York: Macmillan, 1922. Silver Spring, Md.: NASW Classics Edition, 1983.

——— *The Excellent Becomes the Permanent.* New York: Macmillan, 1932.

Addams, Jane, Emily Balch, and Alice Hamilton. *Women at The Hague: The International Congress of Women and Its Results.* New York: Macmillan, 1915.

Albisetti, James C. "Female Education in German-Speaking Austria, Germany, and Switzerland, 1866-1914." Unpublished conference paper, 1990.

Anderson, Bonnie S., and Judith P. Zinsser. *A History of Their Own.* Vol. 2. 2 vols. New York: Harper and Row, 1988.

Banks, Olive. *The Biographical Dictionary of British Feminists.* Vols. 1, 2. 2 vols. New York: New York University Press, 1985-1990.

Benstock, Shari, ed. *The Private Self.* Chapel Hill: University of North Carolina Press, 1988.

Bernstein, Deborah S., ed. *Pioneers and Homemakers: Jewish Women in Pre-State Israel.* Albany: State University of New York Press, 1992.

Biografisch Woordenboek van het Socialisme en de Arbeidersbeweging in Nederland. Ed. P. J. Meertens et al. 6 vols. 1986– .

Biografisch Woordenboek van Nederland. Ed. J. Charité et al. 3 vols. The Hague: Nijhoff, 1979-1994.

Blake, Catriona. *The Charge of the Parasols: Women's Entry to the Medical Profession.* London: Women's Press, 1990.

Bonner, Thomas N. *To the Ends of the Earth: Women's Search for Education in Medicine.* Cambridge: Harvard University Press, 1992.

Bosch, Mineke, with Annemarie Kloosterman. *Politics and Friendship. Letters from the International Woman Suffrage Alliance, 1902–1942.* Columbus: Ohio State University Press, 1990.

Brinkschulte, Eva, ed. *Weibliche Ärzte.* Berlin: Hentrich, 1993.

Brodzki, Bella, and Schenck, Celeste, eds. *Lifelines: Theorizing Women's Autobiography.* Ithaca: Cornell University Press, 1988.

Bussey, Gertrude, and Margaret Tims. *Pioneers for Peace. Women's International League for Peace and Freedom, 1915–1965.* London: WILPF, 1980.

Carroll, Berenice A. "Feminism and Pacifism: Historical and Theoretical Connections." In Ruth Roach Pierson, ed., *Women and Peace: Theoretical, Historical, and Practical Perspectives.* London: Croom Helm, 1987.

Chesler, Ellen. *Woman of Valor: Margaret Sanger and the Birth Control Movement in America.* New York: Simon and Schuster, 1992.

Cook, Blanche Wiesen, ed. *Crystal Eastman on Women and Revolution.* New York: Oxford University Press, 1978.

Cooper, Sandi E. "Women's Participation in European Peace Movements: The Struggle to Prevent World War I." In Ruth Roach Pierson, ed., *Women and Peace: Theoretical, Historical, and Practical Perspectives.* London: Croom Helm, 1987.

——— *Patriotic Pacifism: Waging War on War in Europe, 1815–1914.* New York: Oxford University Press, 1992.

Daalder, H. "Dutch Jews in a Segmented Society." *Acta Historiae Neerlandicae,* vol. 10. The Hague: Martinus Nijhoff, 1978.

David, Katherine. "Czech Feminism and Nationalism in the Late Hapsburg Monarchy: 'The First in Austria.' " *Journal of Women's History* (Fall 1991), 3(2):26–45.

Degen, Marie Louise. *The History of the Women's Peace Party.* Baltimore: Johns Hopkins University Press, 1939.

Dictionary of American Biography. Ed. John A. Garraty and Edward T. James. New York: Scribner's, 1974.

Dictionary of South African Biography. Ed. W. J. de Kock. 5 vols. Capetown: Nasionale Boekhandel, 1968–1987.

Dieteren, Fia. "De geestelijke eenzaamheid van een radicaal-feministe: Wilhelmina Druckers ontwikkeling tussen 1885 en 1898." In *Jaarboek voor Vrouwengeschiedenis 1985.* Nijmegen, Socialistische Uitgeverij Nijmegen.

Douglas, Emily Taft. *Margaret Sanger: Pioneer of the Future.* New York: Holt, Rinehart and Winston, 1970.

Dürkop, Marlis. "Erscheinungsformen des Antisemitismus im Bund Deutscher Frauenvereine." *Feministische Studien* (1984), 1:140–150.

Elwood, R. C. *Inessa Armand: Revolutionary and Feminist.* Cambridge: Cambridge University Press, 1992.

Evans, Barbara. *Freedom to Choose: The Life and Work of Dr. Helena Wright, Pioneer of Contraception.* London: Bodley Head, 1984.

Fassmann, Irmgard Maja. *Jüdische Frauenrechtlerinnen in der deutschen Frauenbewegung 1865–1919.* Hildesheim, 1992.

Feinberg, Harriet. "Aletta Jacobs's *Reisbrieven uit Afrika en Azië.*" Unpublished paper, Cambridge, Mass., 1988.

——— "A Pioneering Dutch Feminist Views Egypt: Aletta Jacobs's Travel Letters." *Feminist Issues* (Fall 1990), 10(2):65–77.

——— "Structure and Texture in Aletta Jacobs's *Herinneringen.*" Unpublished paper, Cambridge, Mass., 1995.

Forkl, Martha, and Elizabeth Koffmahn, eds. *Frauenstudium und akademische Frauenarbeit in österreich.* Vienna, 1968.

Foster, Catherine. *Women for All Seasons: The Story of the Women's International League for Peace and Freedom.* Athens: University of Georgia Press, 1989.

Freidenreich, Harriet Pass. "Jewish Identity and the 'New Woman': Central European Jewish University Women in the Early Twentieth Century." In T. M. Rudavsky, ed., *Gender and Judaism.* New York: New York University Press, 1995.

Gedenkboek bij het 25-jarig bestaan van de Vereeniging voor Vrouwenkiesrecht, 1894–1919. Amsterdam, 1919.

Gelblum, Amira. "Feminism and Pacifism: The Case of Anita Augspurg and Lida Gustava Heymann." *Tel Aviver Jahrbuch für Deutsche Geschichte* (1992), 21:207–225.

Gerritsen, C. V., and Aletta H. Jacobs. *Brieven uit en over Amerika.* Amsterdam: F. van Rossen, 1906.

Gladdish, Ken. *Governing from the Centre: Politics and Policy-Making in the Netherlands.* London: Hurst, 1991.

Gordon, Felicia. *The Integral Feminist: Madeleine Pelletier, 1874–1939.* Minneapolis: University of Minnesota Press, 1991.

Grever, Maria. "Evoking Women's Lives: The Hidden Power of the Internal Struggle in the Historical Work of Dutch Feminist Johanna W. A. Naber, 1859–1941." Paper presented at the eighth Berkshire Conference on the History of Women, Rutgers University, June 9, 1990.

Grossmann, Atina. "Berliner Ärztinnen und Volksgesundheit in der Weimarer Republik: Zwischen Sexualreform und Eugenik." In Christiane Eifert and Susanne Rouette, *Unter allen Umständen: Frauengeschichte(n) in Berlin,* 183–217. Berlin, 1986.

Haighton, Elise. "A Dutch Lady-Doctor." *Phrenological Journal, 1883* 76:199–205, 259–261.

Hall, Ruth. *Passionate Crusader: The Life of Marie Stopes.* New York: Harcourt Brace Jovanovich, 1977.

Heilbrun, Carolyn G. *Writing a Woman's Life.* New York: Ballantyne, 1988.

Heindl, Waltraud, and Marina Tichy. *"Durch Erkenntnis zu Freiheit und Glück": Frauen an der Universität Wien.* Vienna: WUV-Universitätsverlag, 1990.

Hes, Hindle S. *Jewish Physicians in the Netherlands, 1600–1940.* Assen: Van Gorcum, 1980.

Heymann, Lida Gustava, and Anita Augspurg. *Erlebtes—Erschautes. Deutsche Frauenkämpfen für Freiheit, Recht und Frieden, 1850–1940.* Ed. Margrit Twellman. Meisenheim am Glan: Anton Hain, 1972.

International Congress of Women, The Hague, April 28–May 1, 1915. Report.

International Woman Suffrage Alliance. Report of Seventh Congress, Budapest, Hungary, June 15–21, 1913. Manchester: Privately printed, 1913.

Jacobs, Aletta H. *Uit het leven van merkwaardige vrouwen.* Amsterdam: F. van Rossen, 1905.

——— *Reisbrieven uit Afrika en Azië, benevens eenige brieven uit Zweden en Noorwegen.* 2 vols. Almelo: W. Hilarius Wzn., 1913.

Jantsch, Marlene. "Der Aufsteig der österreichischen Ärztin zur Gleichberechtigung." In Martha Forkl and Elizabeth Koffmahn, eds. *Frauenstudium und academische Frauenarbeit in österreich.* Vienna, 1968.

The Jewish Encyclopedia. 12 vols. New York: Funk and Wagnalls, 1906–1917.

Josephson, Harold, Sandi Cooper et al., eds. *Biographical Dictionary of Modern Peace Leaders.* Westport, Ct.: Greenwood Press, 1985.

Kaplan, Marion. *The Jewish Feminist Movement in Germany.* Westport, Ct.: Greenwood Press, 1979.

——— *The Making of the Jewish Middle Class.* New York: Oxford University Press, 1991.

Kuitenbrouwer, Maarten. *The Netherlands and the Rise of Modern Imperialism: Colonies and Foreign Policy, 1870–1902.* Translated by Hugh Beyer. New York: Berg, 1991.

Lange, Cornelie C. de. "Pioneer Medical Women in the Netherlands." *Journal of the American Medical Women's Association* (March 1952), 7(3):99–101. Medical College of Pennsylvania, no. 461.

Leathard, Audrey. *The Fight for Family Planning.* London: Macmillan, 1980.

Leydesdorff, Selma. *We Lived with Dignity: The Jewish Proletariat of Amsterdam, 1900–1940.* Detroit: Wayne State University Press, 1994.

Ligt, Bart de. *The Conquest of Violence.* Trans. by Honor Tracy. With a new introduction by Peter van den Dungen. London: Pluto Press, 1989. [London: George Routledge, 1937.]

Lindeboom, Gerrit Arie. *Dutch Medical Biography: A Biographical Dictionary of Dutch Physicians and Surgeons, 1475–1975.* Amsterdam: Rodopi, 1984.

Lipinska, Melanie. *Histoire des Femmes Médecins depuis l'Antiquité jusqu'à Nos Jours.* Paris: Librairie G. Jacques et Cie., 1900. Medical College of Pennsylvania, no. 158.

McDonnell, Eleanor Kinsella. "Keeping the Stork in His Place." *Pictorial Review* (December 1919), 21(49):55.

McLaren, Angus. *A History of Contraception: From Antiquity to the Present Day.* Oxford: Basil Blackwell, 1990.

Manton, Jo. *Elizabeth Garrett Anderson.* London: Methuen, 1965,

Mensinga, Wilhelm Peter Johann. *Facultative Sterilität.* Reprint, with introduction by Armin Geus. Dusseldorf: Kupka Verlag, 1987.

Michman, Jozeph. "The Jewish Essence of Dutch Jewry." In Jozeph Michman, ed., *Dutch Jewish History, II.* Jerusalem: Hebrew University, 1989.

Michman, Jozeph, ed. *Pinkas HaKehillot: Holland.* Jerusalem: Yad Vashem, 1985.

Morantz-Sanchez, Regina. *Sympathy and Science: Women Physicians in American Medicine.* New York: Oxford, 1985.

Naber, Johanna W. A. "Eerste Proeve van een Chronologisch Overzicht van de Ge-schiedenis der Vrouwenbeweging in Nederland." With an introduction by Ulla Jansz. *Jaarboek voor Vrouwengeschiedenis 1985*, 185–201. [1937.]

Nabrink, Gé. *Seksuele hervorming in Nederland*. Nijmegen: Socialistische Uitgeverij, 1978.

Neumann, Daniela. *Studentinnen aus dem Russischen Reich in der Schweiz*. Zurich: Hans Rohr, 1987.

Nieuw Nederlandsch Biografisch Woordenboek. Ed. P. C. Molhuysen. 10 vols. Leiden: A. W. Sijthoff, 1911–1937.

Notable American Women, 1607–1950: A Biographical Dictionary. Ed. Edward T. James, Janet Wilson James, and Paul S. Boyer. 3 vols. Cambridge: Belknap Press, 1971.

Notable American Women: The Modern Period. Ed. Barbara Sicherman and Carol Hurd Green. Cambridge: Belknap Press, 1980.

Offen, Karen. "Liberty, Equality, and Justice for Women: The Theory and Practice of Feminism in Nineteenth-Century Europe." In Renate Bridenthal et al., eds., *Becoming Visible: Women in European History*. 2d ed. Boston: Houghton Mifflin, 1987.

—— "Defining Feminism: A Comparative Historical Approach." *Signs* (1988), 14(11): 144–145.

Oldfield, Sybil. *Spinsters of This Parish: The Life and Times of F. M. Mayor and Mary Sheepshanks*. London: Virago, 1984.

Outshoorn, Joyce. *Vrouwenemancipatie en socialisme: een onderzoek naar de houding van de SDAP ten opzichte van het vrouwenvraagstuk tussen 1894 en 1919*. Nijmegen: SUN, 1973.

Pethick-Lawrence, Emmeline. *My Part in a Changing World*. London: Gollancz, 1938.

Peyser, Dora. "Alice Salomon, Ein Lebensbild." In *Alice Salomon, Die Begründerin des sozialen Frauenberufs in Deutschland: Ihr Leben und Werk*. Cologne: Carl Heymanns Verlag, 1958.

Pierson, Ruth Roach, ed. *Women and Peace: Theoretical, Historical, and Practical Perspectives*. London: Croom Helm, 1987.

Posthumus-van der Goot, W. H. *Vrouwen vochten voor de vrede*. Arnhem: Van Loghum Slaterus, 1961.

Posthumus-van der Goot, W. H. and Anna de Waal, eds., *Van Moeder op Dochter: De maatschappelijke positie van de vrouw in Nederland vanaf de Franse tijd*. Rev. ed. Nijmegen: SUN, 1977. [1948.]

Potter, Ada. "The History of Dutch Medical Women." *Medical Women's Journal* (January 1923), 30(1):5–6. Medical College of Pennsylvania, no. 66.

Randall, Mercedes M. *Improper Bostonian: Emily Greene Balch, Nobel Peace Laureate 1946*. New York: Twanye, 1964.

Rasmussen, Janet E. "Sisters Across the Sea: Early Norwegian Feminists and Their American Connections." *Women's Studies International Forum* (1982), 5(6):647–654.

Reinalda, Bob, and Natascha Verhaaren. *Vrouwenbeweging en internationale organisaties, 1868–1986. Een vergeten hoofdstuk uit de geschiedenis van de internationale betrekkingen*. De Knipe: Ariadne, 1989.

Riemer, Eleanor S., and John C. Fout. *European Women: A Documentary History*. New York: Schocken, 1980.

Roazen, Paul, *Helene Deutsch: A Psychoanalyst's Life*. Garden City: Anchor, 1989.

Rogow, Faith. *Gone to Another Meeting: The National Council of Jewish Women, 1893–1993*. Tuscaloosa: University of Alabama Press, 1993.

Rohner, Hanny. *Die ersten 30 Jahren des medizinischen Frauenstudiums an der Universität Zürich, 1867–1897*. Zurich, 1972.

Rose, June. *Marie Stopes and the Sexual Revolution*. London: Faber and Faber, 1992.

Rubinstein, David. *A Different World for Women: The Life of Millicent Garrett Fawcett*. New York: Harvester Wheatsheaf, 1991.

Salomon, Alice. "Character Is Destiny: An Autobiography." Unpublished memoir, AR-3875. Leo Baeck Institute, New York.

Sanger, Margaret. *My Fight for Birth Control*. Fairview Park, N.Y.: Maxwell Reprint, 1969.

——— *An Autobiography*. New York, Dover, 1971. [New York: Norton, 1938.]

Schmelzkopf, Christiane. "Rahel Straus." In Heinz Schmitt, ed., *Jüden in Karlsruhe*, 471–480. Karlsruhe: Badenia Verlag, 1988.

Schmidt, Minna Moscherosch. *Four Hundred Outstanding Women of the World and Costumology of Their Time*. Chicago: Minna Moscherosch Schmidt, 1933.

Schreiber, Adele, and Margaret Mathieson. *Journey Towards Freedom. Written for the Golden Jubilee of the International Alliance of Women*. Copenhagen, IAW, 1955.

Shaarawi, Huda. *Harem Years: The Memoirs of an Egyptian Feminist (1879–1924)*. Trans, ed., and with an introduction by Margot Badran. New York: Feminist Press, 1987.

Shepherd, Naomi. *A Price Below Rubies*. Cambridge: Harvard University Press, 1994.

Sicherman, Barbara. *Alice Hamilton: A Life in Letters*. Cambridge: Harvard University Press, 1984.

Smith, Bonnie G. *Changing Lives: Women in European History Since 1700*. Lexington: Heath, 1989.

Sowerwine, Charles. "Women Against the War: A Feminine Basis for Internationalism and Pacifism?" In *Proceedings of the Annual Meeting of the Western Society for French History*, 361–370. Santa Barbara, 1978.

——— *Sisters or Citizens? Women and Socialism in France Since 1876*. New York: Cambridge University Press, 1982.

Stites, Richard. *The Women's Liberation Movement in Russia: Feminism, Nihilism, and Bolshevism, 1860–1930*. Princeton: Princeton University Press, 1978.

Straus, Rahel. *Wir lebten in Deutschland*. Stuttgart, 1966.

Stuurman, Siep. "Samuel van Houten and Dutch Liberalism, 1860–1890." *Journal of the History of Ideas* (1989), 50(1):135–152.

Tiburtius, Franziska. *Erinnerungen einer Achtzigjährigen*. 3d ed. Berlin: C. A. Schwetschke, 1929.

Tilburg, Marja van, et al. *"Op mij rusten grooter en ernstiger plichten": Dr. Aletta Jacobs' zorg voor de wereld*. Vol. 2. Vrouwenstudies Letteren Groningen. Groningen: RUG, Werkgroep Vrouwenstudies Letteren, 1992.

Tuve, Jeanette E. *The First Russian Women Physicians*. Newtonville, Mass.: Oriental Research Partners, 1984.

Usborne, Cornelie. *The Politics of the Body in Weimar Germany*. Ann Arbor: University of Michigan Press, 1992.

Van den Dungen, Peter, and Nick Lewer. "Frauendiplomatie—Ärtzinnen gegen den Krieg." In Thomas M. Ruprecht and Christian Jenssen, eds., *Äskulap oder Mars? Ärzte gegen den Krieg*, 177–194. Bremen: Donat Verlag, 1991.

Van Voris, Jacqueline. *Carrie Chapman Catt: A Public Life*. New York: Feminist Press, 1987.

Verkade, Willem. *Democratic Parties in the Low Countries and Germany: Origins and Historical Developments*. Leiden: Universitaire Pers Leiden, 1965.

Walkowitz, Judith. *Prostitution and Victorian Society*. Cambridge: Cambridge University Press, 1980.

Wenger, Beth S. "Radical Politics in a Reactionary Age: The Unmaking of Rosika Schwimmer, 1914–1930." *Journal of Women's History* (Fall 1990), 2(2):66–99.

Wexler, Alice. *Emma Goldman in Exile*. Boston: Beacon Press, 1989.

Wickert, Christl. "Frauen im Parlament: Lebensläufe sozialdemokratischer Parlamentarierinnen in der Weimarer Republik." In Wilhelm Heinz Schröder, ed., *Lebenslauf und Gesellschaft*, 210–240. Stuttgart: Ernst Klett Verlag, 1985.

—— *Unsere Erwählten: Sozialdemokratische Frauen im Deutschen Reichstag und im Preussischen Landtag 1919 bis 1933*. 2 vols. Göttingen: Sovec, 1986.

Wilde, Inge de. *Aletta Jacobs in Groningen*. Groningen: Studium Generale/Universiteitsmuseum/Rijksuniversiteit, 1979.

—— "De bibliotheek van C. V. Gerritsen, de echtgenoot van Aletta Jacobs." *Jaarboek voor Vrouwengeschiedenis 1982*, 245–255.

—— "Inleiding bij zes brieven van Aletta Jacobs" and (ed.) "Aletta Jacobs, 'Strijdlust is er nog genoeg in mij, maar strijdkracht ontbreekt mij.—Zes brieven.'" *Tijdschrift voor Vrouwenstudies* (1984), 17(5/1):18–26, 27–40.

—— " 'Er is een heilig moeten, waartegen geen bezwaar is bestand.' De betekenis van Hélène Mercier voor de vrouwenbeweging." *Jaarboek voor Vrouwengeschiedenis*, 59–77. 1985.

—— "Betsy Bakker-Nort, 1874–1946." In *249 Vrouwen na Aletta Jacobs*, 29–32. Vrouwelijke gepromoveerden aan de Rijksuniversiteit Groningen 1879–1987. Rijksuniversiteit Groningen, 1987.

—— "Aletta Jacobs als grand old lady." *Hollands Maandblad* (1989), no. 5/6:53–59.

—— "Minder opvallend dan haar 'meer roerige zuster': over de apothekeres Charlotte Jacobs (1847–1916)." In *Groniek: Historisch Tydschrift* (September 1992), 25(118):59–74.

—— " 'Aaneensluiting van de afgestudeerde vrouwen is een eisch van den tijd': Ontstaan en beginjaren van de Nederlandsche Vereeniging van Vrouwen met Academische Opleiding." In *Een verbond van gestudeerde vrouwen*. Verloren: Hilversum, 1993.

Wilde, Inge de, ed. *Brieven van Aletta H. Jacobs aan de familie Broese van Groenou*. Zutphen: Walburg Pers, 1992.

Wiltsher, Anne. *Most Dangerous Women: Feminist Peace Campaigners of the Great War*. Westport, Ct.: Greenwood Press, 1985.

Winkler Prins Encyclopedie "Voor de Vrouw". Ed. Rosa Delrue et al. 2 vols. Amsterdam: Elsevier, 1952.

Winkler Prins Encyclopedie. Ed. J. F. Staal et al. 20 vols. Amsterdam: Elsevier, 1966–1975.

Women in a Changing World. The Dynamic Story of the International Council of Women Since 1888. London: Routledge and Kegan Paul, 1966.

Women's International League for Peace and Freedom. Report of the International Congress of Women, Zurich, May 12 to 17, 1919. Geneva: WILPF, 1919.

Woycke, James. *Birth Control in Germany, 1871–1933*. London: Routledge, 1988.

INDEX